Obesity During Pregnancy in Clinical Practice

Obesity During Pregnancy in Clinical Practice

Editor: Marshalla Ortega

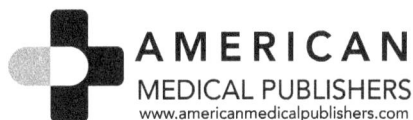

AMERICAN
MEDICAL PUBLISHERS
www.americanmedicalpublishers.com

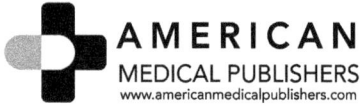

AMERICAN
MEDICAL PUBLISHERS
www.americanmedicalpublishers.com

Cataloging-in-Publication Data

Obesity during pregnancy in clinical practice / edited by Marshalla Ortega.
    p. cm.
Includes bibliographical references and index.
ISBN 978-1-63927-158-0
1. Obesity. 2. Pregnancy--Complications. 3. Maternal health services.
4. Women's health services. I. Ortega, Marshalla.
RG580.O24 O24 2022
618.242--dc23

American Medical Publishers,
41 Flatbush Avenue,
1st Floor, New York,
NY 11217, USA

ISBN 978-1-63927-158-0 (Hardback)

Contents

Preface IX

Chapter 1 **Contribution of prepregnancy body mass index and gestational weight gain to adverse neonatal outcomes: population attributable fractions for Canada** 1
Susie Dzakpasu, John Fahey, Russell S Kirby, Suzanne C Tough, Beverley Chalmers, Maureen I Heaman, Sharon Bartholomew, Anne Biringer, Elizabeth K Darling, Lily S Lee and Sarah D McDonald

Chapter 2 **Obesity and pregnancy outcomes: Do the relationships differ by maternal region of birth?** 13
Miranda Davies-Tuck, Joanne C. Mockler, Lynne Stewart, Michelle Knight and Euan M. Wallace

Chapter 3 **Metformin and dietary advice to improve insulin sensitivity and promote gestational restriction of weight among pregnant women who are overweight or obese** 21
Jodie M. Dodd, Rosalie M. Grivell, Andrea R. Deussen, Gustaaf Dekker, Jennie Louise and William Hague

Chapter 4 **Women's perceptions of discussions about gestational weight gain with health care providers during pregnancy and postpartum** 28
Hara Nikolopoulos, Maria Mayan, Jessica MacIsaac, Terri Miller and Rhonda C. Bell

Chapter 5 **Maternal obesity and its effect on labour duration in nulliparous women** 37
Karen Louise Ellekjaer, Thomas Bergholt and Ellen Løkkegaard

Chapter 6 **Sociodemographic factors and pregnancy outcomes associated with prepregnancy obesity: effect modification of parity in the nationwide Epifane birth-cohort** 47
Julie Boudet-Berquier, Benoit Salanave, Jean-Claude Desenclos and Katia Castetbon

Chapter 7 **Examining the provisional guidelines for weight gain in twin pregnancies** 60
Olha Lutsiv, Adam Hulman, Christy Woolcott, Joseph Beyene, Lucy Giglia, B. Anthony Armson, Linda Dodds, Binod Neupane and Sarah D. McDonald

Chapter 8 **Correlates of poor mental health in early pregnancy in obese European women** 72
Matteo C. Sattler, Judith G. M. Jelsma, Annick Bogaerts, David Simmons, Gernot Desoye, Rosa Corcoy, Juan M. Adelantado, Alexandra Kautzky-Willer, Jürgen Harreiter, Frans A. van Assche, Roland Devlieger, Goele Jans, Sander Galjaard, David Hill, Peter Damm, Elisabeth R. Mathiesen, Ewa Wender-Ozegowska, Agnieszka Zawiejska, Kinga Blumska, Annunziata Lapolla, Maria G. Dalfrà, Alessandra Bertolotto, Fidelma Dunne, Dorte M. Jensen, Lise Lotte T. Andersen, Frank J. Snoek and Mireille N. M. van Poppel

Chapter 9   **Exercise training during pregnancy reduces circulating insulin levels in overweight/obese women postpartum**...**83**
Kirsti K. Garnæs, Siv Mørkved, Kjell Å. Salvesen, Øyvind Salvesen and Trine Moholdt

Chapter 10   **Enablers and barriers to physical activity in overweight and obese pregnant women: an analysis informed by the theoretical domains framework and COM-B model** **94**
C. Flannery, S. McHugh, A. E. Anaba, E. Clifford, M. O'Riordan, L. C. Kenny, F. M. McAuliffe, P. M. Kearney and M. Byrne

Chapter 11   **A retrospective study of gestational weight gain in relation to the Institute of Medicine's recommendations by maternal body mass index in rural Pennsylvania from 2006 to 2015** **107**
Michael L. Power, Melisa L. Lott, A. Dhanya Mackeen, Jessica DiBari and Jay Schulkin

Chapter 12   **Impact of obesity and other risk factors on labor dystocia in term primiparous women**..**116**
Tuija Hautakangas, Outi Palomäki, Karoliina Eidstø, Heini Huhtala and Jukka Uotila

Chapter 13   **Evaluation of an activity monitor for use in pregnancy to help reduce excessive gestational weight gain**..**124**
Paul M. C. Lemmens, Francesco Sartor, Lieke G. E. Cox, Sebastiaan V. den Boer and Joyce H. D. M. Westerink

Chapter 14   **Factors associated with gestational weight gain**..**134**
Edyta Suliga, Wojciech Rokita, Olga Adamczyk-Gruszka, Grażyna Pazera, Elżbieta Cieśla and Stanisław Głuszek

Chapter 15   **Effects of early pregnancy BMI, mid-gestational weight gain, glucose and lipid levels in pregnancy on offspring's birth weight and subcutaneous fat**..**145**
Christine Sommer, Line Sletner, Kjersti Mørkrid, Anne Karen Jenum and Kåre Inge Birkeland

Chapter 16   **Adopting a healthy lifestyle when pregnant and obese**..**154**
Anna Dencker, Åsa Premberg, Ellinor K. Olander, Christine McCourt, Karin Haby, Sofie Dencker, Anna Glantz and Marie Berg

Chapter 17   **Higher maternal leptin levels at second trimester are associated with subsequent greater gestational weight gain in late pregnancy** **164**
Marilyn Lacroix, Marie-Claude Battista, Myriam Doyon, Julie Moreau, Julie Patenaude, Laetitia Guillemette, Julie Ménard, Jean-Luc Ardilouze, Patrice Perron and Marie-France Hivert

Chapter 18   **Maternal super-obesity and perinatal outcomes in Australia**..172
                Elizabeth A. Sullivan, Jan E. Dickinson, Geraldine A Vaughan, Michael J. Peek,
                David Ellwood, Caroline SE Homer, Marian Knight, Claire McLintock,
                Alex Wang, Wendy Pollock, Lisa Jackson Pulver, Zhuoyang Li, Nasrin Javid,
                Elizabeth Denney-Wilson and Leonie Callaway

Chapter 19   **Changes in the biochemical and immunological components of serum and
                colostrum of overweight and obese mothers** 182
                Mahmi Fujimori, Eduardo L. França, Vanessa Fiorin, Tassiane C. Morais,
                Adenilda C. Honorio-França and Luiz C. de Abreu

Chapter 20   **Change in level of physical activity during pregnancy in obese
                women: findings from the UPBEAT pilot trial**..190
                Louise Hayes, Catherine Mcparlin, Tarja I Kinnunen, Lucilla Poston,
                Stephen C Robson and Ruth Bell

Chapter 21   **Pre-pregnancy obesity and non-adherence to multivitamin use: findings from
                the National Pregnancy Risk Assessment Monitoring System (2009–2011)** 198
                Saba W. Masho, Amani Bassyouni and Susan Cha

                Permissions

                List of Contributors

                Index

Preface

Obesity in a mother during pregnancy can have a major impact on offspring development and maternal metabolism. Maternal obesity disrupts the processes of glucose homeostasis, fat oxidation, insulin resistance and amino acid synthesis. Such changes contribute to adverse outcomes, with increased odds of children born with congenital anomalies including spina bifida and neural tube defects. Other anomalies such as cleft lip and palate, anorectal atresia, hydrocephalus, septal anomalies and limb reduction anomalies are other complications associated with this condition. Obesity also affects the mother negatively with an increased risk of gestational diabetes, hypertension and blood clots. An obese mother is at higher risk of going into preterm labor, undergoing a C-section or delivering with shoulder dystocia. This book is compiled in such a manner, that it will provide in-depth knowledge about the impact of obesity during pregnancy in a clinical setting. From theories to research to practical applications, case studies related to all contemporary topics of relevance to this subject have been included in this book. With state-of-the-art inputs by acclaimed experts of this field, this book targets students and professionals.

This book has been the outcome of endless efforts put in by authors and researchers on various issues and topics within the field. The book is a comprehensive collection of significant researches that are addressed in a variety of chapters. It will surely enhance the knowledge of the field among readers across the globe.

It gives us an immense pleasure to thank our researchers and authors for their efforts to submit their piece of writing before the deadlines. Finally in the end, I would like to thank my family and colleagues who have been a great source of inspiration and support.

Editor

Contribution of prepregnancy body mass index and gestational weight gain to adverse neonatal outcomes: population attributable fractions for Canada

Susie Dzakpasu[1*], John Fahey[2], Russell S Kirby[3], Suzanne C Tough[4], Beverley Chalmers[5], Maureen I Heaman[6], Sharon Bartholomew[1], Anne Biringer[7], Elizabeth K Darling[8], Lily S Lee[9] and Sarah D McDonald[10]

Abstract

Background: Low or high prepregnancy body mass index (BMI) and inadequate or excess gestational weight gain (GWG) are associated with adverse neonatal outcomes. This study estimates the contribution of these risk factors to preterm births (PTBs), small-for-gestational age (SGA) and large-for-gestational age (LGA) births in Canada compared to the contribution of prenatal smoking, a recognized perinatal risk factor.

Methods: We analyzed data from the Canadian Maternity Experiences Survey. A sample of 5,930 women who had a singleton live birth in 2005-2006 was weighted to a nationally representative population of 71,200 women. From adjusted odds ratios, we calculated population attributable fractions to estimate the contribution of BMI, GWG and prenatal smoking to PTB, SGA and LGA infants overall and across four obstetric groups.

Results: Overall, 6% of women were underweight (<18.5 kg/m^2) and 34.4% were overweight or obese ($\geq$25.0 kg/m^2). More than half (59.4%) gained above the recommended weight for their BMI, 18.6% gained less than the recommended weight and 10.4% smoked prenatally. Excess GWG contributed more to adverse outcomes than BMI, contributing to 18.2% of PTB and 15.9% of LGA. Although the distribution of BMI and GWG was similar across obstetric groups, their impact was greater among primigravid women and multigravid women without a previous PTB or pregnancy loss. The contributions of BMI and GWG to PTB and SGA exceeded that of prenatal smoking.

Conclusions: Maternal weight, and GWG in particular, contributes significantly to the occurrence of adverse neonatal outcomes in Canada. Indeed, this contribution exceeds that of prenatal smoking for PTB and SGA, highlighting its public health importance.

Keywords: Population attributable fraction, Maternal weight, Preterm birth, Small-for-gestational age, Large-for-gestational age

Background

Low or high prepregnancy body mass index (BMI) and inadequate or excess gestational weight gain (GWG) are linked to an increased risk of adverse neonatal outcomes. Overweight and obese BMI and excess GWG have been associated with large-for-gestational age (LGA) infants, preterm birth (PTB) and stillbirth while underweight BMI and low GWG have been associated with small-for-gestational age (SGA) infants and PTB [1-6]. Although elevated individual-level risks have been documented in numerous studies, less is known about population-level effects of both BMI and GWG on neonatal outcomes.

Population-level effects can be measured using population attributable fractions (PAFs), which reflect the increased risk conferred by a particular determinant and its prevalence in the population. The PAF provides a hypothetical assessment of the proportion of the outcome that

* Correspondence: susie.dzakpasu@phac-aspc.gc.ca
[1]Maternal and Infant Health Section, Health Surveillance and Epidemiology Division, Public Health Agency of Canada, 785 Carling Avenue, 6804A 4th Floor, Ottawa, Ontario K1A 0 K9, Canada
Full list of author information is available at the end of the article

could be avoided if a particular risk factor were eliminated, making it an important outcome measure from a public health perspective. A 2011 systematic review and meta-analysis of risk factors for stillbirth in high-income countries concluded that 8-18% of stillbirths were attributable to maternal overweight and obesity (BMI $\geq$ 25 kg/m^2) [1].

In Canada, based on measured height and weight, the prevalence of obesity among adult women rose from 16% in 1978 to 23% in 2004 [7], reflecting a global trend in increasing overweight and obesity [8]. If this trend continues, as hypothesized by Cnattinguis et al. [9], the public health importance of maternal overweight and obesity may rival prenatal smoking as a modifiable risk factor for adverse pregnancy outcomes. The objective of this study is to examine this hypothesis for Canada, by estimating the contribution of BMI and GWG, as measured by PAFs, to PTB, SGA and LGA and to compare this to the contribution of prenatal smoking, a recognized perinatal risk factor.

Methods
Study population
We used data from the Public Health Agency of Canada's Canadian Maternity Experiences Survey (MES). The MES was a cross-sectional survey of a stratified random sample of women drawn from the 2006 Canadian Census. Women who had a singleton live birth in Canada between November 2005 and May 2006, were at least 15 years of age, living with their infant, and not living on a First Nations reserve or in an institution were eligible to participate. Of 8,244 eligible women, 6,421 (78%) agreed to participate. Data were collected by female interviewers between October 2006 and January 2007 using a computer-assisted telephone interview application. Women had previously been mailed a letter which included information on the survey and asked for their participation. Verbal consent to participate was then obtained at the beginning of each telephone interview. All data in this study were based on women's reports during survey interviews.

For this study, we excluded 491 women who were either missing information on BMI or GWG (the principal determinants of interest), missing information on gestational age (needed for outcome variables) or were less than 18 years old because the BMI classification we used was derived for ages 18 and older. In consideration of the sample design and non-response, each MES participant was assigned a sampling weight. The 5,930 women in this study were thus weighted to a nationally representative population of 71,200 women who had a singleton live birth in Canada between November 2005 and May 2006. Sampling weights took into consideration the probability of each respondent being selected from the stratified sample frame and also adjusted for non-response. Using Census data, comparison of the respondent distribution using the weights to the target population showed a close

approximation on all demographic characteristics investigated (e.g., maternal age and household composition). Detailed information on the survey's development, including the weighting procedure and analysis of respondent characteristics has been reported elsewhere [10,11].

Outcomes
We studied three outcomes: PTB (<37 weeks completed gestation), SGA (weight below the 10th percentile for gestational age) and LGA (weight above the 90th percentile for gestational age). Infants were classified as SGA or LGA using MES data on mother's country of birth and sex-specific growth curves developed by Ray et al. [12]. Ray et al.'s growth curves are specific to mother's country of birth grouped according to seven world regions (Canada, Europe/Western nations, Africa/Caribbean, Middle East/North Africa, Latin America, East Asia/South East Asia/Pacific Islands, South Asia). Accounting for mother's country of birth minimizes the risk of misclassifying newborns of mothers from non-European backgrounds as too small or too large for their gestational age due to recognized non-pathological ethnic differences in birthweight [12,13]. Ray et al.'s growth curves end at 41 weeks gestation and our sample included 90 infants with gestational ages ranging from 42 to 45 weeks. These infants were classified using the 41-week 10th and 90th percentile cut-offs. Fetal growth after 41 weeks gestation could have resulted in a baby being classified in a different growth category (e.g. AGA) than he/she would have been at 41 weeks (e.g., SGA); however any minor misclassification which may have resulted from this approach was deemed preferable to eliminating these records.

Determinants
Prepregnancy BMI and GWG measures were derived from the following questions:

  i) *How tall are you without shoes on?*
  ii) *Just before your pregnancy, how much did you weigh?*
  iii) *How much weight did you gain during your pregnancy?*

We categorized women's prepregnancy weight according to the World Health Organization (WHO) standard as either being underweight (BMI < 18.5 kg/m^2), normal weight (18.5 $\leq$ BMI < 25), overweight (25 $\leq$ BMI < 30) or obese (BMI $\geq$ 30).

We utilized the 2009 Institute of Medicine (IOM) guidelines on GWG to categorize women's weight gain as below, within or above recommended [14]. These guidelines have also been adopted by Health Canada [15]. Because GWG is associated with gestational length, we accounted for gestational length in our calculations. Specifically, we assumed a 2 kg weight gain in the first trimester (as per IOM guidelines) and subtracted this amount from the total reported weight gain to obtain GWG during the remainder of the pregnancy. Next, we subtracted 13 weeks (the first trimester) from the gestational age at birth to obtain the number of weeks in the remainder of the pregnancy. We then compared the GWG in the remainder of the pregnancy to the IOM's recommended GWG during this period, accounting for women's prepregnancy BMI.

Prenatal smoking was determined from the question "During the last 3 months of your pregnancy, did you smoke daily, occasionally, or not at all?" Women who responded either daily or occasionally were categorized as smokers.

Covariates

We studied additional reproductive, health care, sociodemographic and psychosocial characteristics as potential confounders of the association between BMI, GWG and neonatal outcomes. Our selection of covariates was guided by previous studies of risk factors for PTB, SGA and LGA [3,4,6]. Table 1 provides definitions of the variables that are not self-explanatory.

Statistical analysis

Percentages were used to report observed distributions of BMI, GWG, prenatal smoking and other maternal characteristics. Using multivariable logistic regression, we calculated adjusted odds ratios (aORs) separately for each outcome (PTB, SGA and LGA). For SGA analyses, the sample was restricted to infants who were SGA and infants who were average-for-gestational-age (AGA). Similarly, LGA analyses were restricted to infants who were LGA and AGA. BMI, GWG and smoking were included in all multivariable models in order to estimate their independent associations with each outcome. Other covariates were selected purposely into models using the following steps. Based on the Wald test from univariable logistic regression models, we initially included any variable with a p-value below 0.25 [17]. Covariates were then removed from the model if they were statistically non-significant and not a confounder. Significance was evaluated at the 0.05 level and confounding as a

change of 15% or greater in the effect of BMI, GWG or smoking on the outcome being modeled. No adjustment for multiple comparisons was used.

With the exception of maternal age, all variables were treated as categorical in regression models. Records with missing values for covariates other than LICO were excluded from models (<4%). Due to a large number of missing LICO values (8.0%), a missing category was included for this variable. Calculations were carried out overall, and for four mutually exclusive obstetric history groups: primigravidas, multigravidas with a previous PTB, multigravidas without a previous PTB but with a previous early pregnancy loss (miscarriage, abortion, and/or ectopic pregnancy) and multigravidas without a previous PTB or previous early pregnancy loss. Analysis by these groups was based on prior knowledge that pregnancy outcomes differ by parity and for women with antecedent adverse outcomes such as PTB [18,19]. Normal BMI, within recommended GWG and non-smokers were the reference groups.

The contribution of maternal underweight, overweight or obese BMI, less than or more than recommended GWG, and smoking to each outcome was estimated using PAFs. We calculated adjusted PAFs using the sequential and average attributable fraction method [20]. This method involves estimating a logistic regression model with known/available confounders for each outcome, then using this model to compute the adjusted number of cases that would be expected if the risk factor (e.g., excess GWG) were absent in the population. The adjusted PAF is calculated by subtracting this number of expected cases from the number of observed cases, then dividing this value by the number of observed cases.

All analyses were carried out using sampling weights. Results were computed from unrounded weighted components; however weighted sample sizes in results tables were rounded to the nearest hundred, as unrounded estimates overstate precision. We calculated 95% confidence intervals for adjusted ORs and adjusted PAFs using the bootstrap method, which accounts for the variability introduced by the sample design and weighting adjustments [21]. Bootstrap confidence intervals were based on 1,000 samples. We used SAS® Enterprise Guide® software, Version 5.1 [22].

Table 1 Definition of covariate variables

Variable	Definition
Low-income-cut-off (LICO) [16]	A measure of the income threshold below which a family will likely spend 20 percentage points more than the average family on food, shelter and clothing
Medical condition prior to pregnancy	Yes in response to the question "Prior to your pregnancy, did you develop any medical conditions or health problems that required you to take medication for more than 2 weeks, have special care, or extra tests during pregnancy?"
Medical condition during pregnancy	Yes in response to the question "During your pregnancy, did you develop any new medical conditions or health problems that required you to take medication for more than 2 weeks, have special care, or extra tests?"
Depression prior to pregnancy	Yes in response to the question "Before your pregnancy, had you ever been prescribed anti-depressants or been diagnosed with depression?
Short stature	Height of less than 1.55 metres (5 feet 2 inches)

The MES project was presented to Health Canada's Science Advisory Board, Health Canada's Research Ethics Board and the Federal Privacy Commissioner, and was approved by Statistics Canada's Policy Committee [11]. Additional ethical review was not required, as the MES data are anonymous and this study did not generate identifying information.

Results

The distribution of BMI, GWG, smoking and covariates is presented in Table 2. Overall, 6% of women were underweight and 34.4% were either overweight or obese. More than half (59.4%) gained above the recommended weight for their BMI; 18.6% gained less than recommended weight; and smoking was reported by 10.4% of women. The distribution of maternal characteristics varied across obstetric history groups, with women with a previous PTB reporting the highest rates of obesity (19.6%) and prenatal smoking (17.2%) and primigravidas reporting the highest rates of above recommended GWG (61.3%). Among women with above recommended GWG, the average weight gain among primigravidas was also higher (20.4 kg) than that among multigravidas (18.9 kg). Across other characteristics, women with a previous PTB tended to differ from other groups of women. These differences included lower educational achievement, having a household income that was at or below the LICO, having medical conditions prior to pregnancy or during pregnancy, being diagnosed with depression prior to pregnancy and experiencing higher levels of stress and lower social support during their pregnancy. Among the women who reported an early pregnancy loss, 68.2%, 36.4% and 2.7% experienced a miscarriage, abortion and ectopic pregnancy, respectively.

Associations between adverse neonatal outcomes and BMI and GWG

Table 3 presents associations between adverse neonatal outcomes and BMI and GWG.

Preterm birth

The PTB rate among all women was 6.1%, ranging from 4.0% among women with no previous PTB or pregnancy loss to 13.3% among women with a previous preterm birth. Observed rates were highest among women who were underweight or obese, women below or above their recommended GWG and among women who smoked. However, after adjusting for other maternal characteristics, only having above recommended GWG was significantly associated with preterm birth (overall and among primigravidas).

Small-for-gestational-age

The SGA birth rate was 8.1%, ranging from 6.7% among women with no previous PTB or pregnancy loss to 10.5% among primigravidas. Women who were underweight,

were below their recommended GWG and smoked prenatally were significantly more likely to have an SGA baby.

Large-for-gestational-age

The LGA birth rate was 11.3%, ranging from 7.5% among primigravidas to 14.9% among multigravid women with no previous PTB or pregnancy loss. Women who were overweight or obese and were above their recommended GWG were significantly more likely to have an LGA baby. Women whose GWG was below recommendations and women who smoked prenatally were less likely to have an LGA baby.

Generally, the direction of effects for PTB, SGA and LGA remained the same across the four obstetric groups though the magnitude of effects and statistical significance of associations varied. BMI, GWG and smoking were more commonly associated with infant weight (either SGA or LGA) than with PTB. Of the three determinants, only GWG was significantly associated with all outcomes. The small number of women with a previous PTB limited the statistical power to detect significant associations in this group (Table 3).

PAFs for adverse neonatal outcomes

Table 4 presents positive and negative PAFs for adverse neonatal outcomes. Negative PAFs reflect protective ORs in Table 3. We focus on positive PAFs, which estimate the independent contribution of each determinant to PTB, SGA and LGA (i.e., after adjusting for the other two determinants and other covariates).

Preterm birth

Among all women, above recommended GWG contributed to 18.2% of PTB, while low BMI, high BMI and prenatal smoking each contributed to less than 5% of PTB. The pattern among primigravidas and multigravidas with no previous PTB or pregnancy loss was similar to that among all women. Above recommended GWG contributed to over a third of PTB among primigravidas and multigravidas with no previous PTB or pregnancy loss (33.9% and 38.7% respectively). Among women who had experienced a previous PTB, only the PAF of prenatal smoking was positive (5.4%).

Small-for-gestational-age

Among all women, below recommended GWG contributed more (9.2%) to SGA births than prenatal smoking (8.7%) or underweight BMI (5.3%), although the odds of having an SGA baby were higher among women who smoked and were underweight (Table 3). Below recommended GWG, prenatal smoking and underweight BMI contributed to SGA births in all four obstetric groups. The highest PAF due to below recommended weight gain was among multigravidas with no previous PTB or

Table 2 Percent of population with maternal characteristics*

	All women (n = 71,200)	Primigravidas (n = 24,000)	Multigravidas		
			Previous PTB (n = 4,000)	No previous PTB	
				Previous early pregnancy loss[a] (n = 21,300)	No previous early pregnancy loss (n = 21,600)
Percent of sample		33.8	5.7	30.0	30.5
Determinants					
Prepregnancy BMI					
<18.5	6.0	7.1	6.2	5.3	5.4
18.5-24.9	59.7	63.3	51.3	58.1	58.4
25.0-29.9	20.9	17.6	22.9	23.1	22.3
≥30	13.5	12.0	19.6	13.5	13.9
Gestational weight gain					
<recommended	18.6	16.6	18.0	19.4	20.2
=recommended	23.0	22.1	23.2	22.3	24.9
>recommended	59.4	61.3	58.7	58.3	54.9
Smoked 3rd trimester	10.4	7.7	17.2	13.7	10.0
Covariates					
Maternal age					
≤24	15.3	23.6	11.9	12.4	9.5
25-29	34.1	40.4	27.7	29.0	33.5
30-34	33.4	26.1	37.7	35.4	37.8
≥35	17.5	9.8	22.7	23.2	19.3
Maternal education					
Less than high school	6.8	5.1	12.4	7.8	6.7
High school graduate	19.4	17.7	22.7	20.3	19.8
Post-secondary diploma	37.7	38.1	41.6	36.8	37.4
University graduate	36.1	39.2	23.3	35.2	36.1
Low-income-cut-off (LICO)					
≤LICO	18.0	14.9	26.2	19.1	19.1
>LICO	74.0	75.3	69.1	74.1	74.0
Missing	8.0	9.8	4.7	6.9	6.9
Short stature	6.4	5.6	6.8	5.8	7.7
World region of birth					
Canada	76.7	77.8	82.2	76.4	74.9
Europe/Western nations	6.0	5.8	4.4	6.4	5.9
Africa/Caribbean	2.3	2.2	3.4	2.6	1.9
Middle East/North Africa	2.6	2.6	2.3	1.9	3.3
Latin America	2.3	1.8	1.3	2.2	3.2
East Asia/South East Asia/Pacific Islands	5.7	5.4	3.0	6.4	5.7
South Asia	4.5	4.5	3.5	4.1	5.1
Medical conditions prior to pregnancy	15.2	14.3	20.5	16.6	13.8
Medical conditions during pregnancy	24.4	24.8	32.2	25.1	21.8
Depression prior to pregnancy	15.5	13.8	20.2	17.3	14.6

Table 2 Percent of population with maternal characteristics* *(Continued)*

Perceived stress during pregnancy					
Not stressful	43.1	46.4	34.2	41.6	42.6
Somewhat stressful	44.9	44.7	47.6	44.7	45.0
Very stressful	12.0	8.9	18.2	13.8	12.4
No support during pregnancy	12.8	10.0	16.8	14.7	13.3

*Subgroup sample sizes do not add up to the total due to rounding to the nearest 100, as explained in the methods. Abbreviations: PTB – preterm birth, BMI – body mass index.
[a]Early pregnancy loss - miscarriage, abortion and/or ectopic pregnancy.

pregnancy loss (12.3%); the highest PAF due to prenatal smoking was among multigravidas with no previous PTB but with a previous pregnancy loss (13.0%); and the highest PAF due to underweight BMI was among primigravidas (7.5%).

Large-for-gestational-age
Overall, above recommended GWG contributed more (15.9%) to LGA births than being overweight (6.5%) or obese (8.9%). Larger PAFs due to excess GWG were observed among primigravidas and multigravidas with no previous PTB or pregnancy loss, than among multigravidas with a previous pregnancy loss but no previous PTB. Similar to the results for PTB, above recommended GWG contributed to over a third (37.9%) of LGA births in primigravidas. It was not possible to estimate the PAFs for multigravidas with a previous PTB due to the small size of this group (Table 4).

Discussion
The results of this nationally representative study indicate that low or high prepregnancy BMI and inadequate or excess GWG are important contributors to PTB, SGA and LGA infants in Canada. Due to almost 60% of women gaining above the recommended weight for their prepregnancy BMI, excess GWG contributed more to adverse outcomes than high BMI, to 18.2% of PTB and 15.9% of LGA overall. Although the distribution of BMI and GWG was similar across obstetric groups, their impact on studied outcomes was attenuated among women with a previous PTB or early pregnancy loss. The contribution of BMI and GWG to PTB and SGA exceeded that of prenatal smoking. This is the first study to report population-level contributions of maternal weight to PTB, SGA and LGA in Canada.

Our study adds to existing evidence on the association between maternal weight and adverse neonatal outcomes, by estimating the PAFs of PTB, SGA and LGA that could potentially be prevented if all women began their pregnancy with a normal BMI and had a GWG that was within the recommended range. As the PAF is a factor of both the risk associated with a characteristic and the prevalence of that characteristic, we observed

the largest PAFs in subgroups where significant risk and high prevalence converged. For example, the highest odds of LGA (aOR: 2.01[1.12-3.61]) and PTB (aOR: 2.02 [1.13-3.63]) were observed among primigravidas with above recommended GWG and primigravidas also had the highest prevalence of above recommended GWG (61.3%), leading to above recommended GWG contributing to a striking 38.9% of LGA and 33.9% of PTB in these women. A similar pattern was observed among multigravid women with no previous PTB or pregnancy loss. However, the pattern varied among women with a previous PTB or pregnancy loss. Among these women, GWG did not contribute significantly to PTB or LGA although the prevalence of excess GWG was similar to that in other groups. This varied pattern is likely a reflection of differences in the distribution of risk factors across groups. For example, the PTB rate in women with a previous PTB was 13.2%, more than twice the population norm (6.1%), suggesting risk factors for PTB not related to maternal weight. The higher risks associated with excess GWG among primigravidas compared to multigravidas, is likely in part attributable to the fact that on average, primiparous women gained more weight during their pregnancy compared to multiparous women.

The utility of the PAF for informing public health prevention policy is illustrated further by the fact that among all women, even though the risk of having an SGA infant associated with underweight BMI was higher than that associated with below recommended GWG (aOR: 2.04 [1.46-2.52] versus 1.56 [1.20-2.03]); the contribution of underweight BMI to SGA was lower than that of below recommended GWG (5.3% versus 9.2%) because fewer women were underweight than below their recommended GWG (6.0% versus 18.6%). Although PAFs are theoretical, as they are based on a particular risk factor being completely eliminated, our results nevertheless illustrate that maternal weight plays an important role in the incidence of neonatal morbidity at the population level. Studying individual associations of risk alone cannot provide evidence of population-level impacts.

Our findings are difficult to compare to those of other studies due to differences in study methods and underlying characteristics of study populations. For example,

Table 3 Rate (%) and adjusted odds ratios (aORs) of adverse neonatal outcomes associated with BMI, GWG and prenatal smoking*

	PTB		SGA		LGA	
	%	aOR (95% CI)	%	aOR (95% CI)	%	aOR (95% CI)
All women (n = 71,200)	6.1		8.1		11.3	
Prepregnancy BMI						
<18.5	8.4	1.55 [0.96 , 2.52]	20.5	**2.04 [1.46, 2.84]**	4.3	0.64 [0.33, 1.20]
18.5-24.9	5.6	Reference	10.0	Reference	7.5	Reference
25.0-29.9	6.1	0.98 [0.72, 1.33]	8.2	0.95 [0.74, 1.22]	11.4	**1.38 [1.08, 1.75]**
≥30	7.4	1.02 [0.73,1.42]	8.6	0.86 [0.63, 1.15]	14.1	**1.89 [1.45, 2.47]**
Gestational weight gain						
< recommended	6.5	1.35 [0.92, 1.97]	16.1	**1.56 [1.20, 2.03]**	4.6	0.57 [0.39, 0.84]
= recommended	4.5	Reference	10.9	Reference	7.7	Reference
> recommended	6.7	**1.45 [1.06, 1.98]**	7.7	0.70 [0.56, 0.87]	11.0	**1.34 [1.04, 1.72]**
Smoked 3rd trimester						
Yes	8.9	1.31 [0.92, 1.86]	18.4	**2.06 [1.59, 2.67]**	2.8	0.26 [0.16, 0.43]
No	5.8	Reference	9.1	Reference	9.7	Reference
Primigravidas (n = 24,000)	6.8		10.5		7.5	
Prepregnancy BMI						
<18.5	8.7	1.63 [0.77, 3.47]	28.3	**2.47 [1.53, 3.99]**	0.8	0.14 [0.005, 4.69]
81.5-24.9	6.1	Reference	12.2	Reference	6.1	Reference
25.0-29.9	8.6	1.30 [0.80, 2.12]	10.4	0.89 [0.59, 1.34]	7.5	1.12 [0.67, 1.87]
≥30	6.6	0.86 [0.45, 1.66]	12.1	0.97 [0.61, 1.57]	11.4	**1.89 [1.11, 3.21]**
Gestational weight gain						
< recommended	6.6	1.60 [0.78, 3.29]	20.8	1.40 [0.92, 2.12]	2.1	0.49 [0.17, 1.41]
= recommended	3.9	Reference	15.9	Reference	4.1	Reference
> recommended	7.9	**2.02 [1.13, 3.63]**	9.9	0.61 [0.44, 0.86]	8.8	**2.01 [1.12, 3.61]**
Smoked 3rd trimester						
Yes	8.2	1.04 [0.53, 2.04]	27.4	**2.32 [1.49, 3.62]**	2.1	0.29 [0.08, 1.13]
No	6.7	Reference	11.8	Reference	7.0	Reference
Multigravidas, previous PTB (n = 4,000)	13.3		7.4		10.9	
Prepregnancy BMI						
<18.5	8.6	0.70 [0.05, 9.26]	19.7	1.79 [0.20, 15.69]	0	_b
18.5-24.9	15.0	Reference	9.3	Reference	7.2	Reference
25.0-29.9	9.5	0.56 [0.19, 1.67]	6.8	1.14 [0.26, 4.92]	10.6	1.58 [0.33, 7.49]
≥30	14.9	0.89 [0.36, 2.22]	5.9	0.42 [0.08, 2.18]	3.8	0.55 [0.07, 4.34]
Gestational weight gain						
< recommended	13.1	0.83 [0.22, 3.10]	17.1	1.40 [0.35, 5.58]	6.9	1.24 [0.08, 18.45]
= recommended	15.6	Reference	12.8	Reference	4.6	Reference
> recommended	12.5	0.93 [0.33, 2.59]	4.5	0.30 [0.08, 1.14]	7.7	1.01 [0.14, 7.45]
Smoked 3rd trimester						
Yes	16.0	1.45 [0.46, 4.61]	12.8	1.77 [0.43, 7.24]	0	_b
No	12.8	Reference	7.8	Reference	8.3	Reference

Table 3 Rate (%) and adjusted odds ratios (aORs) of adverse neonatal outcomes associated with BMI, GWG and prenatal smoking* *(Continued)*

Multigravidas, no previous PTB, previous loss[a] (n = 21,300)	6.2		7.1		11.8	
Prepregnancy BMI						
<18.5	10.3	1.90 [0.73, 4.93]	14.2	1.75 [0.84, 3.66]	6.7	1.04 [0.37, 2.90]
18.5-24.9	5.7	Reference	9.2	Reference	7.5	Reference
25.0-29.9	5.9	1.00 [0.57, 1.75]	6.4	0.72 [0.44, 1.19]	12.3	1.53 [1.00, 2.36]
≥30	7.2	0.92 [0.47, 1.80]	8.3	0.84 [0.46, 1.54]	16.9	**2.61 [1.61, 4.23]**
Gestational weight gain						
< recommended	8.1	1.14 [0.59, 2.19]	14.2	1.65 [0.96, 2.83]	5.0	0.41 [0.20, 0.81]
= recommended	5.9	Reference	8.2	Reference	9.9	Reference
> recommended	5.7	0.93 [0.53, 1.62]	7.1	0.83 [0.50, 1.36]	11.4	1.02 [0.64, 1.63]
Smoked 3rd trimester						
Yes	8.8	1.77 [0.97, 3.23]	16.3	**2.26 [1.40, 3.64]**	10.8	0.23 [0.10, 0.51]
No	5.8	Reference	7.5	Reference	3.6	Reference
Multigravidas, no previous PTB, no previous loss[a] (n = 21,600)	4.0		6.7		14.9	
Prepregnancy BMI						
<18.5	6.1	2.14 [0.56, 8.20]	15.3	1.81 [0.84, 3.88]	6.9	0.93 [0.31, 2.76]
18.5-24.9	3.5	Reference	8.1	Reference	9.3	Reference
25.0-29.9	3.3	0.75 [0.37, 1.51]	8.3	1.24 [0.76, 2.03]	14.2	1.46 [0.99, 2.14]
≥30	6.5	1.21 [0.59, 2.50]	6.2	0.78 [0.38, 1.61]	16.8	**1.79 [1.14, 2.80]**
Gestational weight gain						
< recommended	3.8	1.98 [0.71, 5.51]	13.6	**1.76 [1.03, 3.03]**	6.2	0.66 [0.34, 1.26]
= recommended	2.1	Reference	8.2	Reference	9.9	Reference
> recommended	4.9	2.52 [0.99, 6.37]	6.4	0.80 [0.49, 1.30]	13.8	1.36 [0.88, 2.08]
Smoked 3rd trimester						
Yes	7.0	1.13 [0.50, 2.59]	15.2	**1.92 [1.10, 3.35]**	3.3	0.29 [0.12, 0.71]
No	3.7	Reference	7.6	Reference	12.1	Reference

*Subgroup sample sizes do not add up to the total due to rounding to the nearest 100, as explained in the methods. Statistically significant aORs are bolded.
Abbreviations: PTB – preterm birth, SGA – small-for-gestational-age, LGA – large-for-gestational-age, BMI – body mass index.
[a]Early pregnancy loss – miscarriage, abortion and/or ectopic pregnancy.
[b]No cases of LGA in these subgroup.

Oteng-Ntim et al. attributed 4.2% of PTB in a hospital-based study in the United Kingdom to obese BMI [23]; and Djelantik et al. attributed 6.6% of PTB in Amsterdam to overweight or obese BMI [24]. However, neither of these studies controlled for GWG. We found that after adjusting for GWG, overweight or obese BMI did not contribute significantly to PTB, whereas more than recommended GWG contributed to almost one in five (18.2%) preterm births. A South Carolina study which investigated independent contributions of BMI and GWG found that inadequate GWG contributed to 8.1% of very low birthweight (VLBW, 500-1,499 g) and underweight, overweight and obese pregnancy BMI contributed to 8.3%, 3.5% and 7.0% of VLBW respectively [25]. But it is not possible to compare our results, as they dichotomized GWG as less than adequate and adequate (i.e., grouped women with recommended GWG with women with excess GWG) and

looked at the impact on low birthweight (LBW) rather than on the constituents of LBW: PTB and SGA, which are known to have different etiologic determinants [6,26]. The importance of looking at PTB and SGA separately, as well as GWG, is highlighted by our findings that excess GWG contributed significantly to PTB but not SGA infants, while underweight BMI and inadequate GWG contributed to both PTB and SGA, but with a larger contribution to SGA. Recognition of such differences facilitates the development of more appropriate preventive interventions for PTB and SGA. Studies have consistently found that obesity contributes significantly to the occurrence of LGA or macrosomia [23,24,27], with PAFs ranging from 7.4% in a UK hospital population in 2004-2008 [23] to 25.7% in Alabama in 1995-1999 [27]. The PAFs of LGA for overweight and obese BMI in our study fell within this range, 6.5% and 8.9% respectively. The large

Table 4 Adjusted population attributable fractions (PAFs) of adverse neonatal outcomes due to BMI, GWG and prenatal smoking*

Characteristic	Prevalence (%) of characteristic	PAF (%, 95 CI)		
		PTB	SGA	LGA
All women (n = 71,200)				
Underweight	6.0	2.6 [2.5, 2.7]	5.3 [5.2, 5.4]	−1.4 [-1.4, -1.3]
Overweight	20.9	−0.4 [-0.6, -0.2]	−0.8 [-0.9, -0.7]	6.5 [6.3, 6.6]
Obese	13.5	0.3 [0.1, 0.4]	−1.6 [-1.7, -1.5]	8.9 [8.8, 9.1]
< recommended GWG	18.6	4.7 [4.4, 5.0]	9.2 [9.0, 9.4]	−6.3 [-6.4, -6.2]
> recommended GWG	59.4	18.2 [17.8, 18.7]	−16.3 [-16.4, -16.1]	15.9 [15.4, 16.3]
Smoked 3rd trimester	10.4	3.2 [3.0, 3.3]	8.7 [8.6, 8.8]	−7.1 [-7.2, -7.0]
Primigravidas (n = 24,000)				
Underweight	7.1	3.3 [3.1, 3.5]	7.5 [7.4, 7.7]	−4.6 [-4.7, -4.5]
Overweight	17.6	4.8 [4.5, 5.1]	−1.4 [-1.6, -1.3]	2.0 [1.7, 2.2]
Obese	12.0	−1.7 [-2.0, -1.5]	−0.1 [-0.2, 0.1]	8.9 [8.6, 9.1]
< recommended GWG	16.6	5.7 [5.5, 6.0]	6.1 [5.8, 6.5]	−5.1 [-5.3, -4.9]
> recommended GWG	61.3	33.9 [33.1, 34.6]	−22.8 [-23.4, -22.3]	37.9 [37.1, 38.6]
Smoked 3rd trimester	7.7	0.3 [0.1, 0.5]	7.5 [7.4, 7.6]	−5.1 [-5.2, -5.0]
Multigravidas, previous PTB (n = 4,000)				
Underweight	6.2	−1.4 [-1.6, -1.2]	4.6 [4.2, 5.1]	−[a]
Overweight	22.9	−10.5 [-11.1, -9.9]	1.9 [1.3, 2.5]	−[a]
Obese	19.6	−2.1 [-2.6, -1.7]	−14.0 [-14.9, -13.2]	−[a]
< recommended GWG	18.0	−3.0 [-3.6, -2.4]	8.0 [7.1, 8.9]	−[a]
> recommended GWG	58.7	−3.6 [-5.1, -2.1]	−54.8 [-57.1, -52.4]	−[a]
Smoked in 3rd trimester	17.2	5.4 [4.9, 6.0]	9.7 [9.0, 10.4]	−[a]
Multigravidas, no previous PTB, previous loss[b] (n = 21,300)				
Underweight	5.3	3.5 [3.3, 3.7]	3.2 [3.1, 3.4]	0.1 [0.0, 0.2]
Overweight	23.1	−0.05 [-0.4, 0.3]	−5.6 [-5.9, -5.4]	8.9 [8.6, 9.2]
Obese	13.5	−1.2 [-1.4, -0.9]	−2.2 [-2.4, -2.0]	13.0 [12.7, 13.2]
< recommended GWG	19.4	2.7 [2.3, 3.1]	11.0 [10.6, 11.4]	−11.4 [-11.6, -11.1]
> recommended GWG	58.3	−3.7 [-4.5, -2.8]	−8.6 [-9.3, -7.9]	1.1 [0.2, 1.9]
Smoked 3rd trimester	13.7	8.0 [7.7, 8.2]	13.0 [12.7, 13.2]	−13.2 [-13.4, -13.0]
Multigravidas, no previous PTB, no previous loss[b] (n = 21,600)				
Underweight	5.4	4.2 [4.0, 4.5]	3.8 [3.7, 4.0]	−0.2 [-0.3, -0.1]
Overweight	22.3	−5.9 [-6.4, -5.5]	3.9 [3.6, 4.2]	7.6 [7.4, 7.8]
Obese	13.9	3.4 [3.0, 3.8]	−2.5 [-2.7, -2.3]	7.9 [7.7, 8.1]
< recommended GWG	20.2	9.5 [9.1, 9.9]	12.3 [11.6, 13.1]	−5.0 [-5.2, -4.8]
> recommended GWG	54.9	38.7 [37.8, 39.5]	−9.3 [-10.0, -8.6]	15.2 [14.6, 15.8]
Smoked 3rd trimester	9.0	1.6 [1.2, 1.9]	7.0 [6.8, 7.2]	−5.4 [-5.4, -5.3]

*Subgroup sample sizes do not add up to the total due to rounding to the nearest 100, as explained in the methods.
Abbreviations: PAF – population attributable fraction, PTB – preterm birth, SGA – small-for-gestational-age, LGA- large-for-gestational-age, BMI – body mass index, GWG – gestational weight gain.
[a]PAFs cannot be estimated due to the small sample size / small number of LGA babies in this group.
[b]Early pregnancy loss – miscarriage, abortion and/or ectopic pregnancy.

PAF reported in the Alabama study reflects the high prevalence of obesity (≥200 lbs) in this population (21.2% versus 13.5% in our study).

The objective of this study was not only to estimate the contribution of BMI and GWG to adverse neonatal outcomes, but to also compare this contribution to that of prenatal smoking for PTB and SGA in particular. We found that overall below recommended and above recommended GWG contributed more to PTB than prenatal smoking (4.7%, 18.2% versus 3.2% respectively), while underweight BMI contributed less (2.6%). Similarly, below recommended GWG contributed more to SGA than prenatal smoking (9.2% versus 8.7%), while underweight BMI contributed less (5.3%). This pattern varied across obstetric groups, with prenatal smoking contributing to a higher proportion of PTB and SGA than BMI or GWG, among women with a previous PTB or pregnancy loss. As stated earlier, this variation in pattern likely reflects differences in the distribution of underlying risk factors for PTB and SGA across groups. Our results are similar to that of a 2003-2004 study in Amsterdam which found that the contribution of pre-pregnancy overweight and obesity (BMI ≥ 25) to PTB exceeded that of prenatal smoking (6.6% versus 5.5%) [24]. This study did not investigate contributions of GWG or underweight BMI.

Recognition of the contribution prenatal smoking makes to adverse pregnancy outcomes has led to considerable efforts to develop smoking cessation interventions during pregnancy [28]. However, the contribution of maternal weight to adverse pregnancy outcomes has not been similarly quantified and less attention has been paid to developing interventions aimed at healthy maternal weight during pregnancy. Our results suggest that due to the much higher prevalence of inadequate GWG (18.6%) and excess GWG (59.4%) compared with prenatal smoking (10.4%), maternal weight in general and GWG in particular contributed significantly more to PTB and SGA than prenatal smoking. Thus, from a public health perspective, the importance of healthy maternal weight for the studied outcomes exceeds that of prenatal smoking. Unfortunately, although there is evidence that counselling from a health care provider regarding GWG is effective in helping women plan to gain the recommended amount of weight [29,30], there is also evidence suggesting that few women receive such counselling [31]. In Canada, as in many other high-income countries, prenatal smoking is decreasing [32], while overweight and obesity are increasing [7]. As this trend continues, the already large PAFs for BMI and GWG are likely to increase while PAFs for prenatal smoking decrease. This was observed by Lu et al. in Alabama between 1980-84 and 1995-99. Although there was no significant change in the risk of LGA associated with obesity (≥200 lbs), the PAF of LGA attributed to obesity increased from 6.5% to 19.1%, as the prevalence of obesity increased from 7.7% to 21.2% [27]. Cnattingius et al. asserted in 2002 that from a public health perspective, maternal overweight and obese BMI was one of the most important modifiable risk factors for pregnancy complications and adverse pregnancy outcomes [9]. Our findings support

and go beyond this assertion to also highlight the importance of underweight BMI and inadequate and excess GWG.

Our study has several limitations. Self-reported data on BMI and GWG are highly correlated with measured values, but they tend to underestimate these measures [33,34]. This could have led to an overestimation of the risk associated with overweight or obese BMI and excess GWG, as women reporting these characteristics are more likely to be at the higher end of the BMI and GWG spectrum and therefore at increased risk of adverse outcomes [33]. Underestimation of these measures could, however, also have led to more conservative PAFs, as PAFs take into consideration the prevalence of the characteristic. Due to a lack of data on per trimester weight gain, as per IOM guidelines, we assumed a 2 kg weight gain in the first trimester and linear weight gain in the remainder of the pregnancy, although some studies suggest alternate patterns [35]. It is possible that if there was excess gain above 2 kg in the first trimester, that could be contributing to adverse outcomes, rather than second or third trimester excess weight gain. There is a need for more research on timing of GWG and neonatal outcomes. Data did not include a breakdown of PTB by aetiology, so we were unable to assess whether the contribution of maternal weight varied by PTB subtypes [36]. The importance of a previous PTB as a risk factor for adverse outcomes in a subsequent pregnancy may vary with the degree of PTB (e.g. at 31 weeks vs at 36 weeks); however we were not able to assess this as data did not include the gestational age of previous PTBs. Data also only included smoking status in the third trimester. Additionally, studying outcomes overall and across four obstetric groups required us to make multiple comparisons which is known to increase the chance of significant findings [37]. However, the associations we noted are plausible and we reported precise confidence intervals to support interpretation. Finally, our data excluded multiple births and infant deaths, making our population healthier than the general population; and some residual confounding may remain due to unmeasured factors. For example, we did not have information on gestational diabetes which is a risk factor for LGA. However, we note that other data found gestational diabetes contributed far less to LGA (2-8%) compared to excess GWG (33.3-37.7%) [38].

Conclusions

Our study provides evidence that maternal weight in general, and GWG in particular, contributes significantly to the occurrence of PTB, SGA and LGA in Canada. The contribution of these modifiable risk factors rivals that of prenatal smoking, and the contributions of high BMI and excess GWG in particular are likely to increase as population rates of overweight and obesity rise. These findings highlight the public health importance of promoting a healthy prepregnancy BMI and appropriate GWG.

Competing interests
The authors declare that they have no competing interests.

Authors' contributions
SD and SDM conceived and guided the study. SD, JF and RSK developed statistical methods and SD carried out statistical analysis. SD and SDM drafted and revised the manuscript on the basis of comments from other authors: JF, RSK, SCT, BC, MIH, SB, AB, EKD and LSL. All authors contributed to the interpretation of the results, critically reviewed all manuscript drafts and approved the final version.

Acknowledgements
We thank the members of the Maternity Experiences Survey Study Group of the Canadian Perinatal Surveillance System who were instrumental to the development of the MES and Statistics Canada for its collaboration with the Public Health Agency of Canada in the implementation of the MES. SDM is supported by a Canadian Institute of Health Research (CIHR) New Investigator Salary Award.

Author details
[1]Maternal and Infant Health Section, Health Surveillance and Epidemiology Division, Public Health Agency of Canada, 785 Carling Avenue, 6804A 4th Floor, Ottawa, Ontario K1A 0 K9, Canada. [2]Reproductive Care Program of Nova Scotia, Halifax, Nova Scotia, Canada. [3]Department of Community and Family Health, College of Public Health, University of South Florida, Tampa, FL, U.S.A. [4]Departments of Paediatrics and Community Health Sciences, Faculty of Medicine, University of Calgary, Calgary, Alberta, Canada. [5]Department of Obstetrics and Gynaecology, Ottawa Hospital Research Institute, University of Ottawa, Ottawa, Ontario, Canada. [6]College of Nursing, Faculty of Health Sciences, University of Manitoba, Winnipeg, Manitoba, Canada. [7]Department of Family and Community Medicine, University of Toronto, Mount Sinai Hospital, Toronto, Ontario, Canada. [8]Midwifery Education Program, Laurentian University, Sudbury, Ontario, Canada. [9]Perinatal Services British Columbia, Provincial Health Services Authority, Vancouver, British Columbia, Canada. [10]Departments of Obstetrics & Gynecology, Radiology, and Clinical Epidemiology & Biostatistics, McMaster University, Hamilton, Canada.

References
1. Flenady V, Koopmans L, Middleton P, Froen JF, Smith GC, Gibbons K, et al. Major risk factors for stillbirth in high-income countries: a systematic review and meta-analysis. Lancet. 2011;377:1331–40.
2. McDonald SD, Han Z, Mulla S, Beyene J, Knowledge Synthesis Group. Overweight and obesity in mothers and risk of preterm birth and low birth weight infants: systematic review and meta-analyses. BMJ. 2010;341:c3428.
3. Bodnar LM, Siega-Riz AM, Simhan HN, Himes KP, Abrams B. Severe obesity, gestational weight gain, and adverse birth outcomes. Am J Clin Nutr. 2010;91:1642–8.
4. Nohr EA, Vaeth M, Baker J, Sorensen T, Olsen J, Rasmussen KM. Combined associations of prepregnancy body mass index and gestational weight gain with the outcome of pregnancy. Am J Clin Nutr. 2008;87:1750–9.
5. Han Z, Mulla S, Beyene J, Liao G, McDonald SD, Knowledge Synthesis Group. Maternal underweight and the risk of preterm birth and low birth weight: a systematic review and meta-analyses. Int J Epidemiol. 2011;40:65–101.
6. Heaman M, Kingston D, Chalmers B, Sauve R, Lee L, Young D. Risk factors for preterm birth and small-for-gestational-age births among Canadian women. Paediatr Perinat Epidemiol. 2012;27:54–61.
7. Tjepkema M. Adult obesity. Health Rep. 2006;17:9–25.
8. Stevens GA, Singh GM, Lu Y, Danaei G, Lin JK, Finucane MM, et al. National, regional, and global trends in adult overweight and obesity prevalences. Popul Health Metr. 2012;10:22.
9. Cnattingius S, Lambe M. Trends in smoking and overweight during pregnancy: Prevalence, risks of pregnancy complications, and adverse pregnancy outcomes. Semin Perinatol. 2002;6:286–95.
10. Public Health Agency of Canada. What mothers say: the Canadian maternity experiences survey. Ottawa: Public Health Agency of Canada; 2009.
11. Dzakpasu S, Kaczorowski J, Chalmers B, Heaman M, Duggan J, Neusy E, et al. The Canadian maternity experiences survey: design and methods. J Obstet Gynaecol Can. 2008;30:207–16.
12. Ray JG, Sgro M, Mamdani MM, Glazier RH, Bocking A, Hilliard R, et al. Birth weight curves tailored to maternal world region. J Obstet Gynaecol Can. 2012;34:159–71.
13. Kierans WJ, Joseph KS, Luo ZC, Platt R, Wilkins R, Kramer MS. Does one size fit all? The case for ethnic-specific standards of fetal growth. BMC Pregnancy Childbirth. 2008;8:1.
14. Institute of Medicine (US) and National Research Council (US) Committee to Reexamine IOM Pregnancy Weight Guidelines, Rasmussen KM, Yaktine AL. Weight gain during pregnancy: reexamining the guidelines. Washington (DC): The National Academies Press (US); 2009.
15. Health Canada. Prenatal Nutrition Guidelines for Health Professionals: gestational weight gain. Health Canada 2010. Available from: http://www.oxfordcounty.ca/Portals/15/Documents/Public%20Health/Healthy%20You/Nutrition/ewba-mbsa-eng.pdf [Accessed 25 September 2014].
16. Statistics Canada. Low income cut-offs. Available from: http://www.statcan.gc.ca/pub/75f0002m/2009002/s2-eng.htm#n1 [Accessed 25 September 2014].
17. Hosmer DW, Lemeshow S. Variable Selection. In: Applied Logistic Regression. New York: John Wiley & Sons; 2000. p. 92–116.
18. Goldenberg RL, Culhane JF, Iams JD, Romero R. Epidemiology and causes of preterm birth. Lancet. 2008;371:75–84.
19. Ota E, Ganchimeg T, Morisaki N, Vogel JP, Pileggi C, Ortiz-Panozo E, et al. Risk factors and adverse perinatal outcomes among term and preterm infants born small-for-gestational-age: secondary analyses of the WHO multi-country survey on maternal and newborn health. PLoS One. 2014;9:e105155.
20. Ruckinger S, von Kries R, Toschke A. An illustration of and programs estimating attributable fractions in large scale surveys considering multiple risk factors. BMC Med Res Methodol. 2009;9:7.
21. Rao JNK, Wu CFJ, Yue K. Some recent work on resampling methods for complex surveys. Surv Methodol. 1992;18:209–17.
22. SAS Institute Inc. SAS EG software, version 5.1 Copyright © 2012 by. SAS Institute Inc, Cary, NC, USA.
23. Oteng-Ntim E, Kopeika J, Seed P, Wandiembe S, Doyle P. Impact of obesity on pregnancy outcome in different ethnic groups: calculating population attributable fractions. PLoS One. 2013;8:e53749.
24. Djelantik AA, Kunst AE, van der Wal MF, Smit HA, Vrijkotte TG. Contribution of overweight and obesity to the occurrence of adverse pregnancy outcomes in a multi-ethnic cohort: population attributive fractions for Amsterdam. BJOG. 2012;119:283–90.
25. Hulsey TC, Neal D, Bondo SC, Hulsey T, Newman R. Maternal prepregnant body mass index and weight gain related to low birth weight in South Carolina. South Med J. 2005;8:411–5.
26. Kramer MS. The epidemiology of adverse pregnancy outcomes: an overview. J Nutr. 2003;133:1592S–6.
27. Lu GC, Rouse DJ, DuBard M, Cliver S, Kimberlin D, Hauth JC. The effect of the increasing prevalence of maternal obesity on perinatal morbidity. Am J Obstet Gynecol. 2001;185:845–9.
28. Chamberlain C, O'Mara-Eves A, Oliver S, Caird JR, Perlen SM, Eades SJ, et al. Psychosocial interventions for supporting women to stop smoking in pregnancy. Cochrane Database Syst Rev. 2013;10, CD001055.
29. Tovar A, Guthrie LB, Platek D, Stuebe A, Herring SJ, Oken E. Modifiable predictors associated with having a gestational weight gain goal. Matern Child Health J. 2011;15:1119–26.
30. Stotland NE, Haas JS, Brawarsky P, Jackson RA, Fuentes-Afflick E, Escobar GJ. Body mass index, provider advice, and target gestational weight gain. Obstet Gynecol. 2005;105:633–8.
31. McDonald SD, Pullenayegum E, Taylor VH, Lutsiv O, Bracken K, Good C, et al. Despite 2009 guidelines, few women report being counseled correctly about weight gain during pregnancy. Am J Obstet Gynecol. 2011;205:333. e1-6.
32. Gilbert NL, Bartholomew S, Raynault MF, Kramer MS. Temporal trends in social disparities in maternal smoking and breastfeeding in Canada, 1992-2008. Matern Child Health J. 2014;18:1905–22.
33. Shields M, Gorber SC, Tremblay MS. Effect of measurement on obesity and morbidity. Health Rep. 2008;19:77–84.

34. Brunner Huber LR. Validity of self-reported height and weight in women of reproductive age. Maternal Child Health J. 2007;11:137–44.

35. Diouf I, Botton J, Charles MA, Morel O, Forhan A, Kaminski M, et al. Specific role of maternal weight change in the first trimester of pregnancy on birth size. Matern Child Nutr. 2014;10:315–26.

36. Nohr EA, Bech BH, Vaeth M, Rasmussen KM, Henriksen TB, Olsen J. Obesity, gestational weight gain and preterm birth: a study within the Danish National Birth Cohort. Paediatr Perinat Epidemiol. 2007;21:5–14.

37. Feise RJ. Do multiple outcome measures require p-value adjustment? BMC Med Res Methodol. 2002;2:8.

38. Kim SY, Sharma AJ, Sappenfield W, Wilson HG, Salihu HM. Association of maternal body mass index, excessive weight gain, and gestational diabetes mellitus with large-for-gestational-age births. Obstet Gynecol. 2014;123:737–44.

2

Obesity and pregnancy outcomes: Do the relationships differ by maternal region of birth?

Miranda Davies-Tuck[1*], Joanne C. Mockler[1,2,3], Lynne Stewart[3], Michelle Knight[2] and Euan M. Wallace[1,2,3]

Abstract

Background: We aimed to determine whether the association between obesity and a range of adverse maternal and perinatal outcomes differed in South Asian and Australian and New Zealand born women.

Methods: A retrospective cohort study of singleton births in South Asian (SA) and Australian/New Zealand (AUS/NZ) born women at an Australian hospital between 2009 and 2013. The interaction between maternal region of birth and obesity on a range of maternal and perinatal outcomes was assessed using multivariate logistic regression.

Results: Obesity was more strongly associated with gestational hypertension/Preeclampsia/HELLP and Gestational Diabetes Mellitus in AUS/NZ born women ($p = 0.001$ and $p < 0.001$, respectively for interaction) and was only associated with shoulder dystocia in SA born women ($p = 0.006$ for interaction). There was some evidence that obesity was more strongly related with admission to NICU/Special care nursery (SCN) ($p = 0.06$ for interaction) and any perinatal morbidity ($p = 0.05$ for interaction) in SA born women.

Conclusions: Interventions targeted at reducing maternal obesity will have different impacts in SA compared to AUS/NZ born women.

Keywords: Obesity, Maternal region of birth and Pregnancy outcomes

Background

Maternal obesity has emerged as one of the key contributors to adverse pregnancy outcomes in high-income nations [1], with no evidence that this trend is likely to reverse in the near future. In these countries almost half of women enter pregnancy with a body mass index (BMI) of 25 or more [1]. Interestingly, many of the adverse outcomes associated with maternal obesity, such as stillbirth, gestational diabetes mellitus (GDM), and operative delivery [1], are also more common in Asian women, with some of the highest rates of poor outcome seen in south Asian(SA) born women with obesity [2, 3]. Not surprisingly, it has been suggested that the associations between obesity and adverse pregnancy outcomes may be additive in some ethnicities [2–4]. For example,

in a study of singleton births in London, UK, obesity in Asian (South and other Asian) women was associated with a stillbirth rate five times higher than in Asian women without obesity. The rate was lower still in Caucasian women, irrespective of obesity [2]. Similarly, obesity appears to be a stronger risk factor for GDM in Asian women than in Caucasian women [3]. However, none of these studies examined possible differential associations between obesity and other maternal and perinatal outcomes by maternal Asian ethnicity. Further, the patterns of Asian migration in the UK have been quite different to that elsewhere in the world and so whether the findings there are equally applicable to Australia is not known. This is potentially quite important because both migration from South Asia to Australia and other high-income countries outside the UK and, quite separately, the rate of obesity among SA born women are increasing internationally [5–8] (http://www.statcan.gc.ca/pub/89-621-x/89-621-x2007006-eng.htm). Accordingly, we

* Correspondence: Miranda.davies@hudson.org.au
[1]The Ritchie Centre, Hudson Institute of Medical Research, Clayton, Vic 3168, Australia
Full list of author information is available at the end of the article

undertook this study to determine whether the association between maternal obesity and a range of adverse maternal and perinatal outcomes differed in South Asian and Australian born women.

Methods

We studied all singleton births ≥24 weeks gestation, free from congenital anomalies at Monash Women's Services, Monash Health, a metropolitan maternity service in Melbourne, Australia, from 2009 to 2013, inclusive. Data were extracted from the Birthing Outcomes System, an electronic database recording all births ≥20 weeks' gestation. For woman the attending midwife, supported by routine data validation, enters 191 data items over the course of pregnancy. For this study, we extracted data from the following fields: maternal age, self reported pre-gravid at booking body mass index (BMI), region of birth, parity, smoking, private or public care, obstetric and intrapartum complications (e.g fetal compromise), onset of labour (spontaneous or induced), augmentation of labour, epidural use, length of first and second stage of labour, blood loss, gestation at birth, birth weight, baby gender, mode of birth (spontaneous/instrumental/caesarean (further defined as Planned or Unplanned), admission to NICU/SCN, perinatal morbidity (e.g. respiratory distress, bradycardia, sepsis, meconium aspiration, birth trauma and birth asphyxia) and stillbirth. Fields were largely complete. Only women who had a pre-gravid BMI at booking recorded were included (98.5 % of AUS/NZ and 99.5 %% of SA women). Other missing data were case-wise excluded. The only fields with missing data were blood loss (0.1 %, $n = 15$) and baby gender (0.015 %, $n = 4$) all other fields were 100 % complete. The birthing outcome system only collects information on self-reported maternal region of birth. Therefore this was then classified, as either Australian and New Zealand (AUS/NZ) region of birth or South Asian (e.g. Afghanistan, Bangladesh, Bhutan, India, Iran, Maldives, Nepal, Pakistan and Sri Lanka) region of birth, according to the United Nations regional groups [9] and was used as a proxy marker for ethnicity.

Women of other nationalities were excluded because the aim of the study was to examine outcomes in South Asian women relative to AUS/NZ women. Obesity was defined as a BMI ≥ 30 kg/m^2. The study was granted an exemption from ethics review by the Monash University Human Research and Ethics Committee, as per section 5.1.22 of the National statement on ethical conduct in Human Research 2007 [10].

Statistical analysis

Maternal demographics, pregnancy, labour and baby outcomes were tabulated by maternal region of birth and obesity. Differences in demographics across groups were determined by a chi^2 test. The univariate association between maternal obesity and region of birth group and pregnancy, labour and birth outcomes were assessed using logistic regression. Known and potential risk factors that were assessed for their inclusion in the final model were maternal age, parity, patient account class, smoking, onset of labour (spontaneous, induced, no labour), gestation, baby birth weight, baby gender, augmentation, epidural, placental abnormality, baby birth weight, onset of labour, birth type (e.g. vaginal/instrumental/operative), episiotomy, length of labour, pre-existing maternal medical conditions and previous caesarean. A number of potential confounders may also reflect steps in the causal pathway, e.g. Obesity to Pre-existing Diabetes to Gestational diabetes, therefore based on the literature potential intermediaries were not included in the final regression models. Potential co-linearity between confounders was also determined prior to the final model being defined. Each of the confounders included in the final model are detailed in the table footnotes. The interaction between maternal region of birth and obesity on each of the outcomes was then assessed by computing an interaction term and including it in the model. Logistic regression was then performed, stratified for maternal country of birth. The likelihood ratio was used to determine the final model. Differential BMI cut offs for SAs have been recommended by the World Health Organisation [11]. Therefore, the analysis was also undertaken defining obesity in South Asian women as ≥26 kg/m^2. Doing so did not change our findings. Therefore, we present results using a BMI cut off of 30 kg/m^2 only. Non-independence is a recognised issue within perinatal datasets, therefore all analyses were also run in nulliparous women only. This did not alter the associations. Due to the rare nature of some of the outcomes we therefore present data on all women to preserve power. Due to the number of hypotheses tested, we also computed a Benjamini–Hochberg false discovery rate corrected p value, after doing this a p-value <0.046 (two-tailed) was regarded as significant. All analyses were performed using the SPSS statistical package (SPSS 20, IBM Corp, Armonk, New York, USA).

Results

Between 2009 and 2013 there were 41 041 singleton births at our institution. Of these, 18 768 (45 %) were to women born either in Australia or New Zealand (AUS/NZ) and 8342 (20 %) were to women born in South Asian countries (SA). Indian women comprised the majority of SA born women (51.4 %), followed by Sri Lankan (21.2 %) and Afghan women (18.6 %). Obesity was seen 27 % of AUS/NZ born women and 10 % of SA born women. The characteristics of the women, stratified by maternal region of birth and obesity, are summarised in Table 1. Associations between pregnancy, labour and perinatal outcomes and maternal region of birth and obesity are summarised in Table 2. Australian born mothers with obesity had the highest rates of gestational hypertension/PE/HELLP, PPH, induced labours and macrosomic babies. Women born in SA with obesity had the highest rates of Gestational Diabetes, Dystocia, unplanned caesarean, fetal compromise, admission to NICU/SCN and any perinatal morbidity. Overall compared to Australian born women without obesity, SA born women with obesity were 7.4 times (95 % CI 6.1–9.02) more likely to have gestational diabetes ($p < 0.001$), twice as likely (95 % CI 1.37–3.01) to experience dystocia ($p < 0.001$), twice as likely (95 % CI 1.66–2.29) to require an unplanned caesarean ($p < 0.001$), 39 % more likely (1.20–1.61) to experience fetal compromise, 53 % (95 % CI 1.31–1.79) more likely to have a baby admitted to the NICU and 39 % (95%CI 1.21–1.59) more likely to have a baby experience a perinatal morbidity ($p < 0.001$) The highest rates of stillbirth were also seen in women born in SA with obesity, although this difference was not statistically significant.

The associations between obesity and pregnancy and labour outcomes, stratified for maternal region of birth, are presented in Table 3. The association between obesity and hypertension/PE/HELLP and GDM was

stronger in AUS/NZ born women than in SA born women ($p = 0.001$ and $p < 0.001$, respectively for interaction). Obesity was associated with a three-fold increased likelihood (95 % CI 2.78–3.54, $p < 0.001$) of gestational hypertension/PE/HELLP in AUS/NZ born women compared to only a 59 % increased likelihood (95 % CI 1.14–2.21, $p = 0.006$) in SA born women. Similarly, GDM was three times more common (OR 3.2, 95 % CI 2.80–3.67, $p < 0.001$) in AUS/NZ born women with obesity and nearly twice as common (OR 1.89(1.57–2.28), $p < 0.001$) in SA born women with obesity. Obesity was also associated with shoulder dystocia in SA born women but not in AUS/NZ born women ($p = 0.006$ for interaction). For all women, irrespective of maternal region of birth, obesity was associated with an increased odds of unplanned caesarean section. There was no evidence of effect modification by maternal region of birth for the association between obesity and preterm birth, severe post-partum haemorrhage, instrumental vaginal birth or unplanned caesarean section.

The associations between obesity and infant outcomes, stratified for maternal region of birth, are presented in Table 4. There was some evidence that obesity was more strongly related with admission to NICU/SCN ($p = 0.06$ for interaction) and any perinatal morbidity ($p = 0.05$ for interaction) in SA born women. Obesity was associated

Table 1 Description of study population

	Australian mothers without obesity ($n = 13,605$)	Australian mothers with obesity ($n = 5163$)	South Asian mothers without obesity ($n = 7467$)	South Asian mothers with obesity ($n = 875$)
Maternal age groups				
< 20 years	621(4.6 %)	139(2.7 %)	34(0.5 %)	4(0.5 %)
20–30years	5846(43.0 %)	2289(44.3 %)	4062(54.4 %)	345(39.4 %)
> 30 years	7138(52.5 %)	2735(53 %)	3371(45.1 %)	526(60.1 %)
Nulliparous	6131(45.1 %)	1887(36.5 %)	3883(52 %)	307(35.1 %)
Past caesarean	1576(11.6 %)	1007(19.5 %)	942(12.6 %)	185(21.1 %)
Private patient	2616(16.2 %)	584(11.3 %)	587(7.9 %)	57(6.5 %)
Smoking				
Smoker	2259(16.6 %)	932(18.1 %)	24(0.3 %)	2(0.2 %)
Non-Smoker	9964(73.2 %)	3625(70.2 %)	7407(99.2 %)	860(98.3 %)
Spontaneous quitter	1382(10.2 %)	606(11.7 %)	36(0.5 %)	13(1.5 %)
Pre-existing hypertension	96(0.7 %)	208(4.0 %)	30(0.4 %)	15(1.7 %)
Pre-existing diabetes	162(1.2 %)	121(2.3 %)	60(0.8 %)	29(3.3 %)
Pre-existing thyroid disease	284(2.1 %)	146(2.8 %)	410(5.5 %)	68(7.8 %)
Baby gender-male	6952(51.1 %)	2676(51.8 %)	3857(51.7 %)	438(50.1 %)
Gestational age				
< 37 weeks	1256(9.2 %)	501(9.7 %)	441(5.9 %)	55(6.3 %)
37–41 + 6 weeks	12,115(89 %)	4570(88.5 %)	6927(92.8 %)	805(92 %)
≥ 42 weeks	234(1.7 %)	92(1.8 %)	99(1.3 %)	15(1.7 %)

Number(%)
Chi^2 test to determine differences across the four groups. All differences were statistically significant at the $p < 0.001$ level
Obesity defined as BMI ≥30 kg/m^2

Table 2 Pregnancy, labour and baby outcomes by maternal region of birth and obesity

	Number(%)	Crude odds ratio (95 % CI)	P value
Gestational Hypertension/PE/HELLP[1] Syndrome			
Australian mothers without obesity	583(4.3 %)	1	-
Australian mothers with obesity	586(11.3 %)	2.86(2.54–3.22)	**<0.001**
South Asian mothers without obesity	264(3.5 %)	0.82(0.71–0.95)	**0.008**
South Asian mothers with obesity	45(5.1 %)	1.21(0.89 to 1.65)	0.23
Gestational Diabetes			
Australian mothers without obesity	433(3.2 %)	1	-
Australian mothers with obesity	491(9.5 %)	3.20(2.80–3.65)	**<0.001**
South Asian mothers without obesity	794(10.6 %)	3.62(3.21–4.08)	**<0.001**
South Asian mothers with obesity	172(19.7 %)	7.44(6.14–9.02)	**<0.001**
Preterm Birth			
Australian mothers without obesity	1256(9.2 %)	1	-
Australian mothers with obesity	501(9.7 %)	1.06(0.95–1.18)	0.32
South Asian mothers without obesity	441(5.9 %)	0.62(0.55–0.69)	**<0.001**
South Asian mothers with obesity	55(6.3 %)	0.66(0.50–0.87)	**0.003**
Dystocia			
Australian mothers without obesity	226(1.7 %)	1	-
Australian mothers with obesity	101(2.0 %)	1.18(0.93–1.50)	0.17
South Asian mothers without obesity	117(1.6 %)	0.94(0.75–1.18)	0.61
South Asian mothers with obesity	29(3.3 %)	2.03(1.37–3.01)	**<0.001**
Postpartum Haemorrhage 1000 ml			
Australian mothers without obesity	661(4.9 %)	1	-
Australian mothers with obesity	372(7.2 %)	1.52(1.33–1.73)	**<0.001**
South Asian mothers without obesity	334(4.5 %)	0.92(0.80–1.05)	0.20
South Asian mothers with obesity	49(5.6 %)	1.16(0.86–1.56)	0.33
Induced Labour			
Australian mothers without obesity	2955(21.7 %)	1	-
Australian mothers with obesity	1496(29 %)	1.47(1.37–1.58)	**<0.001**
South Asian mothers without obesity	1727(23.1 %)	1.09(1.01–1.16)	**0.02**
South Asian mothers with obesity	244(27.9 %)	1.39(1.20–1.62)	**<0.001**
Instrumental Vaginal			
Australian mothers without obesity	1846(13.6 %)	1	-
Australian mothers with obesity	478(9.3 %)	0.65(0.58–0.72)	**<0.001**
South Asian mothers without obesity	1284(17.2 %)	1.32(1.24–1.43)	**<0.001**
South Asian mothers with obesity	97(11.1 %)	0.79(0.64–0.99)	**0.04**
Unplanned Caesarean			
Australian mothers without obesity	1898(14 %)	1	-
Australian mothers with obesity	1003(19.4 %)	1.49(1.37–1.62)	**<0.001**
South Asian mothers without obesity	1398(18.7 %)	1.42(1.32–1.53)	**<0.001**
South Asian mothers with obesity	210(24 %)	1.95(1.66–2.29)	**<0.001**
Small for gestational age(<10th centile)			
Australian mothers without obesity	1449(10.7 %)	1	-
Australian mothers with obesity	367(7.1 %)	0.64(0.57–0.72)	**<0.001**

Table 2 Pregnancy, labour and baby outcomes by maternal region of birth and obesity *(Continued)*

South Asian mothers without obesity	1262(16.9 %)	1.71(1.57–1.85)	**<0.001**
South Asian mothers with obesity	90(10.3 %)	0.96(0.77–1.20)	0.73
Macroscomia(>4 kg)			
Australian mothers without obesity	1575(11.6 %)	1	-
Australian mothers with obesity	994(19.3 %)	1.82(1.67–1.99)	**<0.001**
South Asian mothers without obesity	439(5.9 %)	0.48(0.43–0.53)	**<0.001**
South Asian mothers with obesity	111(12.7 %)	1.11(0.90–1.36)	0.32
Fetal compromise (pregnancy or labour)			
Australian mothers without obesity	3431(25.2 %)	1	-
Australian mothers with obesity	1372(26.6 %)	1.07(1.00–1.15)	0.06
South Asian mothers without obesity	2315(31 %)	1.33(1.25–1.42)	**<0.001**
South Asian mothers with obesity	279(31.9 %)	1.39(1.20–1.61)	**<0.001**
Admission to NICU/SCN[2]			
Australian mothers without obesity	2664(19.5 %)	1	-
Australian mothers with obesity	1238(24.1 %)	1.32(1.22–1.42)	**<0.001**
South Asian mothers without obesity	1455(19.6 %)	1.01(0.94–1.08)	0.85
South Asian mothers with obesity	235(27 %)	1.53(1.31–1.79)	**<0.001**
Any Perinatal Morbidity			
Australian mothers without obesity	5726(42 %)	1	-
Australian mothers with obesity	2341(45.3 %)	1.14(1.07–1.22)	**<0.001**
South Asian mothers without obesity	3197(42.8 %)	1.03(0.97–1.09)	0.31
South Asian mothers with obesity	49(50.2 %)	1.39(1.21–1.59)	**<0.001**
Stillbirth			
Australian mothers without obesity	72(0.5 %)	1	-
Australian mothers with obesity	31(0.6 %)	1.14(0.74–1.73)	0.56
South Asian mothers without obesity	32(0.4 %)	0.81(0.55–1.23)	0.32
South Asian mothers with obesity	6(0.7 %)	1.30(0.56–2.99)	0.54

Number in bold reflect statistical significance
Number(%)
[1]Pre-eclampsia(PE)
[2]Neonatal intensive care unit(NICU)/ Special care nursery(SCN)

with a 66 % increased likelihood of NICU/SCN admission (95 % CI 1.66(1.40–1.97)) in SA born women compared to a 33 % (95 % CI (1.22–1.45)) increase in AUS/NZ born women. Obesity was also associated with a 45 % (95 % CI 1.25–1.68)) increased likelihood of any perinatal morbidity in SA born women compared to a 18 % (95 % CI 1.04–1.27) increased likelihood of any perinatal morbidity in AUS/NZ born women. For all women, irrespective of maternal region of birth, obesity was associated with a reduced likelihood of a Small for Gestational Age (SGA; <10th centile) and an increased likelihood of macrosomia (4.5 kg or more) and fetal distress (Table 4). These findings remained the same when the lower BMI cut off for SA women was used (data not shown). There was no evidence of effect modification by maternal region of birth for obesity and small for gestational age, macrosomia, fetal distress in labour and stillbirth.

Discussion

In this study we have explored the relative impacts of maternal region of birth, as a surrogate for ethnicity, on the association between obesity and rates of maternal and perinatal outcomes. We have shown that important outcomes significantly differed by both maternal region of birth and by obesity. Further, maternal region of birth influenced the association between obesity and hypertensive conditions of pregnancy, GDM, dystocia, admission of baby to NICU/SCN and perinatal morbidity. We believe that these observations can be useful to clinicians, allowing better identification of 'at risk' pregnancies and individualisation of care in pregnancy and childbirth.

To our knowledge, this is the first study to examine the potential effect modification of maternal south Asian region of birth on the well established associations between maternal obesity and a range of maternal and

Table 3 Adjusted odds ratio (95 % CI) for pregnancy and labour outcomes according to maternal obesity

	Australian women odds ratio (95 % CI)	P value	South Asian Women odds ratio (95 % CI)	P value	P for interaction
Gestational Hypertension/PE/HELLP [a]	3.14(2.78–3.54)	**<0.001**	1.59(1.14–2.21)	**0.006**	**0.001**
Gestational Diabetes [b]	3.21(2.80–3.67)	**<0.001**	1.89(1.57–2.28)	**<0.001**	**<0.001**
Preterm Birth [c]	1.04(0.93–1.16)	0.49	1.08(0.81–1.45)	0.60	0.99
Dystocia [d]	1.11(0.87–1.41)	0.16	1.99(1.26–2.96)	**0.002**	**0.006**
PPH1000ml [e]	1.49(1.30–1.71)	**<0.001**	1.32(0.96–1.82)	0.09	0.36
Instrumental Vaginal [f]	0.73(0.65–0.82)	**<0.001**	0.76(0.57–1.01)	*0.05*	0.73
Unplanned Caesarean [g]	1.35(1.23–1.49)	**<0.001**	1.38(1.15–1.66)	**0.001**	0.48

Number in bold reflect statistical significance
[a] Odds ratio for Gestational Hypertension/PE/HELLP according to maternal obesity adjusted for age, parity and smoking status
[b] Odds ratio for gestational diabetes according to maternal obesity adjusted for age, parity and smoking status
[c] Odds ratio for preterm birth according to maternal obesity adjusted for age, parity and smoking
[d] Odds ratio for shoulder dystocia according to maternal obesity adjusted for age, parity, induction, augmentation and epidural
[e] Odds ratio for PPH1000mls according to maternal obesity adjusted age, parity, placental abnormality, baby birth weight, gestational hypertension/PE/HELLP, onset of labour, birth type (e.g. vaginal/instrumental/operative), episiotomy, Length of labour and pre-existing maternal blood disorder
[f] Odds ratio for instrumental delivery according to maternal obesity adjusted for maternal age, parity, onset of birth, epidural, baby birth weight, gestation, head position, augmentation and account class
[g] Odds ratio for Unplanned caesarean delivery according to maternal obesity adjusted for maternal age, parity, account class, previous ceasarean, onset of labour, gestation, birth weight, augmentation, epidural

perinatal outcomes in Australia. As such, our study is the first to explore whether the observations of similar studies previously undertaken in the United Kingdom [2–4] are evident in another international population. This is worth exploring because the ethnic composition of populations of SA women studied in the UK are different to those in Australia, the United States and Canada [6–8] (http://www.statcan.gc.ca/pub/89-621-x/89-621-x2007006-eng.htm). Specifically, the majority of SA born women in the previous UK study were from Pakistan and Bangladesh, with a minority from India [12]. In our study, Indian women comprised the majority of SA born women, followed by Sri Lankan and Afghan women. This is similar to the composition of SA born women in the USA and Canada [8] (http://www.statcan.gc.ca/pub/89-621-x/89-621-x2007006-eng.htm). This is potentially important because the altered rates of

adverse pregnancy outcomes in SA born women have been reported to differ by country within SA [12].

Consistent with previous studies [3, 4] we found that rates of GDM were highest in SA born women with obesity compared to all other women, highlighting the value of appropriate weight management in pregnancy and early GDM testing [13, 14] in these women. However, the association between obesity and GDM was actually stronger in AUS/NZ born women, a finding that does not accord with previous reports from the UK [3, 4]. In those studies the relationship between obesity and diabetes was stronger in Asian and South East/East Asian (oriental) women than in Caucasian women [3, 4]. It is not clear why our findings differ but may reflect biological differences given the compositional make of South Asian born women in our study are different to those in the UK studies, future studies uncovering the mechanisms

Table 4 Adjusted odds ratio (95 % CI) for baby outcomes according to obesity

	Australian women odds ratio (95 % CI)	P value	South Asian Women odds ratio (95 % CI)	P value	P for interaction
Small for gestational age [a]	0.64(0.57–0.72)	**<0.001**	0.64(0.51–0.81)	**<0.001**	0.72
Macroscomia (>4 kg) [b]	1.90(1.73–2.08)	**<0.001**	2.24(1.75–2.83)	**<0.001**	0.10
Fetal Distress (pregnancy or labour) [c]	1.19(1.02–1.28)	**<0.001**	1.31(1.12–1.53)	**0.001**	0.38
Admission to NICU/SCN [d]	1.33 (1.22–1.45)	**<0.001**	1.66(1.40–1.97)	**<0.001**	*0.06*
Any Perinatal Morbidity [e]	1.18(1.04–1.27)	**<0.001**	1.45(1.25–1.68)	**<0.001**	*0.052*
Stillbirth [f]	0.90(0.57–1.42)	0.65	1.42(0.55–3.63)	0.47	0.15

Number in bold reflect statistical significance
[a] Odds ratio for small for gestation age baby according to maternal obesity adjusted for maternal age, parity, smoking and account class
[b] Odds ratio for macrosomia according to maternal obesity adjusted for parity, maternal age, account class, smoking, gestation and baby gender
[c] Odds ratio for Fetal Distress (pregnancy or labour) according to maternal obesity adjusted for maternal age, parity, smoking, gestation and baby gender
[d] Odds ratio for baby admission to NICU/SCN according to maternal obesity adjusted for parity, account class, GDM, gestation, baby gender, onset of labour, birth type
[e] Odds ratio for any perinatal morbidity according to maternal obesity adjusted for maternal age, parity, account class, gestation, baby gender, onset of labour, birth type
[f] Odds ratio for stillbirth according to maternal obesity adjusted for maternal age, parity, previous caesarean, account class, baby gender, gestation and smoking

are needed. Nonetheless, they highlight that maternal obesity is an important risk factor for GDM in all women, irrespective of ethnicity.

The association between obesity and hypertensive disorders of pregnancy was also stronger in AUS/NZ born women than in SA born women, in whom the overall rate was lower. While the precise mechanisms by which obesity increases a woman's risk of hypertension in pregnancy are poorly understood, the association between obesity and pregnancy hypertension has been observed worldwide, in developing and developed countries alike ([1, 15]. Indian women experience decreased rates of hypertension in pregnancy, regardless of obesity [16] suggesting that our finding may reflect a reduced susceptibility in South Asian born women to hypertensive conditions. Preeclampsia remains a major cause of maternal morbidity and mortality and iatrogenic preterm birth. This consistent observation emphasises the maternal and child health benefit opportunities that could be afforded by targeting pre-pregnancy weight and gestational weight gain management. In that regard, our findings suggest that interventions aimed at reducing maternal obesity will have a larger impact in AUS/NZ born women then in SA born women.

While not statistically significantly different, the rate of stillbirth was highest in the SA born women with obesity. Both obesity [1] and SA ethnicity [16–19] are recognised risk factors for stillbirth. This current study suggests that they may interact, an observation previously made by some [4] but not other investigators [2]. Our study was too small, and so underpowered, to be definitive.

The association between maternal obesity and shoulder dystocia is contentious [20]. We found that obesity was only associated with shoulder dystocia in SA born women. To our knowledge this has not been reported before. We identified that obesity was associated with macrosomia in all women regardless of maternal ethnicity suggesting this may not be the sole driver. Pelvimetry studies have demonstrated that South Asian born women have a smaller pelvic inclination than other women [21]. It has also been suggested that obesity leads to an increase in maternal soft tissue inside the pelvis, which narrows the birth canal [22]. These factors combined may explain why obesity was associated with shoulder dystocia in SA born women only. However future work is needed.

We also showed that obesity was more strongly related with admission to NICU/SCN and any perinatal morbidity in SA born women than in AUS/NZ born women. Why this was the case is not clear. The most frequent neonatal morbidities in our study were suspected sepsis, meconium aspiration and birth trauma. It has been previously shown that maternal obesity increases the risk of

neonatal sepsis, patent ductus arteriosus, and/or necrotising enterocolitis [23], possibly through mechanisms of increased systemic inflammation [24, 25]. However, whether maternal ethnicity compounds those risks has not been previously reported.

Regardless of maternal region of birth, we also identified that obesity was associated with suspected fetal compromise, unplanned cesarean section and post partum hemorrhage (PPH) and was protective of instrumental vaginal birth. These findings are not surprising. Obesity has been consistently associated with cesarean section, with fetal compromise being a major driver for that increased risk [1, 26]. That obesity was protective for instrumental vaginal birth in the current study likely reflects the increased rate of caesarean section, resulting in fewer vaginal births overall.

Our study has a number of limitations. Due to how perinatal data are recorded in Australia we are only able to define ethnicity by maternal region of birth. It is possible that some women within the AUS/NZ born group are of south Asian ethnicity. However, this is likely to have underestimated the associations rather than overestimated them. Further, while obesity is an important risk factor, gestational weight gain is increasingly being recognised as an independent risk factor for perinatal outcomes [27–29]. Weight gain is not currently recorded in our electronic database and so we were unable to assess this. The exposures of interest in our study, maternal region of birth and obesity both exist prior to the outcomes occurring however it is possible that our findings only reflect an association not causation. It is also possible that unknown or unmeasured confounding could explain our findings. For example, vitamin D deficiency was not available for women in this study. Vitamin D deficiency is associated with both south Asian region of birth and obesity and has been suggested to be associated with dystocia, although the findings are not consistent [30]. Caution should be made with interpreting this finding.

Conclusion

In summary, we have shown that maternal south Asian region of birth influences the established and well known associations between maternal obesity and hypertensive disorders of pregnancy, GDM, shoulder dystocia, admission of baby to NICU/SCN and perinatal morbidity. Accordingly, interventions targeted at reducing maternal obesity would be expected to have different impacts in SA born compared to AUS/NZ born women. Future research is needed to elucidate the specific mechanisms by which obesity is having differential effects and to assess the efficacy of such interventions on reducing adverse outcomes in women of differing ethnicities. Health economic modelling of cost: benefit analyses assessing interventions aimed at reducing obesity would need to take this into account.

Abbreviations
AUS/NZ: Australian/New Zealand; BMI: Body mass index; GDM: Gestational Diabetes Mellitus; NICU: Neonatal Intensive Care Unit; PE: Preeclampsia; PPH: Post-partum hemorrhage; SA: South Asian; SGA: Small for gestational age

Acknowledgements
We would like to acknowledge Amanda Kendall for her role in retrieving the data.

Funding
MDT receives support from the National Health and Medical Research Council of Australia Fellowship program. EW receives funding form the Victorian Governments' Operational Infrastructure Support Program. None of the funding sources had any involvement in the study design; in the collection, analysis and interpretation of data; in the writing of the report; or in the decision to submit the article for publication.

Authors' contributions
MDT, JM, LS and EW were all involved in the conception and design of the study. MDT and JM were responsible for ethical requirements. MDT and MK were responsible for the data collation and coding. MDT undertook all statistical analyses and interpretations. All authors were involved in manuscript preparation. All authors read and approved the final manuscript.

Competing interests
The authors declare that they have no competing interests.

Consent for publication
Not Applicable.

Author details
[1]The Ritchie Centre, Hudson Institute of Medical Research, Clayton, Vic 3168, Australia. [2]Monash Health, Monash Medical Centre, Clayton, Australia. [3]Department of Obstetrics and Gynaecology, Monash University, Clayton, VIC, Australia.

References
1. Marchi J, Berg M, Dencker A, Olander EK, Begley C. Risks associated with obesity in pregnancy, for the mother and baby: a systematic review of reviews. Obes Rev. 2015;16:621–38.
2. Penn N, Oteng-Ntim E, Oakley LL, Doyle O. Ethnic Variation in stillbirth risk and the role of maternal obesity: analysis of routine data from the London maternity unit. BMC Pregnancy Childbirth. 2014;14:404.
3. Oteng-Ntim E, Kopeika J, Seed P, Wandiembe S, Doyle P. Impact of obesity on pregnancy outcome in different ethnic groups: calculating population attributable fractions. PLoS One. 2013;8(1):e53749.
4. Makgoba M, Savvidou MD, Steer PJ. An analysis of the interrelationship between maternal age, body mass index and racial origin in the development of gestational diabetes mellitus. BJOG. 2011;119:276–82.
5. Chiu M, Maclagan LC, Tu JV, Shah BR. Temporal trends in cardiovascular disease risk factors among white, South Asian, Chinese and black groups in Ontario, Canada, 2001 to 2012: a population-based study. BMJ Open. 2015;5(8):e007232.
6. Laws PJ, Sullivan EA. Australia's mothers and babies 2001. Sydney: Unit ANPS; 2004.
7. Hilder L, Zhichao Z, Parker M, Jahan S, Chambers GM. Australia's mothers and babies 2012. Canberra: AIHW; 2014.
8. State Immigration Data Profiles http://www.migrationpolicy.org/programs/data-hub/state-immigration-data-profiles.
9. UnitedNationsStatisticsDivision.Compositionofmacrogeographical(continental) regions, geographic sub-regions, and selected economic and other groupings
10. The National Statement on Ethical Conduct in Human Research (2007) (National Statement (2007)). https://www.nhmrc.gov.au/book/national-statement-ethical-conducthuman-research.
11. WHO expert Consulation. Appropriate body-mass index for Asian populations and its implications for policy and intervention strategies. Lancet. 2004;363:157–63.
12. Essex HN, Green J, Baston H, Pickett KE. Which women are at an increased risk of a caesarean section or an instrumental vaginal birth in the UK: an exploration within the Millennium Cohort Study. BJOG : an international journal of obstetrics and gynaecology. BJOG. 2013;120(6):724–33.
13. Stewart ZA, Wallace EM, Allan CA. Patterns of weight gain in pregnant women with and without gestational diabetes mellitus: an observational study. Aust N Z J Obstet Gynaecol. 2012;52(5):433–9.
14. Carreno CA, Clifton RG, Hauth JC, Myatt L, Roberts JM, Spong CY, Varner MW, Thorp Jr JM, Mercer BM, Peaceman AM, et al. Excessive early gestational weight gain and risk of gestational diabetes mellitus in nulliparous women. Obstet Gynecol. 2012;119(6):1227–33.
15. Rahman MM, Abe SK, Kanda M, Narita S, Rahman MS, Bilano V, Ota E, Gilmour S, Shibuya K. Maternal body mass index and risk of birth and maternal health outcomes in low-and middle-income countries: a systematic review. Obes Rev. 2015;16:758–70.
16. Dahlen H, Schmied V, Dennis C-L, Thornton C. Rates of obstetric intervention during birth and selected maternal and perinatal outcomes for low risk women born in Australia compared to those born overseas. BMC Pregnancy Childbirth. 2013;13:100.
17. Drysdale H, Ranasinha S, Kendell A, Knight M, Wallace E. Ethnicity and the risk of late-pregnancy stillbirth. MJA. 2012;197:278–81.
18. Gardosi J, Madurasinghe V, Williams M, Malik A, Francis A. Maternal and fetal risk factors for stillbirth: population based study. BMJ. 2013;346:f108.
19. Ravelli ACJ, Tromp M, Eskes M, Droog JC, van der Post JA, Jager KJ, Mol BW, Reitsma JB. Ethnic differences in stillbirth and early neonatal mortality in The Netherlands. J Epidemiol Community Health. 2011;64(8):696–701.
20. Mehta SH, Sokol RJ. Shoulder dystocia: risk factors, predictability, and preventability. Semin Perinatol. 2014;38(4):189–93.
21. Rizk DE, Czechowski J, Ekelund L. *Dynamic assessment of pelvic floor and bony pelvis morphologic condition with the use of magnetic resonance imaging in a multiethnic, nulliparous, and healthy female population.* Am J Obstet Gynecol. 2004;191(1):83.
22. Chu SY, Kim SY, Schmid CH, Dietz PM, Callaghan WM, Lau J, Curtis KM. Maternal obesity and risk of cesarean delivery: a meta-analysis. Obes Rev. 2007;8(5):383–94.
23. Rastogi S, Rojas M, Rastogi D, Haberman S. Neonatal morbidities among full-term infants born to obese mothers. J Matern Fetal Neonatal Med. 2015;28(7):829–35.
24. Ferrante Jr AW. Obesity-induced inflammation: a metabolic dialogue in the language of inflammation. J Intern Med. 2007;262:408–14.
25. Aaltonen R, Heikkinen T, Hakala K, Laine K, Alanen A. Transfer of proinflammatory cytokines across term placenta. Obstet Gynecol. 2005;106(4):802–7.
26. Athukorala C, Rumbold AR, Willson KJ, Crowther CA. The risk of adverse pregnancy outcomes in women who are overweight or obese. BMC Pregnancy Childbirth. 2010;10:56.
27. Park S, Sappenfield WM, Bish C, Salihu H, Goodman D, Bensyl DM. Assessment of the Institute of Medicine recommendations for weight gain during pregnancy: Florida, 2004-2007. Matern Child Health J. 2011;15(3):289–301.
28. Kominiarek MA, Seligman NS, Dolin C, Gao W, Berghella V, Hoffman M, et al. Gestational weight gain and obesity: is 20 pounds too much? Am J Obstet Gynecol. 2013;209(3):e1–11.
29. Gaillard R, Durmuş B, Hofman A, Mackenbach JP, Steegers EAP, Jaddoe VWV. Risk factors and outcomes of maternal obesity and excessive weight gain during pregnancy. Obesity. 2013;21(5):1046–55.
30. Brunvand L, Shah SS, Bergström S, Haug E. Vitamin D deficiency in pregnancy is not associated with obstructed labor. A study among Pakistani women in Karachi. Acta Obstet Gynecol Scand. 1998;77(3):303–6.

3

Metformin and dietary advice to improve insulin sensitivity and promote gestational restriction of weight among pregnant women who are overweight or obese

Jodie M. Dodd[1,2,6*], Rosalie M. Grivell[1,3], Andrea R. Deussen[1], Gustaaf Dekker[1,4], Jennie Louise[5] and William Hague[1,2]

Abstract

Background: Obesity is a significant global health problem, with approximately 50% of women entering pregnancy having a body mass index greater than or equal to 25 kg/m^2. Obesity during pregnancy is associated with a well-recognised increased risk of adverse health outcomes both for the woman and her infant. Currently available data from large scale randomised trials and systematic reviews highlight only modest effects of antenatal dietary and lifestyle interventions in limiting gestational weight gain, with little impact on clinically relevant pregnancy outcomes. Further information evaluating alternative strategies is required.

The aims of this randomised controlled trial are to assess whether the use of metformin as an adjunct therapy to dietary and lifestyle advice for overweight and obese women during pregnancy is effective in improving maternal, fetal and infant health outcomes.

Methods: Design: Multicentre randomised, controlled trial.

Inclusion Criteria: Women with a singleton, live gestation between 10^{+0}-20^{+0} weeks who are obese or overweight (defined as body mass index greater than or equal to 25 kg/m^2), at the first antenatal visit.

Trial Entry & Randomisation: Eligible, consenting women will be randomised between 10^{+0} and 20^{+0} weeks gestation using an online computer randomisation system, and randomisation schedule prepared by non-clinical research staff with balanced variable blocks. Stratification will be according to maternal BMI at trial entry, parity, and centre where planned to give birth.

Treatment Schedules: Women randomised to the *Metformin Group* will receive a supply of 500 mg oral metformin tablets. Women randomised to the *Placebo Group* will receive a supply of identical appearing and tasting placebo tablets. Women will be instructed to commence taking one tablet daily for a period of one week, increasing to a maximum of two tablets twice daily over four weeks and then continuing until birth. Women, clinicians, researchers and outcome assessors will be blinded to the allocated treatment group.

All women will receive three face-to-face sessions (two with a research dietitian and one with a trained research assistant), and three telephone calls over the course of their pregnancy, in which they will be provided with dietary and lifestyle

(Continued on next page)

* Correspondence: jodie.dodd@adelaide.edu.au
[1]Discipline of Obstetrics & Gynaecology, and Robinson Research Institute, The University of Adelaide, Adelaide, South Australia, Australia
[2]Department of Perinatal Medicine, Women's and Children's Hospital, North Adelaide, South Australia, Australia
Full list of author information is available at the end of the article

(Continued from previous page)

advice, and encouraged to make change utilising a SMART goals approach.

Primary Study Outcome: infant birth weight >4000 grams.

Sample Size: 524 women to detect a difference from 15.5% to 7.35% reduction in infants with birth weight >4000 grams ($p = 0.05$, 80% power, two-tailed).

Discussion: This is a protocol for a randomised trial. The findings will contribute to the development of evidence based clinical practice guidelines.

Background

Overweight and obesity represents a significant global health issue, affecting approximately 2.1 billion adults world-wide, [1] with approximately 50% of women entering pregnancy with a body mass index (BMI) in excess of 25 kg/m^2 [2]. The risks associated with obesity during pregnancy and childbirth have been well-documented, and increase with advancing BMI [3]. Immediate pregnancy and birth complications include hypertension and pre-eclampsia, gestational diabetes, need for induction of labour, caesarean section and perinatal death, [3, 4] while infants born to women who are obese are more likely to be macrosomic, require admission to the neonatal intensive care unit, be born preterm, have a congenital anomaly, and require treatment for jaundice or hypoglycaemia [3, 4]. Increasingly, there is recognition of a longer-term health legacy, maternal obesity being associated with a greatly increased risk of both diabetes [5] and cardiovascular disease for the woman, [6] and a significant predictor of obesity in her offspring [7–9].

There is a substantial literature on gestational weight gain during pregnancy summarised by the Institute of Medicine [10]. While these recommendations advocate gestational weight gain of 7–11.5 kg for women who are overweight, and 5-9 kg for women who are obese, [10] a systematic review [11] and large-scale randomised trials [12, 13] highlight only modest effects of antenatal dietary and lifestyle interventions in limiting gestational weight gain, with little impact on clinically relevant pregnancy outcomes [11–13]. Alternative strategies during pregnancy to improve health outcomes for women who are overweight or obese, and their infants, are required.

Increasing maternal BMI is a well-recognised risk factor for the development of gestational diabetes, [3, 4] with the two conditions creating a similar metabolic environment, characterised by insulin resistance, hyperglycaemia, hyperlipidaemia, and a low-grade state of chronic inflammation, all of which influence nutrient availability for fetal growth [14]. Furthermore, women who enter pregnancy overweight or obese have an increased state of insulin resistance when compared with women of normal BMI [15, 16].

Metformin is an oral biguanide, has insulin sensitising properties, and is used increasingly in the treatment of gestational diabetes [17]. Metformin inhibits both gluconeogenesis and glycogenolysis, thereby reducing hepatic glucose production, [18] while increasing insulin mediated skeletal muscle and adipocyte glucose utilisation [19]. Metformin also promotes weight loss in non-pregnant individuals [20, 21].

Given the limited effect of antenatal dietary and lifestyle interventions during pregnancy on both gestational weight gain and clinical pregnancy and birth outcomes, [11–13] there is a need for further evaluation of the role of adjuvant therapies, including metformin, as a strategy to improve health for women who are overweight or obese. The aims of this randomised trial are to evaluate the effects of antenatal metformin and dietary advice among overweight and obese pregnant women on maternal, fetal and infant health outcomes.

The primary hypothesis is that antenatal metformin and dietary advice in overweight and obese pregnant women will reduce the risk of an infant with birth weight greater than 4000 grams.

The secondary hypotheses are that antenatal meltformin and dietary and lifestyle advice in overweight and obese pregnant women will

- Reduce the risk of morbidity from other adverse outcomes for the infant;
- Reduce the risk of maternal morbidity from adverse outcomes;
- Improve maternal quality of life and well-being; and
- Reduce the costs of health care.

Methods

Study design

Multicentre randomised, placebo controlled trial.

Study setting

Public maternity hospitals in metropolitan Adelaide including the Women's and Children's Hospital, The Lyell McEwin Hospital and Flinders Medical Centre.

Inclusion criteria

Women with a singleton, live gestation between 10^{+0}-20^{+0} weeks who are overweight (BMI 25.0 to 29.9 kg/m^2) or obese (BMI ≥30 kg/m^2), at their first antenatal visit will be eligible to participate.

Exclusion criteria

Women with a multiple pregnancy, type 1 or 2 diabetes diagnosed prior to pregnancy, or with significant renal or hepatic impairment such that metformin would be contraindicated will be excluded from participation.

Trial entry

Eligible women will be identified in the antenatal clinic of participating centres, given the trial information sheet and counselled by a researcher, before obtaining informed written consent. Randomisation will occur using the computer based randomisation service of the Discipline of Obstetrics and Gynaecology, The University of Adelaide.

The randomisation schedule will use balanced variable blocks, and will be prepared by an investigator not involved with recruitment or clinical care. There will be stratification of women according to parity (0 versus 1 or more), BMI at booking visit (25 to 29.9 kg/m^2 versus ≥30 kg/m^2), and collaborating centre. Eligible women will be randomised to either the 'Metformin Group' or the 'Placebo Group'.

Supply and blinding of study medication

Metformin tablets 500 mg and placebo tablets identical in appearance will be packed by an independent pharmaceutical packaging company (Pharmaceutical Packaging Professionals, Victoria) and coded according to the randomisation schedule. The women, their caregivers and research staff will be blinded to treatment allocation. Research staff obtaining outcome data will be blinded to treatment allocation. In the unexpected situation where a clinician directly involved in the care of an individual woman considers it essential to ongoing clinical care that treatment group allocation be revealed, this will be performed by an individual not directly involved in the day-to-day management of the trial, and conveyed directly to the clinician.

Treatment schedules

Women who are randomised to the *Metformin Group* will receive a 16 week supply of oral metformin tablets 500 mg, and a further 12 week supply at 28 weeks of their pregnancy. Women will be instructed to commence taking tablets from the time of randomisation, starting with one tablet daily for a period of one week, increasing to a maximum of two tablets twice daily (maximum dose 2000 mg daily) over four weeks as tolerated and then continuing until birth.

Women who are randomised to the *Placebo Group* will receive a 16 week supply of identical appearing placebo tablets, and a further 12 week supply at 28 weeks of their pregnancy. Women will instructed to commence taking tablets from the time of randomisation, starting with one tablet daily for a period of one week, increasing to a maximum of two tablets twice daily over four weeks as tolerated and then continuing until birth.

Treatment compliance will be assessed via completion of a short questionnaire at 36 weeks' gestation in which women will be asked whether they have taken the medication during the previous month. Women who respond 'no' will be considered non-compliant with the treatment, and will be asked to indicate why they are not taking the study medication. All women will be asked if they have experienced symptoms consistent with known side effects of metformin.

Ongoing follow-up of all women in both treatment groups

Over the course of pregnancy, each woman will receive three face-to-face sessions (two with the dietitian shortly after trial entry and again at 28 weeks gestation, and one with a research assistant at 36 weeks gestation) and three telephone calls from the research assistant at 20, 24, and 32 weeks gestation. The intervention has been designed to maximise flexibility and choice for women, while providing advice that can be incorporated into each individual's lifestyle.

Dietary advice provided will be consistent with current Australian dietary standards, [22] and based on our experience with the LIMIT randomised trial [12, 23]. The dietary intervention will maintain a balance of carbohydrates, fat and protein, while specifically encouraging women to reduce their intake of energy dense and non-core foods high in refined carbohydrates and saturated fats, while increasing their intake of fibre, and promoting consumption of two serves of fruit, five serves of vegetables, and three serves of dairy each day [12, 22, 23].

Tailoring of the intervention will be informed by stage theories of health decision making that propose that individuals progress through a series of cognitive phases when undertaking behavioural change [24]. Initially, there will be a planning session with a research dietitian, in which women will be provided with written dietary and activity information, an individual diet and physical activity plan, recipe book and example menu plans. Women will be encouraged to set achievable goals for dietary and exercise change, supported to make these lifestyle changes and to self-monitor their progress, using a SMART goals approach. Women will be encouraged to involve their partner or significant support person in these sessions. These principles will be reinforced at subsequent face-to-face visits with the dietitian and research assistant, and during the telephone contacts [12, 23].

All women will be asked to complete a food frequency questionnaire, exercise diary, and quality of life assessments at trial entry, 28 and 36 weeks gestation, and six months postpartum. Their weight will be recorded at trial entry, at 28 weeks gestation, and at 36 weeks gestation or nearest to birth. All women will be encouraged to attend for a research ultrasound at 28 and 36 weeks gestation that does not constitute routine clinical care, to monitor fetal growth, and in particular the development of small for gestational age infants.

For women who are diagnosed with gestational diabetes, it will be assumed that they are receiving metformin, and further metformin or insulin will be added as required to maintain appropriate glycaemic control as determined by her health care provider. All other care during pregnancy and birth will be according to the practices of the hospital at which the woman is booked to give birth.

After birth, information will be obtained relating to birth and infant outcomes from the case notes by the research assistant and the delivery form completed. Similarly, the postnatal and neonatal forms will be completed for each live born infant after discharge from hospital.

See Table 1 for an outline of timing enrolment, intervention and assessments.

Study endpoints

The primary trial outcome is the incidence of infants with birth weight >4000 grams.

The secondary study outcomes are:

1) Adverse outcomes for the infant including preterm birth (birth before 37 weeks gestation); mortality (either stillbirth (intrauterine fetal death after trial entry and prior to birth), or infant death (death of a live born infant prior to hospital discharge, and excluding lethal congenital anomalies)); infant birth weight <2500 grams; infant birth weight >4500 grams; infant birth weight >90th centile for gestational age and infant sex; infant birth weight <10th centile for gestational age and infant sex; hypoglycaemia requiring intravenous treatment; admission to neonatal intensive care unit, or special care baby unit; hyperbilirubinaemia requiring phototherapy; nerve palsy; fracture; birth trauma; shoulder dystocia.

2) Maternal weight gain outcomes including total gestational weight gain and gestational weight gain classified as below/within/above IoM recommendations [10].

3) Maternal changes in diet and physical activity as measured by questionnaires completed by the woman at trial entry, 28 and 36 weeks gestation, and six and 18 months after birth (Harvard Semi-quantitative Food Frequency Questionnaire, [25, 26] and the Short Questionnaire to Assess Health-enhancing physical activity (SQUASH) [27]).

4) Adverse outcomes for the woman including maternal hypertension and pre-eclampsia (in accordance with recognised Australasian Society for the Study of Hypertension in Pregnancy criteria) [28]; maternal gestational diabetes [29]; need for and length of antenatal hospital stay; antepartum haemorrhage requiring hospitalisation; preterm prelabour ruptured membranes; chorioamnionitis; need and reason for induction of labour; any antibiotic use during labour; caesarean section; postpartum haemorrhage (blood loss ≥600 mL); perineal trauma; wound infection; endometritis; length of postnatal hospital stay; thromboembolic disease; maternal death.

5) Maternal quality of life and emotional wellbeing as measured by questionnaires completed by the woman at trial entry, 28 and 36 weeks of pregnancy and six months postpartum relating to quality of life (as measured using the SF12 Health Survey Questionnaire); [30] preferences for treatment and satisfaction with care (at 6 months postpartum only); anxiety (as measured by the Short Form Spielberger State Trait Inventory [31]) and depression (as measured by the Edinburgh Postnatal Depression Scale [32]). Women will be asked a series of questions about their satisfaction with the intervention, using items modified from a previous childbirth questionnaire [33].

6) Fetal growth and wellbeing at 28 and 36 weeks' gestation assessed by ultrasound (fetal biometry, estimated weight, liquor volume, umbilical artery Doppler waveform, and adiposity) [34].

7) Costs of health care: The primary measure of outcome for the economic analysis will be the cost per live birth. Resource use will include the provision of the dietary intervention and direct costs of health care (expected average clinic fees, the frequency and duration of GP and antenatal visits, as well as in-patient admissions), determined by hospital out-patient visits, in-patient admissions and published data sets including PBS, MBS and Australian Refined Diagnosis Related Groups (AR-DRG) cost weights. Mean costs and effectiveness between treatment groups will be compared and incremental cost effectiveness ratios (ICERs) and confidence intervals presented. For varying threshold values of cost effectiveness, acceptability curves will be presented as described previously [35]. An assessment of the sensitivity of the results to variation in measured resource use, effectiveness and/or unit costs will be undertaken using appropriate one-way and multi-way sensitivity analysis, as described previously [35].

Women will be asked to provide consent to the collection of bio-specimens (including blood/serum at trial entry, 28 weeks gestation and 36 weeks gestation, and cord blood) for potential use in future ancillary studies.

Sample size

The primary clinical endpoint is the incidence of infants born with birth weight >4000 grams, with an estimated

Table 1 Timeline of main activities from recruitment to the end of the clinical trial

		Eligibility screen	Informed consent	Allocation	Commence study medication	Dietary review	Weight	Questionnaires	Fetal ultrasound	Glucose tolerance test (GTT)	Baby measurements	Pregnancy and birth outcomes
	Pre-randomisation	✓	✓				✓					
	Randomisation			✓								
During Pregnancy	As soon as practicable after randomisation				✓	✓		✓				
	28 weeks					✓		✓	✓	✓		
	36 weeks					✓	✓	✓	✓			
	As soon as practicable after birth										✓	
	Six weeks after birth											✓

incidence in women eligible for this trial of 15.5% [12]. To detect a difference from 15.5% to 7.35% (alpha 0.05; power 80%), and accounting for 5% rate of attrition (based on our experience with the LIMIT Study), [12] we will recruit a total of 524 women. This sample size will be powered (80%) to detect the differences in secondary outcomes as detailed in the table below.

Outcome	Difference in Incidence	Difference Detected
Caesarean Section	39.1% to 27.2%	12%
Induction of labour	36.8% to 25.1%	12%
Pre-Eclampsia	14.1% to 6%	8%
Gestational Diabetes	10% to 3.5%	6.5%

Data management

All information obtained from this study will remain strictly confidential. While the results of the study will be published, no data will be presented to allow the identification of individual women. Data will be stored in a locked filing cabinet or on password protected computer file, and accessible only by the study team.

We have previous experience recruiting women for lifestyle intervention trials in this setting [12] and will consider adding further sites as required. Women who withdraw from ongoing participation after randomisation will be asked for consent to utilise the data already collected prior to withdrawal, including birth outcomes where possible.

Analysis and reporting of results

The initial analysis will examine baseline characteristics of all randomised women, as an indication of comparable treatment groups, and include maternal age, parity, race, height, weight, smoking history, past obstetric history, and previous gestational diabetes. Primary and secondary outcomes will be analysed on an "intention to treat" basis, according to treatment allocation at randomisation; multiple imputation by the fully conditional specification (chained equations) method will be used to impute missing outcome data relative risks and 95% confidence intervals will be reported for the major outcomes, and the number needed to treat to benefit or harm calculated. Analyses will be adjusted for stratification variables, and for prespecified prognostic factors identified as potential confounders for particular outcomes. More specific details relating to the proposed analyses, including the handling of missing data will be outlined in the statistical analysis plan to be developed for the trial.

As the lead investigator, JMD will have access to the data, and acts as guarantor to the final data set. The trial manager (ARD) and statistician (JL) will have access to the data, and the statistician (JL) will be responsible for the development of the statistical analysis plan, prior to the conduct of any statistical analyses.

Following completion of the relevant statistical analyses, manuscripts will be prepared for publication, with subsequent presentation of results at relevant scientific and clinical meetings.

Ethics approval

Approval to conduct this study has been obtained from the Women's and Children's Health Network (WCHN) Human Research Ethics Committee's (HREC) and local institutional approval at Women's and Children's Hospital, Flinders Medical Centre and the Lyell McEwin Hospital. Any amendments to the trial protocol will be notified in writing to each of the responsible HREC's, research assistants, and clinicians involved in the study, and where relevant an amendment made to the trial registration.

A data and safety monitoring board (DSMB) will monitor efficacy (or futility) and adverse effects. Based on these considerations, the DSMB may recommend that the protocol be modified or that the GRoW trial be terminated. The DSMB will consist of experts in relevant obstetrics, neonatology and research methodology. All adverse events involving women and infants enrolled in the trial will be reviewed by a multidisciplinary committee, who will be blinded to treatment allocation, in order to clarify cause. These data will be made available for the Data Safety Monitoring Board.

Discussion

This is a protocol for a randomised trial assessing whether the use of metformin in pregnancy, as an adjuvant therapy to dietary and lifestyle advice for women who are overweight or obese is effective in improving maternal, fetal and infant health outcomes. The findings of this trial will contribute to the currently available literature regarding the effect of metformin in pregnancy for women who are overweight and obese, [36, 37] and to the development of evidence based clinical practice guidelines.

Acknowledgements
The authors acknowledge the contribution of staff at study sites in preparation for this study.

Funding
The GRoW Trial is funded by a project grant from the National Health and Medical Research Council (NHMRC), Australia (ID 1043181).
JM Dodd is supported through a NHMRC Practitioner Fellowship (ID 627005).
RM Grivell is supported through a NHMRC Early Career Fellowship (ID 1073514).

Authors' contributions
All authors participated in the study design, JMD wrote the manuscript and the other authors, RMG, ARD, GD, JL and WH, reviewed/edited the manuscript. JL provided statistical expertise for the study design. All authors approved the final version.

Competing interests
The authors declare that they have no competing interests.

Author details
[1]Discipline of Obstetrics & Gynaecology, and Robinson Research Institute, The University of Adelaide, Adelaide, South Australia, Australia. [2]Department of Perinatal Medicine, Women's and Children's Hospital, North Adelaide, South Australia, Australia. [3]Department of Obstetrics & Gynaecology, Flinders Medical Centre and School of Medicine, Flinders University, Adelaide, Australia. [4]Lyell McEwin Hospital, Elizabeth Vale, South Australia, Australia. [5]The University of Adelaide, School of Public Health, Adelaide, South Australia, Australia. [6]Discipline of Obstetrics & Gynaecology, and Robinson Institute, Women's & Children's Hospital, The University of Adelaide, 72 King William Road, North Adelaide, South Australia 5006, Australia.

References

1. Ng M, Fleming T, Robinson M, Thomson B, Graetz N, Margono C, Mullany EC, Biryukov S, Abbafati C, Abera SF, et al. Global, regional, and national prevalence of overweight and obesity in children and adults during 1980–2013: a systematic analysis for the Global Burden of Disease Study 2013. Lancet. 2014;384(9945):766–81.
2. Scheil W, Scott J, Catcheside B, Sage L, Kennare R. In: Health POUS, editor. Pregnancy outcome in South Australia 2012. Adelaide: Government of South Australia; 2015.
3. Dodd JM, Grivell RM, Nguyen A-M, Chan A, Robinson JS. Maternal and perinatal health outcomes by body mass index category. ANZJOG. 2011; 51(2):136–40.
4. Callaway LK, Prins JB, Chang AM, McIntyre HD. The prevalence and impact of overweight and obesity in an Australian obstetric population. MJA. 2006;184(2):56–9.
5. Hedderson MM, Gunderson EP, Ferrara A. Gestational weight gain and risk of gestational diabetes mellitus. Obstet Gynecol. 2010;115(3):597–604.
6. Shah BR, Retnakaran R, Booth GL. Increased risk of cardiovascular disease in young women following gestational diabetes mellitus. Diabetes Care. 2008;31(8):1668–9.
7. Godfrey KM, Inskip HM, Hanson MA. The long-term effects of prenatal development on growth and metabolism. Semin Reprod Med. 2011;29(3):257–65.
8. Wells JC, Haroun D, Levene D, Darch T, Williams JE, Fewtrell MS. Prenatal and postnatal programming of body composition in obese children and adolescents: evidence from anthropometry, DXA and the 4-component model. Int J Obes. 2011;35(4):534–40.
9. Winter JD, Langenberg P, Krugman SD. Newborn adiposity by body mass index predicts childhood overweight. Clin Pediatr. 2010;49(9):866–70.
10. Institute of Medicine (IOM): Weight gain during pregnancy: reexamining the guidelines. In. Edited by Rasmussen KM, Yaktine AL. Washington: National Acedemic Press; 2009.
11. Thangaratinam S, Rogozinska E, Jolly K, Glinkowski S, Roseboom T, Tomlinson JW, Kunz R, Mol BW, Coomarasamy A, Khan KS. Effects of interventions in pregnancy on maternal weight and obstetric outcomes: meta-analysis of randomised evidence. BMJ. 2012;344:e2088.
12. Dodd JM, Turnbull DA, McPhee AJ, Deussen AR, Grivell RM, Yelland LN, Crowther CA, Wittert G, Owens JA, Robinson JS. Antenatal lifestyle advice for women who are overweight or obese: the LIMIT randomised trial. BMJ. 2014;348:g1285.
13. Poston L, Bell R, Croker H, Flynn AC, Godfrey KM, Goff L, Hayes L, Khazaezadeh N, Nelson SM, Oteng-Ntim E, et al. Effect of a behavioural intervention in obese pregnant women (the UPBEAT study): a multicentre, randomised controlled trial. Lancet Diabetes Endocrinol 2015, July 10(http://dx.doi.org/10.1016/S2213-8587(15)00227-2).
14. Catalano PM, Hauguel-De Mouzon S. Is it time to revisit the Pedersen hypothesis in the face of the obesity epidemic? Am J Obstet Gynecol. 2011;204(6):479–87.
15. Challier JC, Basu S, Bintein T, Minium J, Hotmire K, Catalano PM, Hauguel-de Mouzon S. Obesity in pregnancy stimulates macrophage accumulation and inflammation in the placenta. Placenta. 2008;29(3):274–81.
16. Ramsay JE, Ferrell WR, Crawford L, Wallace AM, Greer IA, Sattar N. Maternal obesity is associated with dysregulation of metabolic, vascular, and inflammatory pathways. J Clin Endocrinol Metab. 2002;87(9):4231–7.
17. Rowan JA, Hague WM, Gao W, Battin MR, Moore MP, Investigators. ftMT. Metformin versus insulin for the treatment of gestational diabetes. N Engl J Med. 2008;358(19):2003–15.
18. Bailey CJ, Turner RC. Metformin. N Engl J Med. 1996;334(9):574–9.
19. Wiernsperger NF, Bailey CJ. The antihyperglycaemic effect of metformin: therapeutic and cellular mechanisms. Drugs. 1999;58 Suppl 1:31–9.
20. Yki-Järvinen H, Nikkilä K, Mäkimattila S. Metformin prevents weight gain by reducing dietary intake during insulin therapy in patients with type 2 diabetes mellitus. Drugs. 1999;58 Suppl 1:53–4.
21. Glueck CJ, Fontaine RN, Wang P, Subbiah MT, Weber K, Illig E, Streicher P, Sieve-Smith L, Tracy TM, Lang JE, et al. Metformin reduces weight, centripetal obesity, insulin, leptin, and low-density lipoprotein cholesterol in nondiabetic, morbidly obese subjects with body mass index greater than 30. Metabolism. 2001;50(7):856–61.
22. National Health and Medical Research Council: Australian Dietary Guidelines. In. Canberra: National Health and Medical Research Council; 2013.
23. Dodd JM, Cramp CS, Sui Z, Yelland LN, Deussen AR, Grivell RM, Moran LJ, Crowther CA, Turnbull DA, McPhee AJ, et al. Effects of antenatal lifestyle advice for women who are overweight or obese on maternal diet and physical activity: the LIMIT randomised trial. BMC Med. 2014;12:161. http://www.biomedcentral.com/1741-7015/12/161.
24. Bennett P, Murphy S. Psychology and health promotion. Buckingham: Open University Press; 1997.
25. Willett WC, Reynolds RD, Cottrell-Hoehner S, Sampson L, Browne ML. Validation of a semi-quantitative food frequency questionnaire: comparison with a 1-year diet record. J Am Diet Assoc. 1987;87(1):43–7.
26. Ibiebele TI, Parekh S, Mallitt KA, Hughes MC, O'Rourke PK, Webb PM. Reproducibility of food and nutrient intake estimates using a semi-quantitative FFQ in Australian adults. Public Health Nutr. 2009;12(12):2359–65.
27. Wendel-Vos GC, Schuit AJ, Saris WH, Kromhout D. Reproducibility and relative validity of the short questionnaire to assess health-enhancing physical activity. J Clin Epidemiol. 2003;56:1163–9.
28. Brown MA, Hague WM, Higgins J, Lowe S, McCowan L, Oats J, Peek MJ, Rowan JA, Walters BN, for the Australasian Society for the Study of Hypertension in Pregnancy. The detection, investigation and management of hypertension in pregnancy: full consensus statement. ANZJOG. 2000; 40(2):139–55.
29. SA Maternal & Neonatal Clinical Network: South Australian Perinatal Practice Guidelines: Diabetes mellitus and gestational diabetes. In. South Australia: National Acedemic Press; 2015.
30. Ware JE, Sherbourne CD. The MOS 36 item short form health survey (SF36) conceptual framework and item selection. Med Care. 1992;30:473–83.
31. Marteau TM, Bekker H. The development of a six item form of the State Scale of the Spielberger State Trait Anxiety Inventory (STAI). Br J Clin Psychol. 1992;31:301–6.
32. Cox JL, Holden JM, Sagovsky R. Detection of postnatal depression - development of the 10 item Edinburgh Postnatal Depression Scale (EDPS). Brit J Psych. 1987;154:782–6.
33. Dodd JM, Newman A, Yelland LN, Turnbull DA, Deussen AR, Grivell RM, Moran LJ, Crowther CA, McPhee AJ, Wittert G, et al. Effects of antenatal lifestyle advice for women who are overweight or obese on maternal quality of life: the LIMIT randomised trial. Acta Obstet Gynecol Scand. 2016; 95(3):259–69.
34. Grivell RM, Yelland LN, Deussen A, Crowther CA, Dodd JM. Antenatal dietary and lifestyle advice for women who are overweight or obese and the effect on fetal growth and adiposity: the LIMIT randomised trial. BJOG. 2016;123(2):233–43.
35. Dodd JM, Ahmed S, Karnon J, Umberger W, Deussen A.R., Tran T, Grivell RM, Crowther CA, Turnbull D, McPhee AJ, et al. The economic costs and consequences of providing antenatal lifestyle advice for women who are overweight or obese: the LIMIT randomised trial. BMC Obesity 2015 In press.
36. Chiswick C, Reynolds RM, Denison F, Drake AJ, Forbes S, Newby DE, Walker BR, Quenby S, Wray S, Weeks A, et al. Effect of metformin on maternal and fetal outcomes in obese pregnant women (EMPOWaR): a randomised, double-blind, placebo-controlled trial. Lancet Diabetes Endocrinol. 2015. doi: 10.1016/S2213-8587(15)00219-3.
37. Syngelaki A, Nicolaides KH, Balani J, Hyer S, Akolekar R, Kotecha R, Pastides A, Shehata H. Metformin versus Placebo in Obese Pregnant Women without Diabetes Mellitus. N Engl J Med. 2016;374(5):434–43.

Women's perceptions of discussions about gestational weight gain with health care providers during pregnancy and postpartum

Hara Nikolopoulos[1], Maria Mayan[2], Jessica MacIsaac[1], Terri Miller[3] and Rhonda C. Bell[1*]

Abstract

Background: Maternal body weight is an indicator of the health of a mother and her developing fetus. Risks of poor maternal and fetal health issues increase when women gain too little or too much weight during pregnancy. A study of 600 women from Alberta, Canada, reported approximately 30, 46, 80, and 80% of underweight, healthy weight, overweight, and obese women, respectively, gained in excess of Health Canada gestational weight gain guidelines. Behavioural interventions during pregnancy have shown to be effective at supporting women achieve gestational weight gain (GWG) recommendations and return to their pre-pregnancy weight postpartum, yet few women are counseled about weight gain during pregnancy. A discrepancy exists between health care providers' (HCP) reported counseling behaviours and women's perceptions of counseling by HCPs; most HCPs report counseling women about GWG; conversely, most women report not receiving counseling about GWG. This study explored women's experiences with GWG and their perceptions of discussions about GWG with HCPs during pregnancy and postpartum. This will help to identify gaps in service delivery and highlight areas for improvement that may better support women to achieve GWG recommendations leading to better health outcomes for women and children.

Methods: Five focus groups (*n* = 26) were conducted with women up to 1 year postpartum across the five Alberta health zones. Focus groups were transcribed verbatim and analyzed using qualitative content analysis.

Results: GWG is important to women, for their health and for the health of their baby. In-depth conversations with HCPs about GWG or weight loss do not occur; however, women want the opportunity to discuss weight gain/loss with HCPs. Women would like discussions about gestational weight gain/loss to become part of standard care and offered to all women.

Conclusions: Women suggested that discussions about GWG should occur with all women, and that HCPs should initiate these discussions by asking women how they feel about discussing weight. Conversations should begin early on in pregnancy and continue through to the postpartum period. Interventions assessing discussions about GWG should be implemented and evaluated as this has been identified as a gap in prenatal service delivery.

Keywords: Gestational weight gain, Pregnancy, Postpartum, Healthcare providers, Prenatal care, Antenatal care, Women's perceptions

* Correspondence: rhonda.bell@ualberta.ca
[1]Department of Agricultural, Food and Nutritional Sciences, University of Alberta, 4-126 Li Ka Shing Centre for Health Research Innovation, Edmonton, AB T6G 2E1, Canada
Full list of author information is available at the end of the article

Background

Maternal body weight is an indicator of the health of a mother and her developing fetus. It is well known that the risks of poor maternal and fetal health issues increase when women gain either too little or too much weight during pregnancy [1]. While gaining too little weight is associated with low birth weight and preterm birth, excessive weight gain in pregnancy also contributes to increased rates of maternal and perinatal complications, illness and sometimes even death [2]. The combination of excess weight gain in pregnancy and poor diet quality, followed by less than recommended postpartum weight loss makes pregnancy a major risk factor for obesity and related chronic diseases (e.g. diabetes, certain cancers) in women in later life [3–5].

According to the 2006 Maternity Experiences Survey [6], only 47% of underweight women, 34% of healthy weight women, and 31% of overweight women achieved weights concordant with the 1999 Health Canada gestational weight gain (GWG) guidelines, while 26, 41, and 55% of underweight, healthy weight and overweight women, respectively, exceeded the guidelines. Similar statistics have been reported in several Western countries [7, 8]. Since then, Health Canada has adopted the updated 2009 Institute of Medicine GWG guidelines that reflect the WHO body mass index (BMI) categories and provide ranges of recommended weight gain for underweight, healthy weight, overweight, and obese women [9]. Recent studies indicate that although between 6 and 22% of women gain less weight than is recommended [10], the majority of women to gain in excess of recommended ranges. A study of 600 women living in Alberta, Canada, reported only 64% of underweight, 38% of healthy weight, 16% of overweight, and 14% of obese women met the 2010 Health Canada GWG guidelines, while approximately 30, 46, 80, and 80% of underweight, healthy weight, overweight, and obese women, respectively, gained in excess of the guidelines [11].

Behavioural interventions during pregnancy have shown to be effective at supporting women to achieve GWG recommendations [12] and return to their pre-pregnancy weight postpartum [13], yet few women report being counseled about weight gain during pregnancy [14] despite the fact that most healthcare providers' (HCPs) reported counseling women about GWG [14–16]. It is possible that this discrepancy exists, in part, because little is known about how women perceive their interactions with HCPs when it comes to discussing GWG. For example, it is not known whether women would like to discuss GWG with their HCP, what women consider to be the most acceptable way to approach such discussion, at what point during the pregnancy women would like to discuss GWG, and the frequency that they want discussions to take place. This is important as many pregnant women have poor knowledge of GWG recommendations, and the consequences of inappropriate weight gain and of strategies to support appropriate GWG [17]. Furthermore, a review of the literature shows that behavioural interventions during pregnancy are primarily aimed at overweight and/or obese women but the importance of discussing GWG with women who begin pregnancy with a healthy BMI, between 18.5 and 24.9 kg/m^2, has not been explored. There is a lack of published evidence of interventions that include healthy weight pregnant women, although gaining weight in excess of GWG recommendations is associated with postpartum weight retention [9] which is a strong predictor of overweight/obesity later on [12, 18].

The objective of this study was to gain an understanding of women's experiences with GWG and their perceptions of discussions about GWG with HCPs during pregnancy and postpartum. Understanding women's experiences with GWG will help to identify the supports women perceive are needed to help them achieve health pregnancy weight gain and postpartum weight loss. Findings will contribute to development of interventions aimed at improving interactions between HCP and women to support healthy pregnancy weight gain.

Methods
Study design

This study is one of several studies conducted in the ENRICH research program. ENRICH is a large multi-sector research partnership that uses an ecological framework, with the overall goal of improving maternal health by promoting optimal dietary intake and weight management in pregnancy and postpartum using innovative universal and selected strategies that meet the unique needs of women across Alberta. The present study is the qualitative portion of a study using mixed methods to explore knowledge, beliefs and practices of women in Alberta related to nutrition, physical activity and weight in pregnancy.

Using an exploratory qualitative methodology, focus groups were conducted to learn about women's experiences with weight gain during pregnancy and weight loss during the postpartum period, and to learn about conversations women had with HCPs about GWG during and after pregnancy during routine visits. In exploratory studies, focus groups are useful in providing a variety of perspectives and encourage the exchange of opinions and ideas [19]. Focus groups are useful as, often, participants will build on what is said by others, contributing a wide breadth of experiences that may not otherwise have been explored.

This study was approved by the Health Research Ethics Board – Health Panel at the University of Alberta.

Recruitment

Alberta Health Services provided permission and identified key staff to recruit women from Community/ Public Health Centres in all five Alberta health zones (North, Edmonton, Central, Calgary, and, South). Women who were up to one year postpartum were eligible and were provided information about the study using information sheets, invitation postcards, Facebook posts, or during face-to-face interactions with staff at during "Well Child" immunization visits.. Women indicated their desire to participate in a focus group to Alberta Health Services staff and when ~5–8 women had done so the focus group was scheduled with the research group. This recruitment process helped to open the study to a wider group of potential participants than could have been recruited by the university-based study team.

Data collection

Five focus groups were conducted ($n = 26$) with women across Alberta between July 2014 and September 2014. Focus group questions were semi-structured (including key probing questions), were developed through an iterative process among members of the ENRICH research team, and were pilot tested with a group of five women. All focus groups were conducted by two trained members of the ENRICH research team: the Program Manager (HN) and the Knowledge Translation Coordinator (JT). The Program Manager has formal training in qualitative methods and analyses and several years' experience in this field [20, 21]. The Knowledge Translation Coordinator has experience in helping conduct focus groups in academic settings and within non-governmental organisations. Each focus group lasted approximately 90 min. Written informed consent was obtained from all participants at the beginning of each focus group. Participants were provided with a $25 grocery store gift card and baby bib in appreciation of their time. All participants completed a brief demographic questionnaire prior to beginning the focus group.

Data analysis

Focus groups were digitally recorded, transcribed verbatim by a transcriptionist, and verified for accuracy by the Program Manager (HN) and the Knowledge Translation Coordinator (JT).

All focus group data were analyzed by the ENRICH Program Manager and the Knowledge Translation Coordinator using conventional content analysis: a process of inductively coding and categorizing data [22]. This approach is useful for exploratory studies as it allows for meaning to emerge from the data [23], rather than approaching analysis with preconceived theories, frameworks or ideas. Transcripts were analyzed separately then together by question to get an in-depth understanding of the data.

Transcripts were analyzed independently by a third reviewer external to the ENRICH team for coder reliability and validity of interpretations. Discrepancies were resolved through discussions about interpretation of findings until consensus was reached. Data saturation was achieved for each of the issues discussed.

Results

The average age of participants was 30.4 ± 4.4 years, this was the first child for 80.8% of the women, average pre-pregnancy BMI was 24.4 kg/m^2 ± 4.0, average GWG was 33.9 ± 18.9 lb., and type of HCP seen most often during pregnancy was: Obstetrician/Gynecologist (58.3%), Family Physician (37.5%), Midwife (4.2%). Age, BMI, GWG and type of HCP of this population are consistent with demographic data gathered from the nationally representative Canadian Maternity Experiences Survey (MES) [1].

Overall, the topics women discussed and the issues raised were consistent and reached satuation across the five focus groups. Data regarding women's experiences with weight gain and weight loss, as well as their conversations had with HCPs are organized into three categories: 1) Women are concerned about gestational weight gain, 2) Communication with HCPs about GWG is lacking, and 3) Postpartum weight loss also matters.

Women are concerned about gestational weight gain

Nearly all focus group participants identified that weight gain matters during pregnancy. Women reported that the amount of weight gained during pregnancy had implications for their health, the health of their pregnancy and the health of their baby. Weight gain was seen as a sign that the baby was in good health and that the pregnancy was moving along "on track". Although weight gain was recognized as being important, it was also a source of concern.

Many women believed there was a "right amount" of weight to gain, specifically between 25 and 35 pounds. Women believed that gaining outside of this range (either more or less) may have negative implications for the health of their baby, which was a "big concern" for them.

"...I was gaining way too much, way too fast and I was concerned about the health risk of that, to me and baby. And, yeah, I'm not so active, so...it coming off afterwards...I worried about that."

– Participant E2

Important to note, almost all women were confused about the range of weight gain (i.e., who it applies to and where this range comes from), and what the weight gain range meant in terms of rate and distribution of weight gain. Despite this, they believed this was the weight gain they should aim for, regardless of their pre-pregnancy BMI. Some women questioned the range. As one woman commented,

"I'm just really curious on where the 25 to 35 pound range came from because there's very, very few people that I've talked to who are anywhere near that 25 to 35 range. So I don't know... Because I started to freak out about it, and then when everyone I talked to was like, oh no, I gained 50, 60, 70 pounds, I was like, okay, if everyone's gaining that, then 50 is not too bad then. I'm okay."

– Participant L

As exemplified by the participant above, some participants' expectations of pregnancy-related weight gain were based on past experiences and experiences of family and friends. For example, one participant thought she should gain what her mother had gained, which corresponded with what she had read in popular prenatal books so that is what she aimed for,

"I thought I should gain what my mom gained. That's where I got if from. And, it was right smack in the middle of what the books say, so I had that number in my head."

– Participant E1

When asked about how they were informed of a weight gain range, the majority of women reported accessing various resources, such as the books, *What to Expect When you're Expecting* and *Healthy Parents, Healthy Children - Pregnancy and Birth* (Alberta Health Services); online websites, such as *Baby Centre, Fit Pregnancy, and What to Expect*; and searching "Dr. Google." A few women reported this range was calculated by their HCP based on their pre-pregnancy BMI; however, most participants reported they did not receive information about an appropriate weight gain range from a HCP.

Participants reported varying levels of (dis)satisfaction with the amount of weight gained and their perceived ability to manage weight gain during pregnancy. For some women, gaining more weight than was recommended was frustrating and made them feel out of

control. Some of these women stated that if they understood the implications exceeding recommendations could have on their baby, they would be more motivated to try to keep within GWG recommendations.

One participant noted that she "hated" the way she looked as she kept getting "thicker, thicker, thicker". Some women struggled with changes in body shape (e.g., loss of muscle tone, feeling more "jiggly"). Others resigned themselves to the fact that weight gain was an inevitable part of pregnancy; they would try to lose the weight after the baby was born. Some women found it easy to cope with the amount of weight gained; however, for the few women who were satisfied or not concerned with their weight gain, they gained less than 30 pounds or less weight than they anticipated. They also believed they would be able to lose their weight quickly based on pregnancy experiences of family members and/or lifestyle behaviours (e.g. level of physical activity).

While women's perceptions and experiences regarding weight gain varied, focus group discussions frequently centred on ways women tried to stay healthy and achieve healthy weights during pregnancy. Many women discussed monitoring and tracking their weight outside of doctors' appointments on a frequent basis and almost all participants described modifications to their diet and/ or amounts or types of physical activity. Modifications to diet included eliminating or reducing unhealthy foods, such as sweets, sodas and desserts, and increasing amounts of healthy foods, such as fresh fruits and vegetables. Conversely, some women noted that they "stopped being so strict" with their diet and would occasionally eat fast food because "now is the time to give in to your cravings".

Changes to physical activity included both frequency and type of activity. The majority of women reported that they tried to walk more frequently and for longer periods of time. Others noted reducing the amount of physical activity due to high risk pregnancies (e.g., multiples, in vitro fertilization, extreme nausea), complications (e.g. sciatica, swelling), feeling tired or ill (mainly due to morning sickness), engaging in physical activities that were deemed not safe during pregnancy (e.g., heavy weight lifting), or due to family or social circumstances.

"I didn't want to screw anything up so I stopped running."

– Participant E7

Evident throughout the focus group discussions was stress, both good and bad, that pregnancy can place on a woman. Women talked about feeling stressed because they were "worried" they might do something wrong that could put the baby and pregnancy at risk. Women repeatedly reported experiencing feelings of guilt when they could not fully comply with GWG recommendations; make positive lifestyle changes; or when changes to their normal routine resulted in reducing healthy behaviours, such as exercising less or eating fewer healthy foods. Although women were motivated and aware of the importance of healthy lifestyle behaviours during pregnancy, this was not always simple or possible.

"...it's like, maybe earlier on I wasn't eating the right things and I screwed this up and that's why she's not, you know, growing as much now. So, of course, you know, it kind of sets the wheels spinning... I'm trying to do the best I can here and...I don't want to think I screwed this up..."

– Participant E6

Communication with HCPs about GWG is lacking

Women in all focus groups stated that communication with HCPs about GWG was lacking. An example of this was participants' experiences of being weighed during prenatal appointments. Women described that they were weighed by nurses at nearly every prenatal appointment and that their weight was recorded in their chart but typically not disclosed or discussed with them. This lack of communication about weight gain was confusing, leading some participants to question if GWG was important to their HCPs.

"I thought that maybe the obstetrician didn't really care about the weight I'm gaining because she didn't tell me too much...Every time, just go to the scale, she would look and tell me, 'That's right', every time. I don't know what's good or not."

– Participant C3

"I got weighed at every appointment but no one ever – like, we never discussed whether I was, you know, gaining too much, too little, anything. Like, it was just never really brought up."

– Participant N2

Women who reported that conversations about GWG did occur explained that these conversations were neither timely nor positive. Several women commented that weight gain was discussed by HCPs only after they had gained too much weight or were "out of range". One woman described that her weight was discussed by her physician, "only when I had done something bad" (i.e., gained too much weight in one month). This same

participant expressed that she was "glad that they brought it [weight gain] up because that means they're not ignoring it" but suggested that her doctor could have discussed concerns about weight in a "gentle way...to explore what could be happening". Similarly, another woman recalled that her obstetrician "had this thing about weight gain; she made me feel kind of bad about it, that I had been gaining so much".

Women that reported gaining too much total weight or gained weight too quickly felt that, often, HCPs made assumptions about their lifestyle behaviours resulting in feelings of frustration, humiliation, or distress. One woman, who had been running her entire pregnancy, commented that she was told by her doctor to "jump on the treadmill once in a while" because she had gained 40 pounds by approximately 30 weeks gestation and felt the physician never took the time to inquire about her level of physical activity.

"I tipped the 40 pound scale, and that's when she [the obstetrician] was like, 'Whoa, whoa', like, we hadn't discussed it [GWG] at all up until that point [30 weeks] and then it was, okay, too much weight. But her recommendation was – and as far as I was... 'You should jump on the treadmill once in a while.' And I ran until I was seven months pregnant, outside, because I like to run outside. And then I just – the weather wasn't safe anymore. And so when she said, 'Jump on a treadmill', I was like, seriously? I was running the whole time."

– Participant E6

Again, another woman recalled gaining nine pounds in one month and the doctor "got a little cross with me", telling her "you can't be eating junk food". This approach resulted in some participants experiencing negative emotions, such as guilt, blame, irresponsibility, and feeling out of control as more weight than was recommended was gained. These interactions with HCPs made women feel increasingly frustrated, commenting that the physicians' approach to weight gain was "extreme" and "not helpful", resulting in a lack of trust. As this participant described,

"She [the obstetrician] should have asked me how I felt about my weight gain, not just told me how she felt about it."

– Participant E2

While HCPs communicated when too much weight was gained, many did not offer strategies to help or support women create plans to achieve recommendations, discuss with them how to adjust their expectations when things did not go as planned, or what to do for the remainder of their pregnancy once recommendations were exceeded.

Women wanted to be given the option to talk about weight gain and suggested that discussions about GWG should be done as early on in pregnancy as possible and as part of standard care. To do this, women recommended that HCPs could ease into conversations about weight by simply asking women if it is okay to talk about their weight. One woman stated that,

"Not everyone likes to talk about their weight gain, so I guess they could ask if you like to talk about it."

– Participant C2

Women believe it is the responsibility of HCPs to broach the topic of weight gain and to provide accurate and timely information to women. Women want to discuss weight before exceeding recommendations, to be made aware of recommendations for total and rate of weight gain, their progress at every appointment; and they want regular feedback from their HCPs to assess if they are "on track".

Postpartum weight loss also matters

All women emphasized that it was important to return to their pre-pregnancy weight, with one woman stating "as fast as humanly possible". Women commented that, after delivery, they felt that the focus of postpartum visits by public health nurses and physicians was on the baby; however, moms still matter and women want continued support and education from their HCPs. One woman stated that after the baby is born, "That's the end of it. You're sort of on your own now to deal with whatever". Another woman reflected that HCPs do not discuss weight loss because they are more concerned about postpartum mental health. Another woman mentioned that women's mental wellbeing and weight after pregnancy are often linked and, for that reason alone, physicians should be discussing postpartum weight loss.

Women could not recall ever discussing weight loss with their HCPs before or after giving birth, except for one participant whose midwife talked with her about, "losing the baby weight" while she was still pregnant. While the timing of this conversation was stressful at first, after her baby was born, she found it helpful to remember the midwife's advice to focus on proper eating and not be overly focused about weight loss specifically. This participant wished she could continue discussions about weight loss at all of her postpartum visits; however, since seeing a family doctor, the issue had not been discussed.

The majority of women thought it would be best to have a weight loss discussion during the six week postnatal check-up; alternatively, some women thought it would be helpful to begin these discussions during pregnancy to have the opportunity to start thinking about it early on. Whether weight loss is discussed during or after pregnancy, all women agreed that they want to be given the option to have this discussion and that it should be a part of standard care.

"No matter what size you are, I think every woman should have that [discussing postpartum weight loss] option. ...if your healthcare provider sits there and says, here's your options, it's not like they're telling you you're heavy and you need to lose weight. They're just saying that if you're willing to or if you want to, here you go. And if they're doing it to every woman, then every woman's not going to feel cornered and saying, oh my gosh, you're heavy. If it's like, oh yeah, well, my healthcare provider asked me too, then they're [women] going to be like, oh, okay, well maybe everybody's getting asked. It's not just me. It's a woman thing. It's every woman."

– Participant V1

Discussion

Maternal body weight is simple to measure and widely used in many countries as a general indicator of maternal and fetal health throughout pregnancy [24]. Studies indicate that although maternal weight may be measured at most prenatal visits, between 45 and 80% of women exceed recommended amounts for total weight gain [6–8, 11]. This, in part, may reflect the fact that most women do not have regular, detailed conversations with their HCPs about appropriate GWG [14, 25].

Women reported that they had not had in-depth or regular discussions about GWG with their HCP, but that they would like to. They added further insight by indicating that they believed these conversations to be very important and they perceived HCPs as trusted and credible sources of information during pregnancy. Women believed there was a "right" amount of weight to gain to achieve a healthy pregnancy and that their weight in pregnancy was "more than just a number on a scale". They also believed that the amount of weight gained was important for how they felt about their self-esteem, their health and the health of their baby. Lack of discussion about GWG with their HCP contributed to women's confusion about what the right amount of weight to gain was and how to achieve it. It also contributed to women's feelings of frustration and guilt when HCPs told them that they had gained an inappropriate amount. Our results support and extend the results from the USA [26] in which researchers conducted interviews with 24 overweight and obese women and found that discussions about GWG with HCPs did not occur but that women would like to have these discussions. Focus groups with pregnant women in France also noted that women look to their HCP for direction about health, eating and appropriate weight gain [27].

Women in our study stated that they wanted an opportunity for HCPs to learn about a woman's lifestyle, health behaviours, beliefs and level of motivation so that HCPs could assist them in targeted and supportive ways. Specifically, women wished:

➢ Discussions to begin early in pregnancy and occur regularly throughout pregnancy;
➢ To learn about the weight gain goals based on their pre-pregnancy BMI, including the trajectory of weight gain (i.e., approximate timing and distribution of weight gain);
➢ Regular and constructive updates about GWG to understand how their pregnancy is progressing;
➢ Specific advice and guidance about how to achieve weight gain goals and healthy pregnancies;
➢ Tailored advice about nutrition and physical activity; and
➢ HCP insights into anticipated changes to daily routines and lifestyles. Women in our study identified a large gap in prenatal care since only one woman reported that her HCP discussed postpartum weight loss. Women expressed great interest in wanting to discuss realistic weight loss targets (i.e., amounts and rates of weight loss) along with possible nutrition and physical activity strategies that would be safe and effective. Women suggested that they would welcome discussions about maternal postnatal weight and lifestyle during pregnancy and beginning at approximately 6 weeks postpartum. Relatively few studies have examined approaches to improve postpartum weight loss, although promising results on successful approaches using dietary interventions have recently been reported in Sweden [28–31]. New studies in the USA may shed additional light on how to positively impact on postpartum weight loss in a North American context [32].

Studies report that HCPs may avoid discussing GWG as this may be perceived to be a sensitive topic for women [33, 34]. Results from all of our focus groups were very consistent, with women stating that weight gain in pregnancy is expected and that they perceived weight gain to be an appropriate topic to discuss. Women felt they would be most open to discussions

that began with HCPs asking women if they want to discuss weight gain/loss, and that discussions should be free of assumptions and judgment. Women stated that one way to approach GWG conversations would be for HCPs to ask all women about weight gain/loss, rather than restricting such discussions to women with a pre-pregnancy BMI in the overweight or obese category. Including regular discussions about GWG as part of standard practice with all women may contribute to improving women's perceptions of these conversations. Our findings closely resemble those from [35] whose study was conducted with pregnant and postpartum women from the Boston area. The similarities between these 2 studies suggests that women with a low-risk pregnancy in the USA and Canada may face some similar issues related to GWG support and that they also identify some similar solutions.

Limitations

This was an exploratory study of women's experiences and their perceptions of discussions about GWG with HCPs during pregnancy and postpartum, and as such, only women's perspectives are included. Women self-selected to participate in this study and, therefore, may be more motivated to share either positive or negative experiences than those who did not participate. However, we found that participants genuinely wanted to talk about their positive and challenging experiences with pregnancy. Most participants in this study were having their first child and it is possible that women's perceptions and their needs for support may change in subsequent pregnancies. It was beyond the scope of this study to explore the extent to which women from different pre-pregnancy BMI categories or who experience different amounts or rates of GWG may prefer different types or amounts of support from their HCP, although this could be the focus of additional study.

Results from this study are most applicable in countries where physicians provide primary care to women during pregnancy, and where pregnant women are routinely weighed during prenatal visits. The need for enhancing the relationships between patients and their HCP has been identified in many areas of health care, including prenatal care [36–38]. Finally, although some focus groups were conducted with a small number of participants, findings were similar across the groups and saturation was reached.

Conclusions

Women would like to have more regular and detailed discussions about GWG and postpartum weight loss with HCPs than occurred. Women in our study wanted discussions to be an opportunity for HCPs to learn about their lifestyle, health behaviours, beliefs and level of motivation so that HCPs could assist them in targeted and supportive ways.

This identifies an opportunity to improve prenatal care and could lead to better health outcomes for both women and children. Exceeding weight gain recommendations is a concern among pregnant women and increases the likelihood of retaining excess weight which can lead to chronic diseases in later life [39–41]. Women suggested that discussions about GWG should occur with all women, conversations should begin early in pregnancy as it is difficult to manage weight during pregnancy once weight gain recommendations and/or recommended rates of weight gain have been exceeded, and should continue through to the postpartum period. Interventions to promote healthy, supportive, patient-centred discussions about GWG should be implemented and evaluated to support improvements in perinatal health and practice.

Abbreviations
BMI: Body mass index; GWG: Gestational weight gain; HCPs: Healthcare providers

Acknowledgements
We thank all of the women who took the time to participate in the focus groups and share their personal experiences. We would also like to thank Dawn Phelps, Health Promotion Coordinator with Alberta Health Services who facilitated focus group recruitment. This study, and all of those included in the ENRICH research program, had financial support from Alberta Innovates Health Solutions. In addition to all of the authors, members of ENRICH are: Linda J. McCargar, Paula J. Robson, Dolly Bondarianzadeh, Ilona Czismadi, Venu Jain, Kara Nerenberg, Christian Rueda-Clausen, Arya Sharma, Ellen Toth, Sheila Tyminski, and Yan Yuan.

Funding
This study is funded by a Collaborative Research and Innovation Opportunities grant through Alberta Health Innovates Solutions.

Authors' contributions
RB, HN, MM and TM contributed to the design of the study, the analysis plan, and data interpretation. HN led the data collection and analyses and wrote the first draft of this article. JT contributed to data collection and analyses. All authors commented on multiple drafts and approved the final submission.

Competing interests
The authors declare that they have no competing interests.

Author details
[1]Department of Agricultural, Food and Nutritional Sciences, University of Alberta, 4-126 Li Ka Shing Centre for Health Research Innovation, Edmonton, AB T6G 2E1, Canada. [2]University of Alberta, Community University Partnership, Facility of Extension, 2nd Floor, 2-281 Enterprise Square, 10230 Jasper Avenue, Edmonton, AB T5J 4P6, Canada. [3]Healthy Living, Population, Public and Aboriginal Health, Reproductive Health, Healthy Children and Families, Alberta Health Services, 10101 Southport Road SW cubicle #1740, Calgary, AB T2W 3N2, Canada.

References
1. Chalmers B, Dzakpasu S, Heaman M, Kaczorowski J. The Canadian maternity experiences survey: an overview of findings. J Obstet Gynaecol Can. 2008;30(3):217–28.
2. Davies GA, Maxwell C, McLeod L, Gagnon R, Basso M, Bos H, et al. Obesity in pregnancy. J Obstet Gynaecol Can. 2010;32(2):165–73. Epub 2010/02/26.
3. Nohr EA, Vaeth M, Baker JL, Sorensen TIA, Olsen J, Rasmussen KM. Combined associations of prepregnancy body mass index and gestational weight gain with the outcome of pregnancy. Am J Clin Nutr. 2008;87(6):1750–9.
4. Fraser A, Tilling K, Macdonald-Wallis C, Hughes R, Sattar N, Nelson SM, et al. Associations of gestational weight gain with maternal body mass index, waist circumference, and blood pressure measured 16 y after pregnancy: the Avon longitudinal study of parents and children (ALSPAC). Am J Clin Nutr. 2011;93(6):1285–92.
5. Rasmussen KM, Abrams B. Gestational weight gain and later maternal health: are they related? Am J Clin Nutr. 2011;93(6):1186–7.
6. Lowell H, Miller D. Weight gain during pregnancy: adherence to health Canada's guidelines. Stat Canada Health Rep. 2010;21(2):1–7. no 82-003-XPE.
7. Romano M, Lacaria E, Battini L, Aragona M, Bianchi C, Penno G, et al. How much weight are women gaining during pregnancy? an Italian cohort study. Gynecol Endocrinol. 2015;31(12):942–4. Epub 2015/08/21.
8. Winkvist A, Brantsæter AL, Brandhagen M, Haugen M, Meltzer HM, Lissner L. Maternal prepregnant body mass index and gestational weight gain Are associated with initiation and duration of breastfeeding among Norwegian mothers. J Nutr. 2015;145(6):1263–70.
9. Io M. Weight gain during pregnancy: reexamining the guidelines. Rasmussen KM, yaktine a, editors. Washington: National Academies Press; 2009.
10. Jarman M, Yuan Y, Pakseresht M, Shi Q, Robson PJ, Bell RC, et al. Patterns and trajectories of gestational weight gain: a prospective cohort study. CMAJ open. 2016;4(2):E338–E45.
11. Begum FCI, McCargar LJ. Bell RC and the APrON team gestational weight gain and early postpartum weight retention in a prospective cohort of Albertan women. JOGC. 2012;34:637–47.
12. Asbee SM, Jenkins TR, Butler JR, White J, Elliot M, Rutledge A. Preventing excessive weight gain during pregnancy through dietary and lifestyle counseling: a randomized controlled trial. Obstet Gynecol. 2009;113(2 Pt 1): 305–12. Epub 2009/01/22.
13. Phelan S, Phipps MG, Abrams B, Darroch F, Grantham K, Schaffner A, et al. Does behavioral intervention in pregnancy reduce postpartum weight retention? twelve-month outcomes of the Fit for delivery randomized trial. Am J Clin Nutr. 2014;99(2):302–11. Epub 2013/11/29.
14. McDonald SD, Pullenayegum E, Taylor VH, Lutsiv O, Bracken K, Good C, et al. Despite 2009 guidelines, few women report being counseled correctly about weight gain during pregnancy. Am J Obstet Gynecol. 2011;205(4):333. e1-6. Epub 2011/07/26.
15. Duthie EA, Drew EM, Flynn KE. Patient-provider communication about gestational weight gain among nulliparous women: a qualitative study of the views of obstetricians and first-time pregnant women. BMC Pregnancy Childbirth. 2013;13:231. Epub 2013/12/18.
16. Lutsiv O, Bracken K, Pullenayegum E, Sword W, Taylor VH, McDonald SD. Little congruence between health care provider and patient perceptions of counselling on gestational weight gain. J Obstet Gynaecol Can. 2012;34(6): 518–24. Epub 2012/06/08.
17. Shub A, Huning EY, Campbell KJ, McCarthy EA. Pregnant women's knowledge of weight, weight gain, complications of obesity and weight management strategies in pregnancy. BMC Res Notes. 2013;6:278. Epub 2013/07/23.
18. Olson G, Blackwell SC. Optimization of gestational weight gain in the obese gravida: a review. Obstet Gynecol Clin North Am. 2011;38(2):397–407. xii. Epub 2011/05/18.
19. Patton MQ. Qualitative research and evaluation methods. Integrating theory and practice. 4th edition ed. Thousand Oaks: SAGE Publications, Inc.; 2015.
20. Farmer AP, Nikolopoulos H, McCargar L, Berry T, Mager D. Organizational characteristics and processes are important in the adoption of the Alberta

nutrition guidelines for children and youth in child-care centres. Public Health Nutr. 2015;18(9):1593–601. Epub 2014/10/23.

21.   Nikolopoulos H, Farmer A, Berry TR, McCargar LJ, Mager DR. Perceptions of the characteristics of the Alberta nutrition guidelines for children and youth by child care providers may influence early adoption of nutrition guidelines in child care centres. Matern Child Nutr. 2015;11(2):271–82. Epub 2012/10/02.

22.   Hsieh HF, Shannon SE. Three approaches to qualitative content analysis. Qual Health Res. 2005;15(9):1277–88. Epub 2005/10/06.

23.   Miles MB, Huberman AM, Saldana J. Qualitative data analysis. A methods sourcebook. Third edition ed. Thousand Oaks: SAGE Publications, Inc.; 2013.

24.   Scott C, Andersen CT, Valdez N, Mardones F, Nohr EA, Poston L, et al. No global consensus: a cross-sectional survey of maternal weight policies. BMC Pregnancy Childbirth. 2014;14:167. Epub 2014/06/03.

25.   Daley AJ, Jolly K, Jebb SA, Roalfe AK, Mackillop L, Lewis AL, et al. Effectiveness of regular weighing, weight target setting and feedback by community midwives within routine antenatal care in preventing excessive gestational weight gain: randomised controlled trial. BMC Obes. 2015;3:7. Epub 2016/02/18.

26.   Stengel MR, Kraschnewski JL, Hwang SW, Kjerulff KH, Chuang CH. "What My doctor Didn't tell Me": examining health care provider advice to overweight and obese pregnant women on gestational weight gain and physical activity. Womens Health Issues. 2012;22(6):e535–e40.

27.   Bianchi CM, Huneau JF, Le Goff G, Verger EO, Mariotti F, Gurviez P. Concerns, attitudes, beliefs and information seeking practices with respect to nutrition-related issues: a qualitative study in French pregnant women. BMC Pregnancy Childbirth. 2016;16(1):306. Epub 2016/10/13.

28.   Bertz F, Brekke HK, Ellegård L, Rasmussen KM, Wennergren M, Winkvist A. Diet and exercise weight-loss trial in lactating overweight and obese women. Am J Clin Nutr. 2012;96(4):698–705.

29.   Brekke HK, Bertz F, Rasmussen KM, Bosaeus I, Ellegard L, Winkvist A. Diet and exercise interventions among overweight and obese lactating women: randomized trial of effects on cardiovascular risk factors. PLoS One. 2014;9(2):e88250. Epub 2014/02/12.

30.   Huseinovic E, Bertz F, Leu Agelii M, Hellebo Johansson E, Winkvist A, Brekke HK. Effectiveness of a weight loss intervention in postpartum women: results from a randomized controlled trial in primary health care. Am J Clin Nutr. 2016;104(2):362–70. Epub 2016/07/15.

31.   Huseinovic E, Winkvist A, Bertz F, Hellebo Johansson E, Brekke HK. Dietary assessment among women with overweight and obesity in early postpartum. J hum nutr diet. 2016;29(4):411–7. Epub 2015/12/24.

32.   Rosal MC, Haughton CF, Estabrook BB, Wang ML, Chiriboga G, Nguyen OH, et al. Fresh Start, a postpartum weight loss intervention for diverse low-income women: design and methods for a randomized clinical trial. BMC Public Health. 2016;16:953. Epub 2016/09/11.

33.   Stotland N, Tsoh JY, Gerbert B. Prenatal weight gain: who is counseled? J Womens Health (Larchmt). 2012;21(6):695–701. Epub 2011/11/25.

34.   Heslehurst N, Lang R, Rankin J, Wilkinson JR, Summerbell CD. Obesity in pregnancy: a study of the impact of maternal obesity on NHS maternity services. BJOG. 2007;114(3):334–42. Epub 2007/01/31.

35.   Criss S, Oken E, Guthrie L, Hivert MF. A qualitative study of gestational weight gain goal setting. BMC Pregnancy Childbirth. 2016;16(1):317. Epub 2016/10/22.

36.   de Labrusse C, Ramelet AS, Humphrey T, Maclennan SJ. Patient-centered Care in Maternity Services: A Critical Appraisal and Synthesis of the Literature. Womens Health Issues. 2016;26(1):100–9. Epub 2015/11/10.

37.   Olander EK, Berg M, McCourt C, Carlstrom E, Dencker A. Person-centred care in interventions to limit weight gain in pregnant women with obesity - a systematic review. BMC Pregnancy Childbirth. 2015;15:50. Epub 2015/04/18.

38.   Kornhaber R, Walsh K, Duff J, Walker K. Enhancing adult therapeutic interpersonal relationships in the acute health care setting: an integrative review. J Multidiscip Healthc. 2016;9:537–46. Epub 2016/10/30.

39.   Gunderson EP. Childbearing and obesity in women: weight before, during, and after pregnancy. Obstet Gynecol Clin North Am. 2009;36(2):317–32. ix. Epub 2009/06/09.

40.   Smith DE, Lewis CE, Caveny JL, Perkins LL, Burke GL, Bild DE. Longitudinal changes in adiposity associated with pregnancy. The CARDIA study. Coronary artery risk development in young adults study. JAMA. 1994;271(22):1747–51. Epub 1994/06/08.

41.   Widen EM, Whyatt RM, Hoepner LA, Ramirez-Carvey J, Oberfield SE, Hassoun A, et al. Excessive gestational weight gain is associated with long-term body fat and weight retention at 7 y postpartum in African American and Dominican mothers with underweight, normal, and overweight prepregnancy BMI. Am J Clin Nutr. 2015;102(6):1460–7.

Maternal obesity and its effect on labour duration in nulliparous women

Karen Louise Ellekjaer[1]* (iD), Thomas Bergholt[2] and Ellen Løkkegaard[1]

Abstract

Background: Obesity is increasing among primipara women. We aimed to describe the association between body mass index (BMI) during early-pregnancy and duration of labour in nulliparous women.

Methods: Retrospective observational cohort study of 1885 nulliparous women with a single cephalic presentation from 37 0/7 to 42 6/7 weeks of completed gestation and spontaneous or induced labour at Nordsjællands Hospital, University of Copenhagen, Denmark, in 2011 and 2012.
Total duration of labour and the first and second stages of labour were compared between early-pregnancy normal-weight (BMI <25 kg/m^2), overweight (BMI 25–29.9 kg/m^2), and obese (BMI ≥30 kg/m^2) women. Proportional hazards and multiple logistic regression models were applied.

Results: Early pregnancy BMI classified 1246 (66.1%) women as normal weight, 350 (18.6%) as overweight and 203 (10.8%) as obese. No difference in the duration of total or first stage of active labour was found for overweight (adjusted HR = 1.01, 95% CI 0.88–1.16) or obese (adjusted HR = 1.07, 95% CI 0.90–1.28) compared to normal weight women. Median active labour duration was 5.83 h for normal weight, 6.08 h for overweight and 5.90 h for obese women.
The risk of caesarean delivery increased significantly for overweight and obese compared to normal weight women (odds ratios (OR) 1.62; 95%CI 1.18–2.22 and 1.76; 95%CI 1.20–2.58, respectively). Caesarean deliveries were performed earlier in labour in obese than normal-weight women (HR = 1.80, 95%CI 1.28–2.54).

Conclusion: BMI had no significant effect on total duration of active labour. Risk of caesarean delivery increased with increasing BMI. Caesarean deliveries are undertaken earlier in obese women compared to normal weight women following the onset of active labour, shortening the total duration of active labour.

Background

Average body mass index (BMI) has increased over the past 30 years and obesity has become a global health issue [1, 2]. This tendency has a wide range of implications in the field of obstetrics as women with a higher BMI are at risk of various complications during pregnancy such as gestational diabetes, preeclampsia, macrosomia, dystocia, and stillbirths [3, 4]. Furthermore, increasing BMI is associated with an increased rate of caesarean delivery due in part to failure of labour-progression [5–7].

Previously published studies have not clarified the extent to which BMI influences the duration of labour. One study showed no significant effect [8] whereas others describe prolonged duration of labour with increasing BMI [9–11]. It is pertinent to consider the effect of maternal BMI on the progress and duration of labour in order to facilitate decision-making on potential obstetric interventions. In order to ensure proper labour management, perceptions about labour progression in obese women should be evidence-based and not guided by assumptions.

The objective of this study was to describe the association between BMI during early-pregnancy and the duration of labour.

* Correspondence: Karen.ellekjaer@gmail.com
[1]Department of Obstetrics and Gynaecology, Nordsjællands Hospital, University of Copenhagen, Dyrehavevej 29, 3400 Hillerød, Denmark
Full list of author information is available at the end of the article

Methods

The study population included women who gave birth at the Department of Gynaecology and Obstetrics, Nordsjællands Hospital, University of Copenhagen, Denmark, between January 1, 2011 and December 31, 2012.

Data were obtained through electronically based hospital charts (Doculive, DLEPR v. 4.9.3.0) describing all prenatal obstetric consultations and ultrasound scans as well as labour, delivery, and the postnatal period. Data were listed according to the Danish 10-digit personal identification number (dd-mm-yy-xxxx).

Data was extracted for women allocated to group 1 or 2a of Robsons 10 group classification system [12]. Hence, the study population included all nulliparous women with a single cephalic presentation from 37 0/7 to 42 6/7 weeks of completed gestation who were either induced or entered labour spontaneously. Multiparous women, multiple pregnancies, pre-term pregnancies, elective caesarean deliveries as well as breeches, transverse- or oblique presentations were excluded. Standard protocol for labour induction in our institution comprised prostaglandin-induced cervical ripening or induction with oxytocin. No transcervical catheters were used for induction of labour.

Maternal first trimester height and weight was recorded at the first prenatal consultation. Early pregnancy BMI was calculated and the women were grouped in BMI categories of <25 kg/m^2, 25–29.9 kg/m^2, and ≥30 kg/m^2.

Gestational age was assessed with a dating ultrasound scan. Maternal age was calculated from the woman's date of birth. Weight of the baby was recorded after birth. Hypertensive disease was grouped to reflect all women who had hypertensive diseases prior to pregnancy or who developed hypertension or preeclampsia during pregnancy. Manual chart review provided information on smoking status, labour induction, use of cardiotocography (CTG), augmentation using oxytocin, and epidural analgesia.

The primary outcome was duration of active labour. This was recorded as the total duration then subdivided into phases. Total duration of labour was calculated from the beginning of active labour until time of delivery. The beginning of active labour was defined as the onset of regular contractions combined with a dilated cervical orificium >3 cm. Women who had a cervical orificium dilated further upon arrival at the labour ward were defined as being in active labour from the time of admittance.

The total duration of labour was subdivided into phases 1 and 2. Phase 1 was defined as the period from active labour until the cervix was fully dilated, while phase 2 was defined as the remaining time from full dilatation until birth.

The secondary outcome comprised route of delivery, maternal post-partum complications, neonatal morbidity, and neonatal mortality. Apart from vaginal and caesarean delivery, mode of delivery included the level of urgency for caesarean deliveries. Level 1 required delivery within 15 min compared with 30 min for level 2 and 60 min for level 3. Maternal post-partum complications comprised post-partum haemorrhage (PPH) with bleeding in excess of 1000 ml. A 1000 ml limit for PPH was chosen from a clinical perspective as local protocol requires that women with PPH > 1000 ml should be referred to an operating theatre in case of a potential need of anaesthesia which is associated with higher risk among obese women. Foetal outcome was assessed by Apgar score at 5 min, arterial cord pH, and admission to the neonatal intensive care unit (NICU).

The study was approved by the Danish Data Protection Agency (case number: HIH-2013-012, I-Suite no: 02208).

Statistical analysis

Baseline characteristics between the three categories of BMI (<25 kg/m^2, 25–29.9 kg/m^2, and ≥30 kg/m^2) during early-pregnancy were compared using Chi-squared test. Cox proportional hazards regression was used for analyses regarding duration of labour. Models were fitted with two separate outcome measures. Firstly, an event was defined as vaginal delivery, whereas caesarean delivery was censored. Secondly, an event was defined as caesarean delivery, whereby vaginal birth was the censoring criteria.

Univariate Cox-regression models were performed. In multivariate analyses, adjustments were made for maternal height and age, birth weight, epidural analgesia, induction of labour and administration of oxytocin during labour. In our study we differentiated augmentation with oxytocin from induced labor oxytocin as follows: if oxytocin was administered before the onset of regular contractions in combination with a dilated cervical orifice >3 cm it was considered as an attempt at induction. If oxytocin was administered after the onset of regular contractions in combination with a dilated cervical orifice >3 cm it was considered as labour augmentation. As all cases were evaluated manually this reduced the risk of incorrect data due to coding errors.- All of the above-mentioned factors were chosen due to their independent effect on either labour duration or rates of caesarean delivery. In addition, we wished to adjust for maternal race, however, as this information was not registered in labour charts, we were unable to extract data to include in our mutivariate analysis. Backwards elimination by stepwise regression eliminated hypertensive disease and gestational diabetes, which was therefore not accounted for in the final analysis.

Survival curves depicted the number of deliveries over time within each BMI category. The proportional hazard assumption was checked graphically. For the secondary outcome variables, univariate logistic regressions were carried out followed by multivariate analysis, with adjustment for potential confounders. P-values <0.05 were considered statistically significant.

The database was established using Microsoft Access 2010. Statistical analysis was performed using IBM SPSS Statistics version 19.

Results

Data was extracted for a total of 1907 women. Of these, 22 non-Danish citizens were not eligible for inclusion, as they did not possess a permanent Danish personal identification number (CPR), which was necessary for comparable data. Hence, a total of 1885 women were included in the study (Fig. 1).

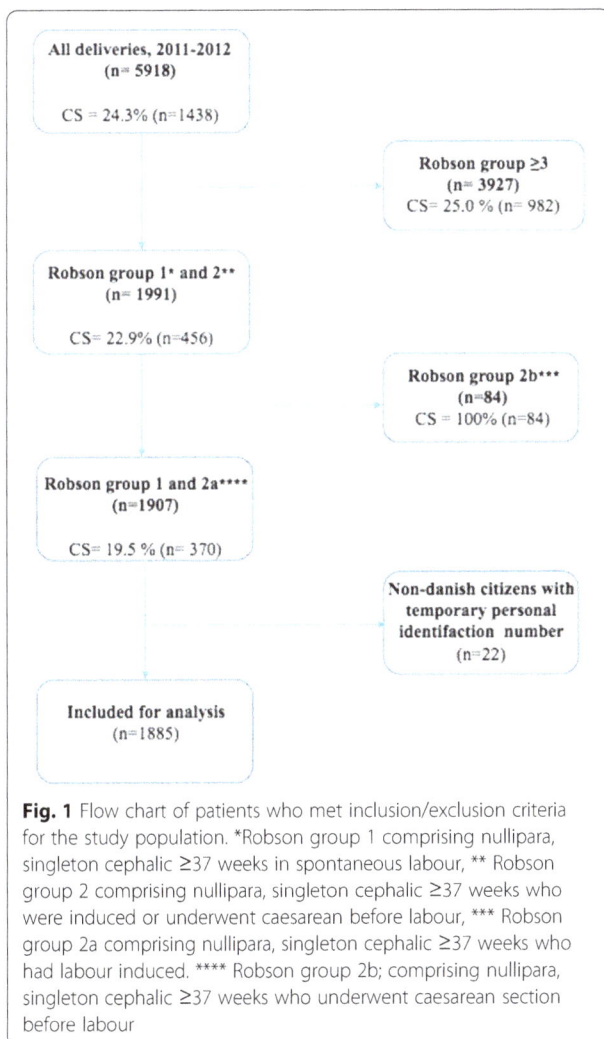

Fig. 1 Flow chart of patients who met inclusion/exclusion criteria for the study population. *Robson group 1 comprising nullipara, singleton cephalic ≥37 weeks in spontaneous labour, ** Robson group 2 comprising nullipara, singleton cephalic ≥37 weeks who were induced or underwent caesarean before labour, *** Robson group 2a comprising nullipara, singleton cephalic ≥37 weeks who had labour induced. **** Robson group 2b; comprising nullipara, singleton cephalic ≥37 weeks who underwent caesarean section before labour

Women of normal weight comprised 66.1% of the population (n = 1246), overweight 18.6% (n = 350), and obese 10.8% (n = 203). Only 4.5% (n = 86) did not have BMI recorded, most often due to lack of attendance at prenatal hospital visits. BMI was equally distributed according to maternal age, height, or gestational age, whereas an association between BMI and hypertensive disease and gestational diabetes was found ($p < 0.01$) (Table 1). The proportion of induced births increased with increasing BMI, as did the use of oxytocin for augmentation of labour, epidural analgesia, and CTG monitoring. Birth weight was associated with BMI.

Labour duration could be determined for 1808 women. Fifty-eight women (3.1%) had caesarean sections due to a failed attempt of labour induction, whereas 19 women did not have the onset of regular contractions recorded. The number of women who were already in active labour upon admittance to the hospital was equally distributed with regard to BMI (p = 0.09). All 1808 women with determined labour duration gave birth within 24 h of the onset of active labour. Median active labour duration was 5.83 h for normal weight, 6.08 h for overweight and 5.90 h for obese women.

From univariate Cox analysis, we found a hazard ratio (HR) of vaginal delivery of 0.83 (95% confidence interval [CI] 0.73–0.96) for overweight (BMI 25–29.9 kg/m^2) compared to normal weight women, implying a longer duration of active labour for overweight women compared with those with normal-weight (Table 2). However, after adjustment for confounders this association was not significant (HR = 1.01, 95% CI 0.88–1.16). There was no significant difference in total duration of active labour among obese women (BMI ≥30 kg/m^2) compared to normal weight women, either before or after adjustment for confounders (Fig. 2).

The total duration of labour was subdivided into phases. In total, 155 obese women (76.4%) reached phase 2 with full dilation of the orifice, whereas the same applied to 284 (81.1%) overweight and 1112 (89.2%) normal weight women ($p < 0.01$) (Table 4). No significant difference in the duration of phase 1 was found between the BMI groups. However, phase 2 showed a more accelerant course of labour in obese than normal weight women, with a HR of 1.29 (95%CI 1.07–1.55) after adjustment (Table 2).

There were 353 (19.5%) caesarean deliveries in the study population comprising 1808 women who had labour duration recorded succesfully. The rate of caesarean deliveries was unequally distributed over the BMI strata, including 16.0% (n = 199) of normal weight, 26.3% (n = 92) of overweight, and 30.5% (n = 62) of obese women being delivered by caesarean ($p < 0.01$). The number of caesarean deliveries was equally distributed between phases 1 and 2 of labour depending on

Table 1 Distribution of covariates at baseline among women in different body mass index groups

Covariates	p-value	Maternal BMI [a]:		
		<25	25–29.9	≥30
		(n = 1246; 66.1%)	(n = 350; 18.6%)	(n = 203; 10.8%)
Maternal age	p = 0.92			
< 25		317 (25.4%)	86 (24.6%)	54 (26.6%)
25–30		429 (34.4%)	126 (36.0%)	74 (36.4%)
30–35		376 (30.2%)	100 (28.5%)	59 (29.1%)
> 35		124 (10.0%)	38 (10.9%)	16 (7.9%)
Height	p = 0.75			
< 160 cm		124 (10.0%)	36 (10.3%)	15 (7.4%)
160-169 cm		595 (47.7%)	178 (50.9%)	106 (52.2%)
170–179 cm		477 (38.3%)	124 (35.4%)	73 (36.0%)
≥ 180 cm		50 (4.0%)	12 (3.4%)	9 (4.4%)
Hypertensive disease	p < 0.01			
No		1132 (90.9%)	271 (77.4%)	158 (77.8%)
Yes		114 (9.1%)	79 (22.6%)	45 (22.2%)
Gestational Diabetes	p < 0.01			
No		1218 (97.8%)	335 (95.7%)	188 (92.6%)
Yes		28 (2.2%)	15 (4.3%)	15 (7.4%)
Gestational age	p = 0.27			
37–38 weeks		173 (13.9%)	46 (13.1%)	36 (17.7%)
39–40 weeks		635 (51.0%)	180 (51.4%)	98 (48.3%)
≥ 41 weeks		438 (35.1%)	124 (35.5%)	69 (34.0%)
Labour Induced	p < 0.01			
Yes		363 (29.1%)	131 (37.4%)	98 (48.3%)
No		831 (70.9%)	219 (62.6%)	105 (51.7%)
CTG	p < 0.01			
Yes		906 (72.7%)	285 (81.4%)	176 (86.7%)
No		340 (27.3%)	65 (18.6%)	27 (13.3%)
Oxytocin	p = 0.03			
Yes		744 (59.7%)	232 (66.3%)	135 (66.5%)
No		502 (40.3%)	118 (33.7%)	68 (33.5%)
Epidural analgesia	p < 0.01			
Yes		501 (40.2%)	170 (48.6%)	114 (56.2%)
No		745 (59.8%)	180 (51.4%)	89 (43.8%)
Birthweight	p < 0.01			
<3.0 kg		187 (15.0%)	41 (11.7%)	11 (5.5%)
3.0–3.5 kg		439 (35.3%)	111 (31.8%)	80 (39.8%)
3.5–4.0 kg		456 (36.7%)	141 (40.4%)	69 (34.3%)
>4.0 kg		162 (13.0%)	56 (16.1%)	41 (20.4%)

Values are numbers (percentages)
86 women (4.5%) did not have BMI recorded and were therefore not accounted for in analysis

BMI (p = 0.30). There was no difference in the use of vacuum extraction.

From logistic regression analysis, we found significantly increased odds ratios (OR) of caesarean delivery with increasing BMI (OR = 1.62, 95%CI 1.18–2.22 among overweight women and OR = 1.76, 95%CI 1.20–2.58 among obese women versus women of normal weight) (Table 4). Adjustments were made for maternal height and age, birth weight, labour induction, epidural analgesia, and administration of oxytocin during labour.

Table 2 Cox regression showing the hazard ratio (HR) of vaginal birth in the defined body mass index (BMI) groups, with and without adjustment for covariates

Covariates	Total duration [a]			
	Crude HR	95% CI	Adjusted HR	95% CI
BMI				
< 25	1		1	
25–29.9	0.83	[0.73–0.96]	1.01	[0.88–1.16]
≥ 30	0.94	[0.78–1.12]	1.07	[0.90–1.28]
Height				
< 160 cm	1		1	
160–169 cm	1.31	[1.08–1.59]	1.32	[1.09–1.61]
170–179 cm	1.44	[1.18–1.76]	1.61	[1.32–1.98]
≥ 180 cm	1.66	[1.21–2.26]	1.73	[1.26–2.38]
Age				
< 25	1		1	
25–29	0.87	[0.77–0.99]	1.04	[0.91–1.19]
30–34	0.82	[0.72–0.94]	0.97	[0.84–1.11]
≥ 35	0.62	[0.51–0.77]	0.68	[0.54–0.84]
Birthweight				
< 3.0 kg	1		1	
3.0–3.5 kg	0.77	[0.66–0.90]	0.66	[0.56–0.78]
3.5–4.0 kg	0.53	[0.46–0.62]	0.49	[0.42–0.58]
> 4.0 kg	0.38	[0.31–0.46]	0.38	[0.30–0.47]
Epidural				
No	1		1	
Yes	0.29	[0.26–0.32]	0.33	[0.29–0.37]
Augmentation with oxytocin:				
No	1		1	
Yes	0.31	[0.28–0.35]	0.40	[0.36–0.45]
Induced labour:				
No	1		1	
Yes	0.91	[0.82–1.02]	1.68	[1.48–1.90]
Phase 1				
	Crude HR	95% CI	Adjusted HR	95% CI
BMI				
< 25	1		1	
25–29.9	0.99	[0.86–1.14]	1.11	[0.96–1.28]
≥ 30	1.01	[0.85–1.21]	1.04	[0.86–1.24]
Phase 2				
	Crude HR	95% CI	Adjusted HR	95% CI

Table 2 Cox regression showing the hazard ratio (HR) of vaginal birth in the defined body mass index (BMI) groups, with and without adjustment for covariates (Continued)

BMI				
< 25	1		1	
25–29.9	0.90	[0.96–1.28]	0.99	[0.86–1.14]
≥ 30	1.06	[0.96–1.28]	1.29	[1.07–1.55]

Phase 1 was defined as the period of time from active labour until the cervix was fully dilated
Phase 2 was defined as the period of time from when the cervix was fully dilated to the actual birth. Caesarean deliveries censored
A hazard ratio (HR) >1 indicates an increased number of vaginal deliveries over time compared to the reference group; a shorter duration of labour.
A HR < 1 indicates a decreased number of vaginal deliveries over time compared to the reference group; a longer duration of labour
[a]77 women (4.1%) did not have duration measures recorded and were therefore not accounted for in analysis

In univariate Cox analysis, we found an increased HR of caesarean delivery, resulting in a shorter duration from onset of active labour until caesarean with increasing BMI. Compared with normal weight women, the HR of caesarean delivery was 1.39 (95%CI 1.06–1.81) for overweight and 1.94 (95%CI 1.40–2.69) among obese women (Table 3). After adjustment, the results remained significantly increased only for obese women (HR = 1.80, 95%CI 1.28–2.54) (Fig. 3).

Post-partum haemorrhage (PPH) occurred in 122 women (6.5%). The risk of PPH in the obese women was increased compared with normal weight women (OR = 2.04, 95%CI 1.23–2.38). However, after adjustment for birth weight, epidural analgesia, and caesarean delivery, the association was no longer significant (OR = 1.54, 95%CI 0.90–2.61) (Table 4).

There was no difference in neonatal morbidity assessed by Apgar score less than 8 after 5 min and number of admissions to the NICU according to maternal BMI. However, the incidence of an arterial cord pH <7.05 was 4.3% (n = 8) in the infants of obese women compared with 2.1% (n = 7) in overweight women and 1.6% (n = 18) in normal-weight women (p = 0.04). The OR of an arterial cord pH <7.05 within the obese group was increased (OR = 2.85, 95%CI 1.22–6.65) compared with the normal-weight group (Table 4).

One neonatal death occurred in the overweight group.

Discussion

This retrospective cohort study of nulliparous women demonstrated a slight decrease in labour duration during the second phase of active labour, but not in the total duration of active labour, for obese women compared with normal-weight women. Furthermore, caesarean deliveries were performed sooner in obese women following the onset of active labour than in

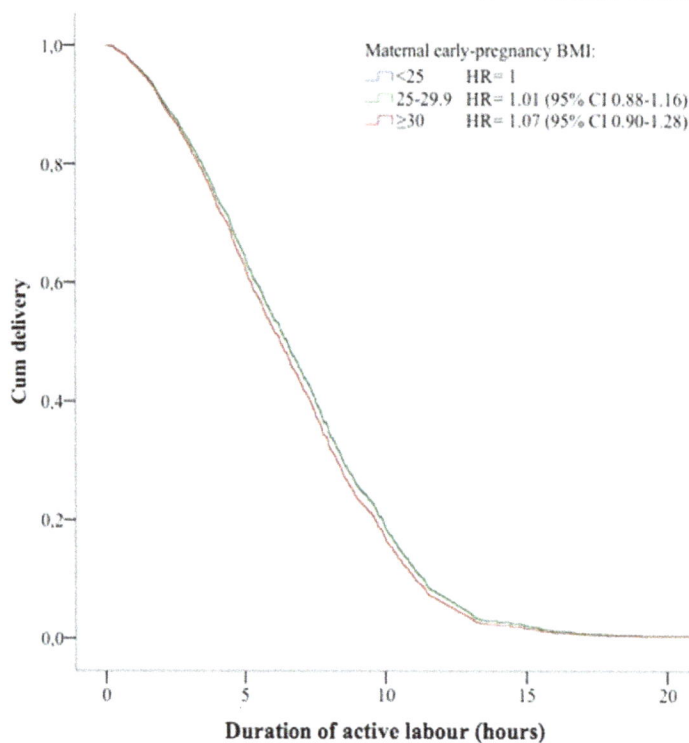

Fig. 2 Survival plot as a function of time from onset of active labour until vaginal delivery. Event was defined as delivery. Women were censored at the time of caesarean delivery. Adjustments were made for maternal age, height, birth weight, labour induction, augmentation with oxytocin, and epidural analgesia. A hazard ratio (HR) >1 illustrates a shorter duration of labour while a HR <1 illustrates a longer duration of labour compared to the reference group consisting of normal-weight women

normal-weight women undergoing caesarean, thereby shortening the total duration of active labour in obese women.

A few previous studies suggested no association between labour progression and increasing BMI. A British study of 8350 nulliparous women compared labour progression in obese versus non-obese women, observing no significant difference within the first or second stages of labour [8]. Contrary to our findings, a majority of previous studies report an independent effect of BMI on total duration of active labour. These studies specifically identify the duration of the first stage of labour as being increased, further supporting an overall increase in labour duration [9–11, 13–15]. A study by Kominiarek et al. included 118,978 nulli- and multiparous women in separate analyses. This study found a significant increase in total duration of labour with increasing BMI among nulliparous women [11]. However, the definition of active labour differed from that of most other studies, as a cervical dilatation of only 1 cm was accepted when defining the onset of labour, thereby including what was considered as the latent phase in the current study.

A study by Carlhäll et al. included 63,829 nulliparous women and found a significantly slower progression of labour but reduced duration of the second stage of labour in obese women compared with women with normal BMI [9]. The latter finding is in agreement with that of our study. However, their definition of the second stage of labour was confined to the initiation of pushing efforts and can therefore not be directly compared to the results of our study, as we defined the second stage of labour as the time when the cervical orificium was fully dilated. In contrast to our study, Carlhäll et al. did not include augmentation by oxytocin and the use of epidural analgesia as confounders. Because these parameters have an independent effect on the duration of labour [16] and both appear to be unequally distributed with regard to BMI, this could possibly have distorted the outcomes.

A greater number of censored cases within the obese group during the second stage of labour could have explained our findings of a decreased duration of phase 2. However, this was not the case because caesarean deliveries were less frequently performed in obese women after entering the second stage of labour compared to women of normal BMI. Nevertheless, fewer obese

Table 3 Cox regression showing the hazard ratio (HR) of caesarean delivery comparing the defined BMI groups, with and without adjustment for covariates

Covariates	Total labour [a]			
	Crude HR	95% CI	Adjusted HR	95% CI
BMI				
< 25	1		1	
25–29.9	1.39	[1.06–1.81]	1.28	[0.97–1.69]
≥ 30	1.94	[1.40–2.69]	1.80	[1.28–2.54]
Height				
< 160 cm	1		1	
160–169 cm	0.83	[0.60–1.15]	0.77	[0.55–1.09]
170–179 cm	0.74	[0.52–1.05]	0.64	[0.44–0.93]
≥ 180 cm	0.67	[0.31–1.41]	0.50	[0.23–1.08]
Age				
< 25	1		1	
25–29	0.99	[0.72–1.37]	0.97	[0.69–1.37]
30–34	1.22	[0.88–1.68]	1.31	[0.94–1.84]
≥ 35	1.57	[1.08–2.29]	1.82	[1.22–2.69]
Birthweight				
< 3.0 kg	1		1	
3.0–3.5 kg	0.89	[0.56–1.41]	0.98	[0.59–1.61]
3.5–4.0 kg	1.03	[0.67–1.59]	1.13	[0.71–1.82]
> 4.0 kg	1.39	[0.87–2.18]	1.43	[0.87–2.36]
Epidural				
No	1		1	
Yes	1.16	[0.88–1.53]	0.96	[0.72–1.29]
Augmentation with oxytocin				
No	1		1	
Yes	1.21	[0.85–1.72]	0.96	[0.65–1.42]
Induced labour				
No	1		1	
Yes	1.80	[1.43–2.27]	1.67	[1.33–2.17]
Phase 1				
	Crude HR	95% CI	Adjusted HR	95% CI
BMI				
< 25	1		1	
25–29.9	1.68	[1.07–2.66]	1.55	[0.97–2.48]
≥ 30	1.56	[0.86–2.84]	1.56	[0.84–2.89]
Phase 2				
	Crude HR	95% CI	Adjusted HR	95% CI

Table 3 Cox regression showing the hazard ratio (HR) of caesarean delivery comparing the defined BMI groups, with and without adjustment for covariates (Continued)

BMI				
< 25	1		1	
25–29.9	1.22	[0.77–1.94]	1.08	[0.67–1.74]
≥ 30	1.56	[0.86–2.84]	1.56	[0.84–2.89]

Phase 1 defined as the period of time from active labour until fully dilated
Phase 2 defined as the period of time from when fully dilated until actual birth. Vaginal deliveries censored
A HR > 1 illustrates an increased number of caesarean deliveries over time compared to the reference group; A shorter duration of labour. A HR < 1 illustrates a decreased number of vaginal deliveries over time compared to the reference group; A longer duration of labour
[a]77 women (4.1%) did not have duration measures recorded and were therefore not accounted for in analysis

women entered the second stage of labour compared with women of normal weight, thus decreasing the number of women available for the analysis.

We found a significant increase in caesarean deliveries with increasing BMI. This is in accordance with the findings of several larger studies [3–5]. A review by Wispelwey et al. summarized the main risk modulators of caesarean delivery in obese women, including difficulty in initiation of labour and increased induction rates [17]. Since our study only describes women who initiated active labour, and we adjusted for medical induction in statistical analyses it seems likely that there is an independent effect of obesity on the risk of caesarean delivery.

We found that obese women were granted fewer hours of active labour before a caesarean was performed compared with women of normal weight. This could be explained by a possible earlier onset of labour complications within the obese population. However, since there was no difference in the numbers within the different levels of emergency caesareans, this seems unlikely (data not shown). Alternatively, an increased consciousness amongst healthcare staff concerning the issue of maternal obesity may have had an indirect influence on treatment. A more cautious approach to managing these women might have been unknowingly adopted, resulting in an earlier decision to perform a caesarean delivery [18].

The occurrence of PPH >1000 mL was associated with increasing early-pregnancy BMI. In multiple logistic regression analyses, the association was no longer significant, but the estimate still indicated an increased risk of PPH with higher BMI. Accordingly, most other studies found an isolated effect of obesity on the risk of PPH [19].

A slight increase in the incidence of arterial cord pH values <7.05 was associated with increasing early-pregnancy BMI, which could indicate a neonatal

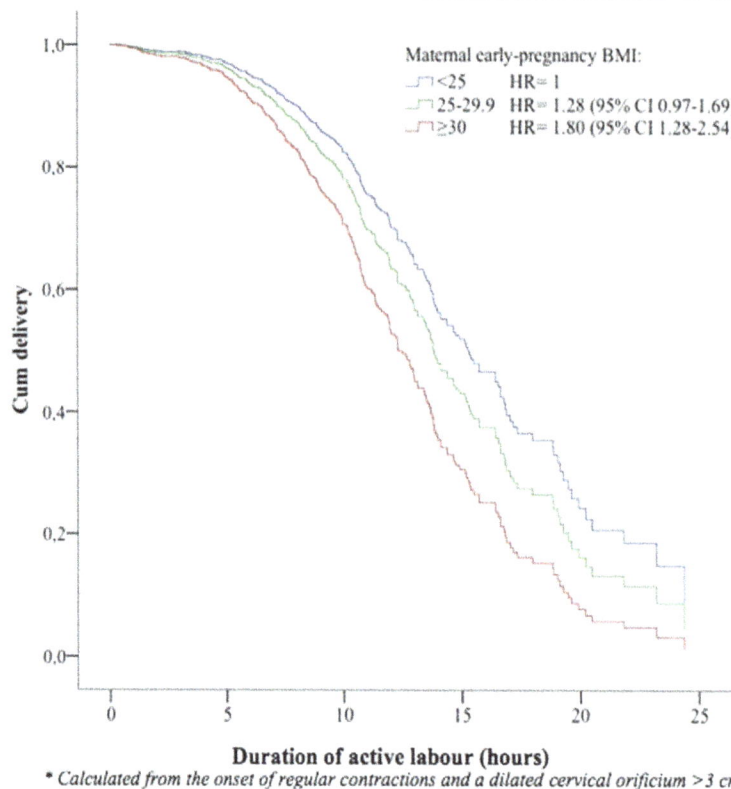

Fig. 3 Survival plot as a function of time from the onset of active labour until caesarean delivery. Event was defined as delivery. Women were censored at the time of vaginal delivery. Adjustments were made for maternal age, height, birth weight, labour induction, augmentation with oxytocin, and epidural analgesia. A hazard ratio (HR) >1 illustrates a shorter duration of labour while a HR <1 illustrates a longer duration of labour compared to the reference group consisting of normal-weight women

outcome that was less positive [20]. The remaining foetal outcome measurements were not associated with maternal BMI.

Conclusion

We found no association between BMI and the total duration of labour; however, an increased risk of a shorter second stage of labour was apparent for obese women. Our results suggest an overall increased risk of caesarean delivery with increasing BMI. Furthermore, caesarean deliveries performed on obese women were carried out earlier in the course of labour, giving obese women a shorter time of active labour compared with normal-weight women delivering by caesarean.

The risk of PPH in excess of 1000 mL increased with increasing BMI, but only in unadjusted analysis. Additionally, an increased risk of arterial cord blood with pH <7.05 was identified. The remaining neonatal outcome measures were unaffected by BMI.

The results of this study provide valuable information on the expected progression of labour in overweight and obese women and should aid obstetric care providers in deciding if and when to intervene in the labour process. Defining the normal progression of labour for

overweight and obese women can help eradicate non-scientific misconceptions about the influence of obesity, resulting in more appropriate treatment of women in this weight group. Finally, the results will aid obstetric health care providers in counselling women on the effect of their overweight.

Strengths

- Consecutive sampling of women over a 2-year period reduces the selection bias of the cohort
- The sampling of data reveals results that depict everyday practice.
- All charts were manually scrutinized and data for all variables were validated, enhancing the quality of our data
- Adjustments for multiple important confounders were performed.

Limitations

- The size of the study population.
- BMI was recorded in early pregnancy and this study can therefore not account for the effect of

Table 4 Descriptive and logistic regression analysis regarding secondary outcome variables. Values of odds ratios are presented as crude estimates as well as after adjustment

Secondary outcome variables	p-value			Crude OR	95% CI	Adjusted OR	95% CI
Total number of caesarean deliveries [a]	(p < 0.01)	No	Yes				
BMI < 25		1047 (84.0%)	199 (16.0%)	1		1	
BMI 25–29.9		258 (73.7%)	92 (26.3%)	1.88	[1.42–2.49]	1.62	[1.18–2.22]
BMI ≥ 30		141 (69.5%)	62 (30.5%)	2.31	[1.66–3.23]	1.76	[1.20–2.58]
Caesarean prior to onset of active labor [a]	(p < 0.01)	No	Yes				
BMI < 25		22 (1.8%)	1211 (98.2%)	1		1	
BMI 25–29.9		19 (5.4%)	331 (94.6%)	1.99	[1.12–3.52]	1.64	[0.90–2.98]
BMI ≥ 30		18 (8.9%)	185 (91.1%)	3.37	[1.87–6.07]	2.75	[1.47–5.16]
Reached 2nd stage of labour [a]	(p < 0.01)	No	Yes				
BMI < 25		134 (10.8%)	1112 (89.2%)	1		1	
BMI 25–29.9		66 (18.9%)	284 (81.1%)	1.85	[1.38–2.48]	0.61	[0.45–0.84]
BMI ≥ 30		48 (23.6%)	155 (76.4%)	2.13	[1.50–3.03]	0.59	[0.40–0.85]
Vacuum delivery [b]	(p = 0.39)	No	Yes				
BMI < 25		1068 (85.7%)	178 (14.3%)	1		1	
BMI 25–29.9		304 (86.9%)	46 (13.1%)	0.91	[0.64–1.27]	0.83	[0.58–1.18]
BMI ≥ 30		181 (89.2%)	22 (10.8%)	0.73	[0.46–1.17]	0.65	[0.40–1.06]
Post-partum haemorrhage ≥ 1000 mL [c]	(p = 0.02)	No	Yes				
BMI < 25		1176 (89.1%)	70 (10.9%)	1		1	
BMI 25–29.9		325 (92.9%)	25 (7.1%)	1.29	[0.81–2.07]	1.04	[0.64–1.70]
BMI ≥ 30		181 (89.2%)	22 (10.8%)	2.04	[1.23–3.38]	1.54	[0.90–2.61]
Arterial cord pH < 7.05 [d]	(p = 0.04)	No	Yes				
BMI < 25		1128 (98.4%)	18 (1.6%)	1			
BMI 25–29.9		323 (97.9%)	7 (2.1%)	1.36	[0.56–3.28]		
BMI ≥ 30		187 (95.7%)	8 (4.3%)	2.85	[1.22–6.65]		

[a]Adjustments made for: Age, height, birthweight, labour induction, epidural analgesia and use of oxytocin during labour
[b]Adjustments made for: Age and use of oxytocin during labour
[c]Adjustments made for: Birthweight, epidural analgesia and caesarean delivery
[d]No Adjustments were made

gestational weight gain on labour duration or outcome.

- Gestational age at the first prenatal visit was not recorded; however, most women attended visits early in their pregnancy, as is standard practice
- Measurements of cervical dilation were subjective and were based on examinations performed by numerous midwives
- The results of this study are only applicable to women who reach the active stage of labour as it does not take into consideration the duration of the preliminary latent phase.
- The uniformity of labour management cannot be ensured due to the number of different care providers. However, all personnel are required to follow established guidelines, which should eliminate any substantial differences in the management of care

Abbreviations
BMI: Body mass index; CI: Confidence interval; CTG: Cartiotocography; HR: Hazard ratio; NICU: Neonatal intensive care unit; OR: Odss ratio; PPH: Post partum haemorrhage

Acknowledgments
A special thanks to Dr. Jørgen G. Berthelsen, Nordsjællands Hospital, for providing data extracts.

Funding
This work was supported by "The Research Fund", Nordsjællands Hospital, University of Copenhagen. The funding sources had no involvement in any part of this study.

Authors' contributions
KLE has made substantial contributions to the conception, design of the work, the acquisition, the analysis and the interpretation of data for the work. KLE has drafted the work and approved the final version to be published. EL, TB has made substantial contributions to the conception, the design of the work and the interpretation of data for the work. EL has critically revised the work for important intellectual content and approved

of the final version to be published. TB has critically revised the work for important intellectual content and approved of the final version to be published. KLE, EL, TB agree to be accountable for all aspects of the work in ensuring that questions related to the accuracy or integrity of any part of the work are appropriately investigated and resolved. All authors read and approved the final manuscript.

Competing interests
The authors declare that they have no competing interests.

Source of study
Department of Obstetrics and Gynaecology, Nordsjællands Hospital, University of Copenhagen, Denmark.

Author details
[1]Department of Obstetrics and Gynaecology, Nordsjællands Hospital, University of Copenhagen, Dyrehavevej 29, 3400 Hillerød, Denmark. [2]Department of Obstetrics and Gynaecology, Rigshospitalet, University of Copenhagen, Blegdamsvej 9, 2100 Copenhagen, Denmark.

References
1. World Health Organization. Global Health Observatory Data Repository. Available at: http://apps.who.int/gho/data/node.main.A903?lang=en. Accessed 6 Nov 2014.
2. Fisher SC, Kim SY, Sharma AJ, Rochat R, Morrow B. Is obesity still increasing among pregnant women? Prepregnancy obesity trends in 20 states, 2003-2009. Prev Med. 2013;56:372–8.
3. Cedergren MI. Maternal morbid obesity and the risk of adverse pregnancy outcome. Obstet Gynecol. 2004;103:219–24.
4. Davies GA, Maxwell C, McLeod L, Gagnon R, Basso M, Bos H, et. al. Obesity in pregnancy. J Obstet Gynaecol Can 2010;32:165-173.
5. Bergholt T, Lim LK, Jorgensen JS, Robson MS. Maternal body mass index in the first trimester and risk of caesarean delivery in nulliparous women in spontaneous labour. Am J Obstet Gynecol. 2007;196:163.e1–5.
6. Poobalan AS, Aucott LS, Gurung T, Smith WC, Bhattacharya S. Obesity as an independent risk factor for elective and emergency delivery in nulliparous women–systematic review and meta-analysis of cohort studies. Obes Rev. 2009;10:28–35.
7. Cedergren MI. Non-elective caesarean delivery due to ineffective uterine contractility or due to obstructed labour in relation to maternal body mass index. Eur J Obstet Gynecol Reprod Biol. 2009;145:163–6.
8. Usha Kiran TS, Hemmadi S, Bethel J, Evans J. Outcome of pregnancy in a woman with an increased body mass index. BJOG. 2005;112:768–72.
9. Carlhall S, Kallen K, Blomberg M. Maternal body mass index and duration of labour. Eur J Obstet Gynecol Reprod Biol. 2013;171:49–53.
10. Norman SM, Tuuli MG, Odibo AO, Caughey AB, Roehl KA, Cahill AG. The effects of obesity on the first stage of labour. Obstet Gynecol. 2012;120:130–5.
11. Kominiarek MA, Zhang J, Vanveldhuisen P, Troendle J, Beaver J, Hibbard JU. Contemporary labour patterns: the impact of maternal body mass index. Am J Obstet Gynecol. 2011;205:244.e1–8.
12. Robson MS. Can we reduce the caesarean section rate? Best Practice Res Clin Obstet Gynaecol. 2001;15(1):179–94.
13. Vahratian A, Zhang J, Troendle JF, Savitz DA, Siega-Riz AM. Maternal prepregnancy overweight and obesity and the pattern of labour progression in term nulliparous women. Obstet Gynecol. 2004;104:943–51.
14. Hilliard AM, Chauhan SP, Zhao Y, Rankins NC. Effect of obesity on length of labour in nulliparous women. Am J Perinatol. 2012;29:127–32.
15. Pevzner L, Powers BL, Rayburn WF, Rumney P, Wing DA. Effects of maternal obesity on duration and outcomes of prostaglandin cervical ripening and labour induction. Obstet Gynecol. 2009;114:1315–21.
16. Anim-Somuah M, Smyth RM, Jones L. Epidural versus non-epidural or no analgesia in labour. Cochrane Database Syst Rev. 2011;(12):CD000331.
17. Wispelwey BP, Sheiner E. Cesarean delivery in obese women: a comprehensive review. J Matern Fetal Neonatal Med. 2013;26(6):547–51. doi:10.3109/14767058.2012.745506.
18. Foy AJ, Filippone EJ. The case for intervention bias in the practice of medicine. Yale J Biol Med. 2013;86(2):271–80.
19. Blomberg M. Maternal obesity and risk of postpartum haemorrhage. Obstet Gynecol. 2011;118:561–8.
20. Malin GL, Morris RK, Khan KS. Strength of association between umbilical cord pH and perinatal and long term outcomes: systematic review and meta-analysis. BMJ. 2010;340:c1471.

Sociodemographic factors and pregnancy outcomes associated with prepregnancy obesity: effect modification of parity in the nationwide Epifane birth-cohort

Julie Boudet-Berquier[1]*, Benoit Salanave[1], Jean-Claude Desenclos[2] and Katia Castetbon[3]

Abstract

Background: In light of the adverse outcomes for mothers and offspring related to maternal obesity, identification of subgroups of women at risk of prepregnancy obesity and its related-adverse issues is crucial for optimizing antenatal care. We aimed to identify sociodemographic factors and maternal and neonatal outcomes associated with prepregnancy obesity, and we tested the effect modification of parity on these associations.

Methods: In 2012, 3368 mothers who had delivered in 136 randomly selected maternity wards were included just after birth in the French birth cohort, Epifane. Maternal height and weight before and at the last month of pregnancy were self-reported. Maternal and neonatal outcomes were collected in medical records. Prepregnancy Body Mass Index (pBMI) was classified into underweight (<18.5), normal (18.5-24.9), overweight (25.0-29.9) and obesity (≥30.0). Since we found statistically significant interactions with parity, the multinomial logistic regression model estimating associations of pBMI class with sociodemographic characteristics and pregnancy outcomes was stratified on parity (1335 primiparous and 1814 multiparous).

Results: Before pregnancy, 7.6% of women were underweight, 64.2% were of normal weight, 18.0% were overweight and 10.2% were obese. Among the primiparous, maternal age of 25-29 years (OR = 2.09 [1.13-3.87]; vs. 30-34 years), high school level (OR = 2.22 [1.33-3.73]; vs. university level), gestational diabetes (OR = 2.80 [1.56-5.01]) and hypertensive complications (OR = 3.80 [1.83-7.89]) were independently associated with prepregnancy obesity. Among the multiparous, primary (OR = 6.30 [2.40-16.57]), junior high (OR = 2.89 [1.81-4.64]) and high school (OR = 1.86 [1.18-2.93]) education levels (vs. university level), no attendance at antenatal classes (OR = 1.77 [1.16-2.72]), excess gestational weight gain (OR = 1.82 [1.20-2.76]), gestational diabetes (OR =5.16 [3.15-8.46]), hypertensive complications (OR = 8.13 [3.97-16.64]), caesarean delivery (OR = 1.80 [1.18-2.77]) and infant birth weight ≥ 4 kg (OR = 1.70 [1.03-2.80]; vs. birth weight between 2.5 kg and 4 kg) were independently associated with prepregnancy obesity.

Conclusion: Obesity before pregnancy is associated with a set of sociodemographic characteristics and adverse pregnancy outcomes that differ across parity groups. Such findings are useful for targeted health policies aimed at attaining healthy prepregnancy weight and organizing perinatal care.

Keywords: Adverse pregnancy outcomes, Maternal obesity, National birth cohort, Social inequalities

* Correspondence: julie.boudet-berquier@univ-paris13.fr
[1]Nutritional Surveillance and Epidemiology Team (ESEN), French Public Health Agency, Paris-13 University, Centre de Recherche en Epidémiologie et Statistiques, COMUE Sorbonne Paris Cité, SMBH Building, 1st floor, door 136, 74 rue Marcel Cachin, 93017 Bobigny Cedex, France
Full list of author information is available at the end of the article

Background

Since women entering pregnancy with obesity may face adverse health issues affecting themselves and their offspring [1], maternal obesity is now a crucial public health problem worldwide [2]. Studies have provided strong evidence of the association of maternal obesity with risk of gestational diabetes mellitus (GDM), pre-eclampsia, caesarean delivery and large-for-gestational-age newborns [3–6]. Moreover, pre-existing type 2 diabetes [7] may be involved in higher risk of congenital malformations associated with maternal obesity [8]. Preterm birth and small- and large-for-gestational-age birth might also partially mediate the association observed between maternal obesity and higher risk of stillbirth and infant death [9]. In addition, recent observational studies suggested the involvement of maternal obesity in the risk, for the offspring, to develop obesity during adulthood independently of their adult lifestyle factors [10], and to suffer from premature mortality related to cardiovascular events [11].

In view of these adverse health issues, identification of sociodemographic characteristics associated with maternal obesity is useful for implementing targeted preventive actions and improving their efficacy. However, the relationship between sociodemographic factors and prepregnancy body mass index (pBMI) appears inconsistent across studies. Poor socioeconomic conditions (living in a low income household [5] or in a deprived area [12, 13]) have consistently been found to be risk factors in maternal obesity. In contrast, inconsistent results have been found in the association of maternal obesity with age at giving birth [12, 14] and educational level [5, 12].

A number of studies have indicated that parity was a risk factor in maternal obesity [5, 12, 14]. Several authors have investigated underlying mechanisms involved in the relationship between childbearing and development of obesity, including post-partum weight retention [15–17]. Excessive gestational weight gain (GWG) and a short time lapse between pregnancies have been shown to be independently associated with postpartum weight retention and further maternal obesity [16]. Weight gained during pregnancy and after birth might depended not only on prepregnancy body weight and hormonal changes, but also on modifications in lifestyle due to child-rearing and socioeconomic factors [18]. Such considerations suggest that the association of sociodemographic characteristics with the risk of maternal obesity may differ by parity. In addition, the pattern of adverse health outcomes associated with prepregnancy weight have been shown to differ between primiparous and multiparous women [19]. A better understanding of the role of parity in the relationship between maternal obesity and adverse pregnancy issues would therefore optimize perinatal care.

However, studies investigating the effect modification of parity in the association between maternal obesity and sociodemographic factors and maternal and neonatal outcomes are scarce. Using data from the French nation-wide birth cohort Epifane, performed in 2012, our objectives were: (1) to assess sociodemographic characteristics and maternal, fetal and neonatal outcomes associated with maternal obesity; and (2) to investigate the effect modification of parity by testing the interaction between parity and sociodemographic and medical factors. Our hypotheses were that: (1) in France, in 2012, sociodemographic characteristics and maternal and neonatal outcomes in obese mothers differ from those of normal-weight women; (2) such associations vary between primiparous and multiparous women.

Methods

Study design

We have previously described the study methods [20]. Briefly, Epifane was a nation-wide birth cohort based on two-stage random sampling. First, 136 maternity wards in mainland France were randomly selected proportionally to the yearly number of deliveries and stratified on the private/public status, equipment level of the maternity hospital and five geographic areas. Then, after verifying eligibility criteria, 25 mother-infant dyads per maternity ward were included one or two days after delivery. Eligibility criteria for mothers were the following: age over 18, not institutionalized, able to speak, read or write French or to get help from someone who did. The newborn had to be born at 33 amenorrhea weeks (AW) or later, without severe pathology requiring hospitalization, and had not been transferred to a unit other than the maternity ward in the days following birth. A total of 3368 dyads from 136 maternity wards were included between January and April 2012. Mothers and midwives filled out a questionnaire at the maternity ward, and each mother-infant dyad was then followed up during the child's first year. Thus, mothers were contacted by phone at 1, 4, 8 and 12 months post-partum. The Epifane cohort project was approved by the Committee for Data Processing in Health Research (CCTIRS, registration n°11.335) and the French Data Protection Authority (CNIL, authorization n°911,299).

Prepregnancy body mass index (pBMI)

Our outcome of interest was the pBMI. It was calculated using self-reported height and weight before pregnancy: weight before pregnancy (kg)/height (m^2). The pBMI was grouped into 4 classes according to the WHO classification [21]: underweight (<18.5), normal weight (18.5-24.9), overweight (25.0-29.9) and obesity (≥30.0).

Parity status

At 1 month post-partum, mothers indicated the total number of their biological children, comprising the newborn included in the Epifane cohort. Based on this information, we categorized parity as primiparous women (the women for whom the newborn included in the Epifane cohort was the first child) and multiparous women (the women for whom the newborn included in Epifane was at least the second).

Covariates

We studied the association of the pBMI with a set of different factors, including sociodemographic characteristics, health behaviors, and maternal and neonatal outcomes.

Gestational weight gain during pregnancy (GWG) according to IOM recommendations

GWG was defined as the difference between prepregnancy weight and weight in the last month of pregnancy, declared by mothers. The 2009 Institute of Medicine (IOM) recommendations [22] define adequate GWG based on pBMI as follows: between 12.7 and 18.1 kg for women with prepregnancy underweight; 11.3 and 15.9 kg for women of normal weight; 6.8 and 11.3 kg for those who are overweight; 5.0 and 9.7 kg for women with prepregnancy obesity. In accordance with these recommendations, a three-category variable indicated whether the woman met these recommendations: GWG within IOM recommendations, GWG lower than IOM recommendations and GWG higher than IOM recommendations.

Demographic and socioeconomic factors

Maternal age, maternal country of birth, marital status (married/not married), education level (primary school, junior high school, high school, university) and occupation (farmer/craftswoman/merchant, manager, intermediate occupation, manual worker, unemployed) were collected using a questionnaire completed by the mothers at the maternity ward. We categorized maternal age using classes already used in national [23] and international [3] studies: 18-24 years, 25-29 years, 30-34 years and ≥35 years.

At each phone interview during the child's first year, mothers were asked if they had returned to work. If so, they specified the exact date in days and months. We used a categorical variable: return to work before the infant was 4 months old, between 4 and 6 months old, between 6 and 12 months old, or did not return to work 12 months after child's birth.

Health behaviors during pregnancy

Tobacco consumption (did not smoke before and during pregnancy; smoked before but not during pregnancy, smoked before and during pregnancy), any alcohol consumption during pregnancy (yes/no) and attendance at antenatal classes (yes/no) were also self-reported at the maternity ward.

Maternal, fetal and neonatal outcomes

Maternity midwives collected information on pregnancy and birth conditions from health records. We selected maternal, fetal and neonatal outcomes which had been found to be associated with maternal obesity in the literature [1, 3–5]. Maternal and fetal conditions included maternal hypertensive complications during pregnancy (including hypertension and/or pre-eclampsia during pregnancy), other complications during pregnancy (premature delivery threat, fetal growth restriction, bleeding, preterm rupture of membranes, etc.), congenital defects and mode of delivery. In addition, diagnosis of GDM was declared by the mother and by the midwife at the maternity ward. In case of inconsistent answers between the mother and the midwife, mothers were considered as suffering from GDM when the midwife reported it; or when the mother reported suffering from GDM and subsequently described the medical care received to manage it. French guidelines concerning GDM were updated in 2010, recommending targeted screening of high-risk women, including women with pBMI higher than 25 kg/m^2 [24]. The screening process comprises a fasting blood glucose tolerance test during the first trimester of pregnancy and a 75 g Oral Glucose Tolerance Test (OGTT) between 24 and 28 gestational weeks. Diagnostic criteria for GDM include a fasting blood glucose level ≥ 0.92 g/L (5.1 mmol/L), and/or a 1-h-after-OGTT blood glucose level ≥ 1.80 g/L (10.0 mmol/L) and/or a 2-h-after-OGTT blood glucose level ≥ 1.53 g/L (8.5 mmol/L). Based on the Epifane cohort, however, 15.3% of overweight women and 9.8% of obese women were not screened [25]. Neonatal outcomes included gestational age at birth, sex, birth weight and Apgar score 5 min after birth collected in the health record.

Statistical analyses

In total, 18.6% of questionnaires in our sample (n = 628) had missing values for occupation; "missing information" was retained as a full category. To address missing data on sociodemographic characteristics with a rate of missing data above 5% (maternal country of birth, education, and parity), logistic regression models were performed, including, when appropriate, maternal age, marital status, parity, education, occupation and partner's education. Missing values for tobacco consumption before and during pregnancy (n = 12) were imputed using the mode "no smoking before and during pregnancy." We did not impute missing data concerning pregnancy outcomes (n = 59); thus, only dyads with available information concerning pregnancy and delivery outcomes were included in analyses.

Weights were first calculated so as to take into account inclusion probabilities. To provide statistical estimates representative of the source population, marginal calibration was then performed on maternal age, matrimonial status, level of education (as a binary variable, level of education equal or lower than high school or higher high school graduation) and type of pregnancy (multiple or single). Percentages observed in the French National Perinatal Survey 2010 were used as references, since they had been validated against vital statistics [23]. To take into account the random complex sampling design, the stratification variable and final weights were taken into account in all analyses using the "svyset" command, (Stata° V12.1).

We used multinomial logistic regression to identify factors associated with pBMI, normal weight status (pBMI between 18.5 and 24.9) being the reference class. In bivariate analyses, demographic and socioeconomic factors, health behaviors during pregnancy and maternal, fetal and neonatal outcomes were compared by pBMI category using the adjusted Wald test. Variables associated with pBMI with a p-value < 0.20 were included in the initial multinomial logistic regression model. The final model included covariates selected after using a manual back stepwise procedure, and significantly associated with pBMI with a p-value < 0.05. Nonetheless, a covariate was retained if its removal led to a variation in the odds ratio (OR) above 10%.

In order to assess an effect modification of parity (primiparous/multiparous) with each covariate of the pBMI categories, we performed multinomial logistic regression models, including interaction terms such as "parity * sociodemographic covariate" and "parity * pregnancy or delivery outcome". Interaction p-values in the adjusted model are presented in the Additional file 1: Table S1. Since interactions of parity with maternal age (p-value = 0.02), maternal education (p-value = 0.08), and tobacco consumption (p-value = 0.08) could be considered statistically relevant (p-value < 0.10 [26]), in the final model, we stratified the adjusted multinomial on parity. Analyses were performed using Stata (version 12.1). Odds ratios were estimated with a 95% confidence interval.

We ran a set of sensitivity analyses. First, analyses were carried out in a sample of women with available information concerning parity status (n = 2888). Secondly, in order to address the issue of possible overadjustment in the association between maternal obesity and caesarean section, multivariate models excluding infant birthweight, hypertensive complications and GDM were estimated. Indeed, these factors themselves have been found to be associated with caesarean section [27].

Results

Study sample

Among 3368 mothers included, 3220 completed information on prepregnancy weight and height (Fig. 1). Twelve were excluded from the present analyses because they suffered from pre-existing diabetes (n = 10) or their child had cleft lip and/or palate (n = 2), leading to 3208 dyads included in bivariate analyses. Further, 3149 mothers were included in multivariate analyses due to missing values for some maternal and neonatal outcomes.

Subject characteristics

Most mothers were 25-34 years old, born in France, with university level education (Table 1). About half were first-time mothers. Before pregnancy, 7.6% were underweight (n = 240), 64.2% of normal weight (n = 2067), 18.0% overweight (n = 583) and 10.2% had obesity (n = 318). Medians of pBMI and interquartiles ranges in each pBMI class defined by the WHO classification are presented for primiparous and for multiparous women in Fig. 2. Thirty-seven percent of women gained more weight during pregnancy than IOM recommendations (Table 2). Slightly less than 80% of women delivered vaginally. Approximately 90% gave birth to newborns weighing between 2.5 kg and 4 kg. Gestational diabetes occurred in 7.7% of women and hypertensive complications in 3.5% (Table 2).

Except for alcohol consumption, all demographic, socioeconomic and health behavior characteristics were associated with pBMI categories in bivariate analyses, with a p-value under 0.20 (Table 1). In addition, GWG, GDM, hypertensive complications, delivery mode and birth weight were associated with pBMI category with a p-value under 0.20 (Table 2). In preliminary multivariate analyses, maternal age and birthplace, parity, education level, occupation, tobacco status, attendance at antenatal classes, GWG, GDM, hypertensive complications, mode of delivery and birth weight were significantly associated (p-value < 0.05) with pBMI class (Data not shown). Since we found a statistically significant interaction (p-value < 0.10) between parity and maternal age (p-value = 0.02), parity and maternal education (p-value = 0.08), and parity and tobacco consumption (p-value = 0.08) we present here only the adjusted model stratified on parity (Tables 3 and 4).

Sociodemographic factors associated with maternal obesity

Among the primiparous, women aged 25-29, when compared to those aged 30-34, were more likely to have obesity before pregnancy than to be of normal weight (p-value < 0.05). Those with a high school level were more likely to have obesity than to be of normal weight before pregnancy, compared to women with a university level.

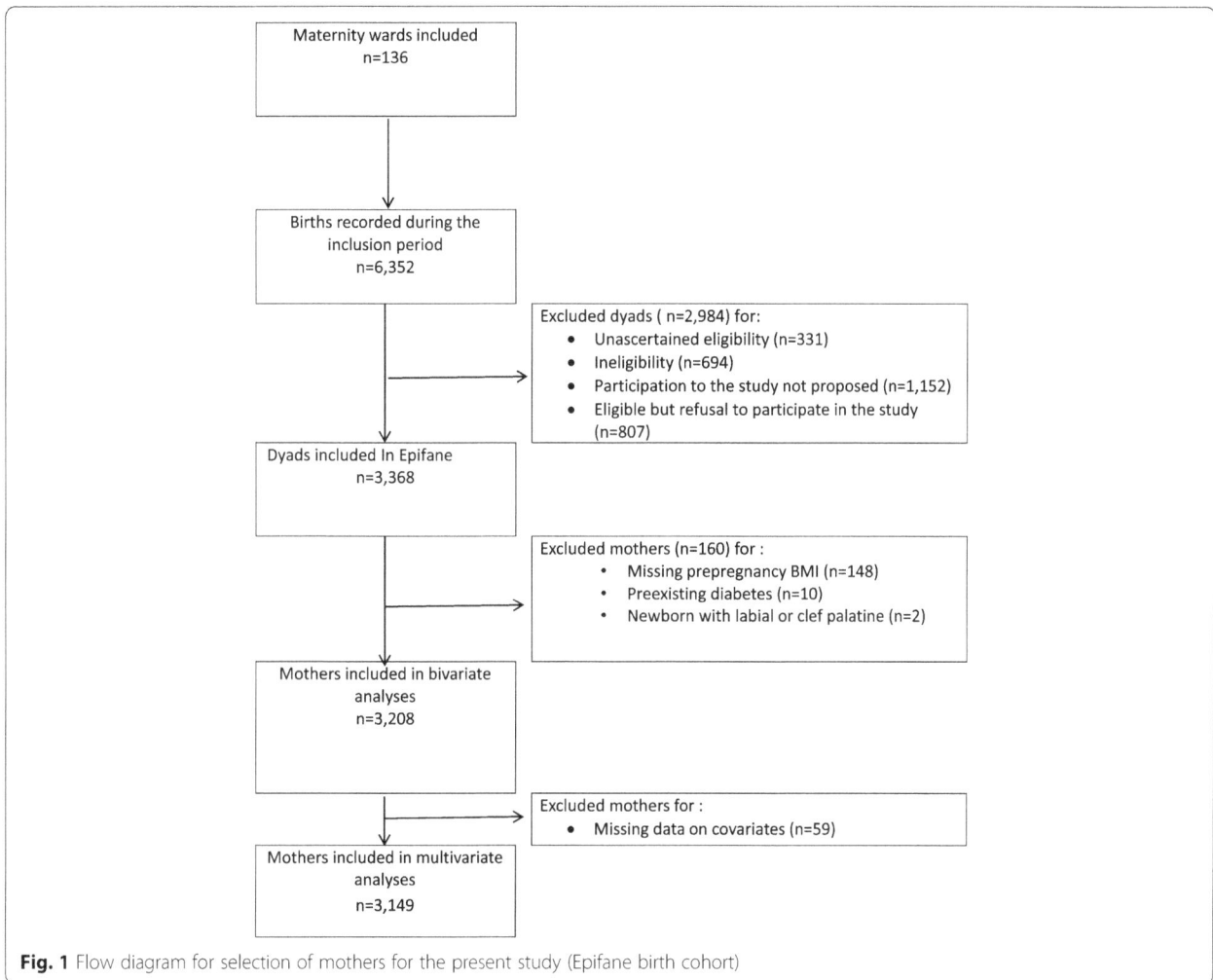

Fig. 1 Flow diagram for selection of mothers for the present study (Epifane birth cohort)

Among the multiparous, women with a primary, junior high or high school level were more likely to have obesity than to be of normal weight before pregnancy compared to women with a university level (p-value < 0.05). Women who did not attend antenatal classes during pregnancy were more likely to have obesity before pregnancy than to be of normal weight.

Maternal and fetal outcomes associated with maternal obesity

Among the primiparous, obesity before pregnancy, compared to a normal weight before pregnancy, was positively associated with GDM and hypertensive complications during pregnancy (p-value < 0.05). Among the multiparous, the odds of GDM, hypertensive complications, excessive GWG (vs GWG within IOM recommendations), caesarean section (vs. vaginal delivery) and infant birth weight ≥ 4 kg (vs. infant birth weight comprised between 2.5 and 4 kg) were higher for women with a pBMI ≥ 30.0 kg/m^2 before pregnancy than for those with a pBMI comprised between 18.5 and 24.9 kg/m^2 (p-value < 0.05).

As part of multinomial logistic regression, results for underweight and overweight women are also presented in Tables 3 (sociodemographic factors) and 4 (pregnancy outcomes).

Sensitivity analyses

In the sample with non-imputed information concerning parity status, the same results were found (Additional file 2: Table S2 and Additional file 3: Table S3), excepting: (1) among the multiparous (n = 1648), the association was no longer statistically significant (p-value > 0.05) for birth weight ≥ 4 kg (OR = 1.67 [0.99-2.81], vs. 2.5 kg – 4.0 kg) (Additional file 3: Table S3); (2) among the primiparous (n = 1240), maternal age above 35 became significantly associated (p-value < 0.05) with prepregnancy obesity (OR = 2.27 [1.03-5.00], vs. 30-34 years) (Additional file 2: Table S2).

After removing covariates, infant birth weight, hypertensive complications and GDM, maternal obesity was still significantly associated (p-value < 0.05) with caesarian section (OR = 1.64 [1.09-2.46]) among multiparous

Table 1 Maternal sociodemographic characteristics and health behavior, overall and across-prepregnancy body mass index classes ($n = 3208$)

| | All | Prepregnancy BMI | | | | p-value[a] |
| | | Underweight | Normal weight | Overweight | Obesity | |
	$n = 3208$	$n = 240$	$n = 2067$	$n = 583$	$n = 318$	
%						
Maternal age (years) ($n = 3208$)						
18-24	17.0	28.6	15.9	16.2	16.9	$<10^{-3}$
25-29	32.9	34.2	32.1	34.2	34.5	
30-34	31.1	26.6	33.0	30.8	22.9	
≥ 35	19.0	10.7	19.0	18.8	25.7	
Maternal country of birth ($n = 3208$)						
France (mainland and overseas)	83.8	83.3	84.9	82.7	79.1	0.03
Africa	8.7	5.0	7.9	11.8	11.4	
Europa, Asia, America, Oceania	7.5	11.7	7.2	5.5	9.5	
Parity ($n = 3208$)						
1 child	43.3	48.1	45.4	37.3	37.3	$<10^{-3}$
2 children or more	56.7	51.9	54.6	62.7	62.7	
Marital status ($n = 3208$)						
Married	47.7	42.0	47.0	51.7	49.7	0.08
Unmarried	52.3	58.0	53.0	48.3	50.3	
Maternal education ($n = 3208$)						
Primary school	2.4	5.4	1.2	4.0	5.1	$<10^{-3}$
Junior high school	20.7	22.6	18.5	21.8	30.7	
High school	23.6	21.2	22.5	25.7	29.5	
University	53.3	50.8	57.8	48.5	34.7	
Maternal occupation ($n = 3208$)						
Farmer, craftswoman, merchant	2.1	2.2	2.5	0.8	2.4	$<10^{-3}$
Management profession	15.6	13.0	18.5	10.6	8.2	
Intermediate profession	47.1	44.9	46.6	51.4	43.2	
Manual worker	7.3	6.8	7.0	6.4	10.9	
Unemployed	6.8	4.0	5.8	9.8	10.1	
Missing	21.1	29.1	19.5	21.0	25.2	
Time of return to work[b] ($n = 3208$)						
<= 4 months	34.4	32.5	37.1	29.9	27.5	$<10^{-3}$
]4 months-6 months]	12.5	14.4	13.2	10.0	11.3	
]6 months-12 months]	24.4	26.9	23.9	27.1	20.9	
Did not go back at 12 months	28.7	26.2	25.9	32.9	40.3	
Smoking before/during pregnancy ($n = 3208$)						
No smoking before or during	67.6	62.0	66.8	70.4	71.3	0.07
Smoking before but not during	15.7	14.8	16.7	13.5	14.1	
Smoking before and during	16.7	23.2	16.5	16.1	14.7	
Alcohol during pregnancy ($n = 3198$)						
No consumption	93.9	94.9	93.6	94.1	93.9	0.87
Consumption	6.1	5.1	6.4	5.9	6.1	
Antenatal classes ($n = 3205$)						
Attended	53.2	51.2	56.8	48.8	39.0	$<10^{-3}$
Not attended	46.8	48.8	43.2	51.2	61.0	

[a]Adjusted Wald test P-value for comparisons across pBMI classes
[b]Defined as time when the mother returned to work after birth

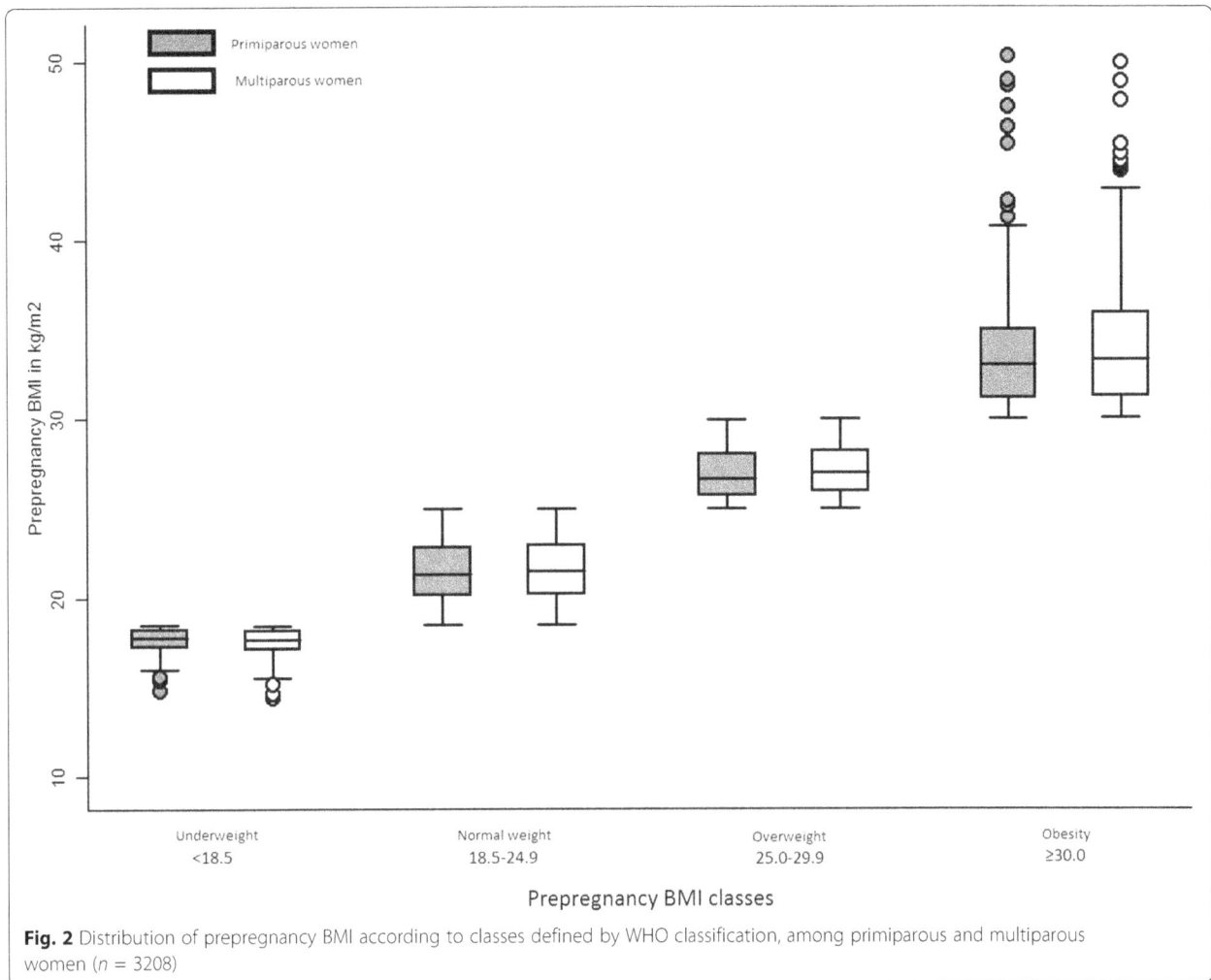

Fig. 2 Distribution of prepregnancy BMI according to classes defined by WHO classification, among primiparous and multiparous women (*n* = 3208)

women. Among primiparous women, maternal obesity was then significantly associated (*p*-value < 0.05) with caesarian section (OR = 1.69 [1.03-2.77]).

Discussion

Our study identifies an extensive range of sociodemographic characteristics, health behaviors and maternal and neonatal outcomes independently associated with maternal obesity before pregnancy. Parity modulated the relationship between pBMI categories and numerous characteristics. Among primiparous women, maternal obesity was associated with a maternal age of 25-29 years, a high school education, and with GDM and hypertensive complications during pregnancy. Among the multiparous, maternal obesity was associated with primary, junior high and high school levels, and absence of attendance at antenatal classes. In this group, obesity before pregnancy was also associated with GDM, hypertensive complications, excess weight gain during pregnancy, caesarean section and infant birth weight ≥ 4 kg.

In our study, 10.2% of mothers had obesity before pregnancy. This prevalence is very close to the 9.9% prevalence observed in the French National Perinatal survey performed in 2010 [23]. The French National Perinatal survey was a nationwide survey that collected information on births after 22 weeks of amenorrhea, and also used self-reported prepregnancy weight and height several days after delivery [23]. However, the two studies, the French National Perinatal survey and the Epifane cohort, potentially underestimated the prevalence of obesity among French childbearing women. Indeed, several studies performed at the beginning of pregnancy [28, 29] showed that women who were overweight or with obesity before pregnancy tended to underestimate their weight. In addition, in Epifane, only dyads with a live infant born after 33 weeks were included. Since maternal obesity has been shown to be associated with greater risk of miscarriage [30] and premature delivery [31], obesity before pregnancy may have been underrepresented in Epifane. Compared to other studies performed in Western countries using self-reported anthropometric

Table 2 Maternal and neonatal outcomes, overall and across-prepregnancy body mass index (n = 3208)

		Prepregnancy BMI				
	All	Underweight	Normal weight	Overweight	Obesity	p-value[a]
	n = 3208	n = 240	n = 2067	n = 583	n = 318	
%						
Type of pregnancy (n = 3208)						
Multiple	1.3	0.9	1.3	1.5	1.6	0.86
Single	98.7	99.1	98.7	98.5	98.4	
Mean of GWG (in kg) (n = 3162)						
	13.2	14.5	13.9	12.6	8.7	$<10^{-3}$
Gestational weight gain (n = 3162)[b]						
Within IOM	35.5	48.8	36.5	29.5	29.0	$<10^{-3}$
Below IOM	27.5	35.5	31.5	12.1	23.5	
Above IOM	37.0	15.7	32.0	58.3	47.5	
Gestational diabetes mellitus (n = 3204)						
No	92.3	98.6	94.4	88.8	80.7	$<10^{-3}$
Yes	7.7	1.4	5.6	11.2	19.3	
Hypertensive complications[c] (n = 3204)						
No	96.5	98.4	97.6	96.8	87.4	$<10^{-3}$
Yes	3.5	1.6	2.4	3.2	12.6	
Delivery mode (n = 3200)						
Vaginal	81.4	89.6	82.9	77.5	73.2	$<10^{-3}$
Cesarean	18.6	10.4	17.1	22.5	26.8	
Gestational age at birth (n = 3183)						
≥ 37 amenorrhea weeks	96.4	94.3	96.5	96.8	96.3	0.50
33-36 amenorrhea weeks	3.6	5.7	3.5	3.2	3.7	
Infant's sex (n = 3200)						
Male	49.4	48.6	49.6	49.6	47.8	0.95
Female	50.6	51.4	50.4	50.4	52.2	
Infant's birth weight (n = 3202)						
[2.5 kg-4 kg[	89.0	85.7	89.8	89.1	86.4	$<10^{-3}$
≥4 kg	7.4	3.8	6.8	8.8	11.1	
<2.5 kg	3.6	10.5	3.4	2.2	2.6	
Apgar score at 5 min (n = 3181)						
10	94.7	96.5	95.2	93.2	93.6	0.40
8-9	4.6	3.1	4.4	5.9	4.8	
≤7	0.7	0.3	0.4	1.0	1.6	

[a]Adjusted Wald test P value for comparisons across pBMI classes
[b]Gestational weight gain in agreement with recommendations defined in 2009 by the IOM
[c]Hypertensive complications including hypertension and/or preeclampsia during pregnancy

measures, the rate of obesity before pregnancy was close to that reported in Norway (8.8%) [32], but much lower than that reported in the US (24%) [33] or Australia (20%) [34].

For first-time mothers, we showed that a maternal age of 25-29 years compared to 30-34-year-old women was associated with obesity before pregnancy. A possible explanation would be that age at first birth might also reflect socioeconomic status. In Epifane, among primiparous women, 52.9% of women aged 25-29 had a university education, while this was the case for 65.5% of 30-34-year-old women. A positive association between maternal education and maternal age at first birth has been previously reported [35]. In addition, in Epifane, 12.3% of primiparous 25-29-year-old women held managerial positions, compared to 21.6% of 30-34–year-old

Table 3 Association of sociodemographic factors with prepregnancy BMI category (multinomial regression model stratified on parity) (n = 3149)

	Primiparous (n = 1335)						Multiparous (n = 1814)					
	Underweight		Overweight		Obesity		Underweight		Overweight		Obesity	
	n = 107		n = 214		n = 114		n = 130		n = 357		n = 197	
	OR	[95% CI]	OR	[95% CI]	OR	[95% CI]	OR	[95% CI]	OR	[95% CI]	OR	[95% CI]
Maternal age (years)												
18-24	2.07	[0.97-4.39]	0.80	[0.48-1.32]	1.27	[0.57-2.85]	3.03	[1.57-5.87]	0.73	[0.39-1.37]	0.98	[0.49-1.97]
25-29	1.55	[0.85-2.82]	0.69	[0.46-1.04]	2.09	[1.13-3.87]	1.28	[0.80-2.05]	1.39	[1.01-1.93]	1.11	[0.72-1.72]
30-34	1		1		1		1		1		1	
≥ 35	0.84	[0.30-2.35]	0.70	[0.37-1.33]	2.01	[0.94-4.28]	0.74	[0.42-1.32]	1.04	[0.73-1.48]	1.45	[0.93-2.25]
Maternal country of birth												
France (mainland and overseas)	1		1		1		1		1		1	
Maghreb and Sub-Saharan Africa	1.09	[0.34-3.49]	0.99	[0.37-2.67]	0.81	[0.25-2.61]	0.54	[0.17-1.67]	1.31	[0.78-2.20]	0.77	[0.43-1.38]
Europe, Asia, America, Oceania	3.16	[1.52-6.54]	0.75	[0.34-1.67]	0.78	[0.22-2.79]	1.21	[0.50-2.89]	0.49	[0.22-1.09]	1.64	[0.79-3.41]
Maternal education												
Primary school	3.73	[1.10-12.68]	1.77	[0.53-5.91]	0.69	[0.09-5.38]	3.21	[1.01-10.17]	4.59	[1.89-11.16]	6.30	[2.40-16.57]
Junior high school	1.42	[0.74-2.72]	0.96	[0.56-1.62]	1.59	[0.83-3.07]	0.54	[0.29-1.00]	1.42	[0.96-2.10]	2.89	[1.81-4.64]
High school	0.93	[0.49-1.78]	1.52	[1.01-2.29]	2.22	[1.33-3.73]	0.79	[0.46-1.35]	0.98	[0.68-1.41]	1.86	[1.18-2.93]
University	1		1		1		1		1		1	
Maternal occupation												
Farmer, craftswoman, merchant, entrepreneur	0.92	[0.25-3.39]	0.31	[0.08-1.14]	1.15	[0.26-5.04]	0.83	[0.22-3.14]	0.25	[0.08-0.75]	0.71	[0.17-2.86]
Management profession	0.97	[0.50-1.87]	0.61	[0.37-1.00]	1.12	[0.51-2.49]	0.64	[0.35-1.19]	0.67	[0.42-1.06]	0.47	[0.22-1.05]
Intermediate profession	1		1		1		1		1		1	
Manual worker	0.78	[0.27-2.23]	0.49	[0.21-1.14]	0.84	[0.34-2.05]	0.97	[0.46-2.04]	0.71	[0.41-1.20]	1.42	[0.83-2.45]
Unemployed	0.55	[0.18-1.76]	1.82	[0.84-3.93]	1.85	[0.75-4.57]	0.30	[0.08-1.08]	1.29	[0.70-2.39]	1.48	[0.76-2.88]
Missing	1.36	[0.74-2.51]	0.67	[0.40-1.13]	1.57	[0.92-2.69]	1.39	[0.84-2.30]	0.94	[0.67-1.33]	0.96	[0.62-1.50]
Smoking before/during pregnancy pregnancy)												
No smoking before or during	1		1		1		1		1		1	
Smoking before, but not during	0.92	[0.51-1.66]	0.91	[0.60-1.38]	0.77	[0.42-1.42]	0.99	[0.55-1.80]	0.47	[0.30-0.73]	0.61	[0.36-1.05]
Smoking before and during	1.24	[0.67-2.27]	0.50	[0.31-0.79]	0.56	[0.30-1.05]	1.27	[0.74-2.16]	0.99	[0.68-1.43]	0.65	[0.40-1.05]
Antenatal classes												
Attended	1		1		1		1		1		1	
Not attended	1.25	[0.70-2.22]	1.30	[0.83-2.03]	1.36	[0.80-2.31]	0.99	[0.65-4.52]	1.02	[0.76-1.38]	1.77	[1.16-2.72]

The model was also adjusted for gestational weight gain, gestational diabetes mellitus, hypertensive complications, delivery mode and infant's birth weight (see Table 4)

primiparous women. We have adjusted analyses on such characteristics; however maternal education and occupation at birth might be insufficient to entirely capture the effect of socioeconomic status. Thus, unmeasured confounders and residual confounding cannot be ruled out, especially regarding women's living conditions over life [36].

A low maternal education level was a risk factor of obesity before pregnancy, in accordance with previous studies [5, 37]. This result is also consistent with a study performed in the general French population, in which a low education level was associated with increased risk of obesity among adult women [38]. Women who are better educated and grow up under more favorable socioeconomic conditions may have had better nutritional knowledge and developed healthier behavior during child- and adulthood. Furthermore, mothers with a low education level may also be more likely to live in disadvantaged areas, shown in North America to be more obesogenic environments than affluent neighborhoods [39].

Parity also had an effect on the relationship between maternal obesity and attendance at antenatal classes. In Epifane, 76.2% of primiparous women and 35.9% of

Table 4 Association of maternal and neonatal outcome with prepregnancy BMI category (multinomial regression model stratified on parity) (n = 3149)

	Primiparous (n = 1335)						Multiparous (n = 1814)					
	Underweight		Overweight		Obesity		Underweight		Overweight		Obesity	
	n = 107		n = 214		n = 114		n = 130		n = 357		n = 197	
	OR	[95% CI]	OR	[95% CI]	OR	[95% CI]	OR	[95% CI]	OR	[95% CI]	OR	[95% CI]
Gestational weight gain												
Within IOM	1		1		1		1		1		1	
Below IOM	0.70	[0.42-1.16]	0.47	[0.26-0.85]	0.81	[0.44-1.50]	0.97	[0.63-1.51]	0.39	[0.26-0.60]	0.84	[0.53-1.32]
Above IOM	0.20	[0.10-0.38]	2.87	[1.93-4.26]	1.39	[0.82-2.37]	0.64	[0.37-1.10]	2.27	[1.68-3.06]	1.82	[1.20-2.76]
Gestational diabetes mellitus												
No	1		1		1		1		1		1	
Yes	0.27	[0.06-1.26]	1.51	[0.80-2.87]	2.80	[1.56-5.01]	0.27	[0.06-1.15]	3.43	[2.17-5.43]	5.16	[3.15-8.46]
Hypertensive complications												
No	1		1		1		1		1		1	
Yes	0.74	[0.16-3.37]	1.46	[0.62-3.43]	3.80	[1.83-7.89]	0.51	[0.06-4.14]	0.72	[0.28-1.88]	8.13	[3.97-16.64]
Delivery mode												
Vaginal	1		1		1		1		1		1	
Caesarean	0.77	[0.43-1.37]	1.38	[0.92-2.07]	1.33	[0.80-2.23]	0.39	[0.19-0.81]	1.28	[0.90-1.82]	1.80	[1.18-2.77]
Infant's birth weight												
[2.5 kg-4 kg[	1		1		1		1		1		1	
≥ 4 kg	0.43	[0.06-2.94]	1.40	[0.70-2.77]	1.18	[0.36-3.86]	0.84	[0.38-1.87]	0.80	[0.52-1.22]	1.70	[1.03-2.80]
< 2.5 kg	2.47	[1.14-5.33]	1.03	[0.37-2.90]	0.83	[0.28-2.47]	4.93	[2.36-10.32]	0.48	[0.16-1.41]	0.56	[0.14-2.18]

The model was also adjusted for maternal age, maternal country of birth, education, occupation, smoking before and during pregnancy and antenatal class attendance (see Table 3)

multiparous women attended antenatal classes. In France, seven antenatal classes are reimbursed by health insurance, in order to "contribute to the improvement of women, expectant mothers and newborn health" and to "encourage active involvement of the woman and the couple in their birth plan" [40]. Such classes provide comprehensive information on female physiology, conditions of delivery (position and gestures), and essential care during the infant's first months (feeding, sleeping…), and proposed several approaches: obstetric psychoprophylaxis, yoga, aquatic gym, sophrology and so on. However, as in other countries [41, 42], participation in antenatal education has been shown to be closely related to socioeconomic status in France [43]. Single women [41], born in foreign countries [41, 42], with a low education level or occupational status [43] are less likely to participate in antenatal classes. However, after adjusting for sociodemographic factors, maternal obesity was still significantly associated with antenatal classes among multiparous women, suggesting another underlying mechanism. It was previously shown that obese women were more likely to have a negative perception of their bodies [44]. We may assume that obese multiparous women might have experienced uncomfortable feelings when attending such classes in a previous

pregnancy, and subsequently decided to avoid them. Furthermore, we hypothesize that obese multiparous women may have suffered from complications such as the threat of premature delivery or fetal growth restrictions that were not addressed in our study, and felt these classes were less appropriate to their situation.

In studies performed among Danish [45] and American [46] women, mean weight gain during pregnancy was higher in primiparous than in multiparous women; in both strata of parity, women with higher BMI gained less on an average during their pregnancy than other pBMI groups. Due to the period during which these two cohorts were carried out (1996-2002 and 2005-2007, respectively), authors did not use 2009 IOM recommendations for GWG. These recommendations were updated in 2009, taking into account pBMI, and were aimed at decreasing the risk of post-partum weight retention, preterm birth, non-elective caesarean, GDM and pre-eclampsia [22]. In our study, primiparous gained more weight than multiparous (data not shown), and the average weight gain during pregnancy was the lowest in the highest pBMI categories. Nevertheless, although women with obesity before pregnancy gained less weight during their pregnancy than normal-weight women, they more often exceeded 2009 IOM recommendations, probably due to the lower threshold for meeting these guidelines when pBMI is high. We suggest that obese women who were less well educated confronted living conditions in which implementation of a healthy diet and regular physical activity is a challenge. Surprisingly, despite the same rate of obese women exceeding IOM recommendations among primiparous and multiparous women (47.5%), maternal obesity was associated with excessive GWG according to IOM recommendations only among multiparous women. This might be explained by the GWG in normal-weight women, which differs between primiparous and multiparous women. Indeed, 35.2% of normal-weight women exceeded IOM recommendations among primiparous women, while this was the case for 29.3% of normal weight women among the multiparous.

Maternal obesity before pregnancy was associated with infant birth weight ≥ 4 kg, but this association was statistically significant only among multiparous women. Both maternal obesity before pregnancy [4] and multiparity [3] are considered independent risk factors for infant birth weight above 4 kg. In the Epifane cohort, only newborns not transferred to another unit in the days following birth were included. A birth weight above 4,0-4,5 kg has been shown to be associated with increased risk of adverse perinatal issues, such as shoulder dystocia and perinatal asphyxia [47], requiring transfer to a neonatal intensive care unit. Thus, we probably underestimated the proportion of macrosomia in Epifane, as well as the association between maternal obesity and macrosomia.

Maternal obesity was also associated with caesarean delivery; however, this association was statistically significant only among multiparous women in the final model including infant birth weight, hypertensive complications and GDM. After removing these covariates in the sensitivity analyses, maternal obesity was also significantly associated with caesarean section among primiparous women. This suggests that they may be intermediate factors in the association of maternal obesity with caesarean section among primiparous women. We were unable to distinguish pre-labor caesarean section from emergency section, but a recent French study found an increased risk of pre-labor caesarean delivery for women with obesity only among the multiparous [48]. As those authors pointed out, this might be related to reluctance by the obstetrician to attempt vaginal delivery in women with obesity, in particular, multiparous women with previous caesarean section, for whom the rate of successful vaginal delivery is lower than for normal-weight women [49].

Consistent with other studies [3–5], obesity before pregnancy was associated with GDM and hypertensive complications in both primiparous and multiparous women. A meta-analysis performed in 2007 found that women with obesity had an unadjusted OR of 3.56 [3.05-4.21] for developing GDM compared to women of normal weight [50]. Many factors are involved in the relationship of maternal obesity with hypertensive complications and pre-eclampsia, such as insulin resistance, genetic factors, immunologic and infectious processes, but also lifestyle factors [51].

Limits and strengths of our study should be mentioned. First, based on the interaction test results, we stratified analyses on parity, thus sustaining its effect modification. However, this may have led to a decrease in statistical power. In order to limit the decrease in statistical power and bias selection due to non-random missing values, we imputed parity status. Sensitivity analyses without imputation showed only a few differences in results. Secondly, prepregnancy weight and height were collected at delivery, leading to an unmeasured level of recall bias. As previously mentioned, the fact that the mothers self-reported their prepregnancy weight and height may have led to misclassification, with risk of underestimating some associations. Nevertheless, it is difficult to correctly measure prepregnancy weight at a reasonable period before pregnancy. Weight at the first prenatal appointment (often occurring at the end of the first trimester of pregnancy in France) may reflect gestational weight gain at the beginning of pregnancy, which varies among women. The strength of our study lays in our sample analysis from a recent nation-wide birth cohort. In addition, we disposed of an extensive set of sociodemographic factors and high-quality data concerning outcomes, collected by midwives from health records.

Conclusions

France has been confronted with an increase in prepregnancy body mass index since the seventies [52]; thus, identification of sociodemographic risk factors in maternal obesity is useful for implementing specific preventive action. Our study helps identify sociodemographic factors and health behavior related to prepregnancy obesity among primiparous and multiparous women. We have also highlighted an effect modification of parity in the association of prepregnancy obesity with maternal and neonatal outcomes, with higher risk in multiparous women. It has been shown that increased body mass index between the first and second pregnancy is associated with higher risk of maternal issues during the second pregnancy [53] and higher risk of stillbirth and infant mortality for the second newborn [54]. Our study design did not enable us to assess weight gain between the first and second pregnancy; longitudinal cohorts performed during a longer period will be useful for assessing changes in body mass index between the first and subsequent pregnancies. Identifying sociodemographic subgroups at risk of maternal obesity will enable targeting intervention aimed at reducing prepregnancy weight and maintaining healthy BMI between pregnancies. Maternal obesity is linked not only to lifestyle habits such as dietary intake and physical activity, but also to the social and physical environment. Development of effective actions, along with organization of pre- and postnatal care for primiparous and multiparous women with obesity, must take these factors into consideration.

Additional files

Additional file 1: Table S1. Interactions between parity and covariates in their association with maternal pre-pregnancy BMI.

Additional file 2: Table S2. Sensitivity analyses estimating the association of sociodemographic factors with prepregnancy BMI category in the sample with non-imputed information concerning parity status: multinomial regression model stratified by parity ($n = 2888$).

Additional file 3: Table S3. Sensitivity analyses estimating the association of maternal and neonatal outcome with prepregnancy BMI category in the sample with non-imputed information concerning parity status: multinomial regression model stratified on parity ($n = 2888$).

Acknowledgments
The authors are grateful to the midwives who contributed to data collection in the maternity wards and to parents who participated in the survey. They are also grateful to Catherine de Launay and Caroline Guerrisi, who contributed to data monitoring and descriptive analyses, and to Jerri Bram, who edited the manuscript.

Funding
This survey was funded by the French Public Health Agency (Agence nationale de santé publique) and Paris-13 University. Julie Boudet-Berquier is the recipient of a doctoral grant from the Ministère de l'Enseignement Supérieur et de la Recherche, Paris, France and the Ecole des Hautes Etudes en Santé Publique (EHESP, Rennes, France).

Authors' contributions
KC and BS designed and conducted the research. JBB analyzed data and wrote the initial manuscript. KC, BS and JCD critically reviewed the manuscript. JBB had primary responsibility for final content. All authors read and approved the final manuscript.

Competing interests
The authors have no conflicts of interest to disclose. The authors have no financial relationships to disclose relevant to this article.

Author details
[1]Nutritional Surveillance and Epidemiology Team (ESEN), French Public Health Agency, Paris-13 University, Centre de Recherche en Epidémiologie et Statistiques, COMUE Sorbonne Paris Cité, SMBH Building, 1st floor, door 136, 74 rue Marcel Cachin, 93017 Bobigny Cedex, France. [2]French Public Health Agency (Agence nationale de Santé publique), Saint Maurice, France. [3]Centre de Recherche « Epidémiologie, Biostatistique et Recherche clinique », School of Public Health, Université libre de Bruxelles (ULB), Brussels, Belgium.

References
1. Poston L, Caleyachetty R, Cnattingius S, Corvalán C, Uauy R, Herring S, et al. Preconceptional and maternal obesity: epidemiology and health consequences. Lancet Diabetes Endocrinol. 2016;4(12):1025–36.
2. Black RE, Victora CG, Walker SP, Bhutta ZA, Christian P, de Onis M, et al. Maternal and child undernutrition and overweight in low-income and middle-income countries. Lancet. 2013;382(9890):427–51.
3. Nohr EA, Vaeth M, Baker JL, Sørensen TI, Olsen J, Rasmussen KM. Combined associations of prepregnancy body mass index and gestational weight gain with the outcome of pregnancy. Am J Clin Nutr. 2008;87(6):1750–9.
4. Heude B, Thiébaugeorges O, Goua V, Forhan A, Kaminski M, Foliguet B, et al. Pre-pregnancy body mass index and weight gain during pregnancy: relations with gestational diabetes and hypertension, and birth outcomes. Matern Child Health J. 2012;16(2):355–63.
5. Gaillard R, Durmuş B, Hofman A, Mackenbach JP, Steegers EAP, Jaddoe VWV. Risk factors and outcomes of maternal obesity and excessive weight gain during pregnancy. Obesity (Silver Spring). 2013;21(5):1046–55.
6. Roman H, Goffinet F, Hulsey TF, Newman R, Robillard PY, Hulsey TC. Maternal body mass index at delivery and risk of caesarean due to dystocia in low risk pregnancies. Acta Obstet Gynecol Scand. 2008;87(2):163–70.
7. Grundy SM. Obesity, metabolic syndrome, and cardiovascular disease. J Clin Endocrinol Metab. 2004 Jun;89(6):2595–600.
8. Correa A, Marcinkevage J. Prepregnancy obesity and the risk of birth defects: an update. Nutr Rev. 2013;71(Suppl 1):S68–77.
9. Bodnar LM, Siminerio LL, Himes KP, Hutcheon JA, Lash TL, Parisi SM, et al. Maternal obesity and gestational weight gain are risk factors for infant death: pregnancy weight gain, obesity, and infant death. Obesity (Silver Spring). 2016;24(2):490–8.
10. Reynolds RM, Osmond C, Phillips DIW, Godfrey KM. Maternal BMI, parity, and pregnancy weight gain: influences on offspring adiposity in young adulthood. J Clin Endocrinol Metab. 2010;95(12):5365–9.
11. Reynolds RM, Allan KM, Raja EA, Bhattacharya S, McNeill G, Hannaford PC, et al. Maternal obesity during pregnancy and premature mortality from cardiovascular event in adult offspring: follow-up of 1 323 275 person years. BMJ. 2013;347:f4539.
12. Kim SY, Dietz PM, England L, Morrow B, Callaghan WM. Trends in pre-pregnancy obesity in nine states, 1993-2003. Obesity (Silver Spring). 2007;15(4):986–93.
13. Heslehurst N, Rankin J, Wilkinson JR, Summerbell CD. A nationally representative study of maternal obesity in England, UK: trends in incidence and demographic inequalities in 619 323 births, 1989-2007. Int J Obes(Lond). 2010;34(3):420–8.
14. Heslehurst N, Ells L, Simpson H, Batterham A, Wilkinson J, Summerbell C. Trends in maternal obesity incidence rates, demographic predictors, and health inequalities in 36 821 women over a 15-year period. BJOG. 2007;114(2):187–94.
15. Gunderson EP. Childbearing and obesity in women: weight before, during, and after pregnancy. Obstet Gynecol Clin N Am. 2009;36(2):317–32.
16. Davis EM, Babineau DC, Wang X, Zyzanski S, Abrams B, Bodnar LM, et al. Short inter-pregnancy intervals, parity, excessive pregnancy weight gain and risk of maternal obesity. Matern Child Health J. 2014;18(3):554–62.
17. We J-S, Han K, Kwon H-S, Kil K. Effect of maternal age at childbirth on obesity in postmenopausal women: a Nationwide population-based study in Korea. Medicine (Baltimore). 2016;95(19):e3584.
18. Gunderson EP, Murtaugh MA, Lewis CE, Quesenberry CP, West DS, Sidney S. Excess gains in weight and waist circumference associated with childbearing: the coronary artery risk development in young adults study (CARDIA). Int J Obes. 2004;28(4):525–35.
19. Cnattingius S, Bergström R, Lipworth L, Kramer MS. Prepregnancy weight and the risk of adverse pregnancy outcomes. N Engl J Med. 1998;338(3):147–52.
20. Boudet-Berquier J, Salanave B, De Launay C, Castetbon K. Introduction of complementary foods with respect to French guidelines:description and associated socio economic factors in a nation-wide birth cohort (Epifane survey). Matern Child Nutr. 2016; doi:10.1111/mcn.12339. [Epub ahead of print]
21. World Health Organization. Obesity: preventing and managing the global epidemic. Report of a WHO consultation. World Health Organ Tech Rep Ser. 2000;894:i–xii. 1-253
22. IOM (Institute of Medicine) and NRC (National Research Council). Weight

Gain During Pregnancy: Reexamining the Guidelines. Washington, DC: The National Academies Press; 2009.

23. Blondel B, Lelong N, Kermarrec M, Goffinet F. National Coordination Group of the National Perinatal Surveys. Trends in perinatal health in France from 1995 to 2010. Results from the French National Perinatal Surveys. J Gynecol Obstet Biol Reprod(Paris). 2012;41(4):e1–15.

24. Senat M-V, Deruelle P. Gestational diabetes mellitus. Gynecol Obstet Fertil. 2016;44(4):244–7.

25. Regnault N, Salanave B, Castetbon K, Cosson E, Vambergue A, Barry Y. Gestational diabetes in France in 2012: screening, prevalence, and treatment modalities during pregnancy. Bull Epidemiol Hebd. 2016;9:164–73. Available from: http://www.invs.sante.fr/beh/2016/9/2016_9_2.html.

26. Selvin S. Statistical analysis of epidemiologic data. 3rd ed. New York: Oxford University Press; 2004.

27. Yang X, Hsu-Hage B, Zhang H, Zhang C, Zhang Y, Zhang C. Women with impaired glucose tolerance during pregnancy have significantly poor pregnancy outcomes. Diabetes Care. 2002;25(9):1619–24.

28. Yu SM, Nagey DA. Validity of self-reported pregravid weight. Ann Epidemiol. 1992;2(5):715–21.

29. Holland E, Moore Simas TA, Doyle Curiale DK, Liao X, Waring ME. Self-reported pre-pregnancy weight versus weight measured at first prenatal visit: effects on categorization of pre-pregnancy body mass index. Matern Child Health J. 2013;17(10):1872–8.

30. Talmor A, Dunphy B. Female obesity and infertility. Best Pract Res Clin Obstet Gynaecol. 2015;29(4):498–506.

31. Marchi J, Berg M, Dencker A, Olander EK, Begley C. Risks associated with obesity in pregnancy, for the mother and baby: a systematic review of reviews. Obes Rev. 2015;16(8):621–38.

32. Haugen M, Brantsæter AL, Winkvist A, Lissner L, Alexander J, Oftedal B, et al. Associations of pre-pregnancy body mass index and gestational weight gain with pregnancy outcome and postpartum weight retention: a prospective observational cohort study. BMC Pregnancy Childbirth. 2014;14:201.

33. Hauff LE, Leonard SA, Rasmussen KM. Associations of maternal obesity and psychosocial factors with breastfeeding intention, initiation, and duration. Am J Clin Nutr. 2014;99(3):524–34.

34. Donath SM, Amir LH. Maternal obesity and initiation and duration of breastfeeding: data from the longitudinal study of Australian children. Matern Child Nutr. 2008;4(3):163–70.

35. Martin JA, Hamilton BE, Ventura SJ, Osterman MJK, Wilson EC, Mathews TJ. Births: final data for 2010. Natl Vital Stat Rep. 2012;61(1):1–72.

36. Novak M, Ahlgren C, Hammarström A. A life-course approach in explaining social inequity in obesity among young adult men and women. Int J Obes. 2006;30(1):191–200.

37. Bogaerts A, Van den Bergh B, Nuyts E, Martens E, Witters I, Devlieger R. Socio-demographic and obstetrical correlates of pre-pregnancy body mass index and gestational weight gain: correlates of pre-pregnancy BMI and GWG. Clin Obes. 2012;2(5–6):150–9.

38. Vernay M, Malon A, Oleko A, Salanave B, Roudier C, Szego E, et al. Association of socioeconomic status with overall overweight and central obesity in men and women: the French nutrition and health survey 2006. BMC Public Health. 2009;9(1):215.

39. Harrington DW, Elliott SJ. Weighing the importance of neighbourhood: a multilevel exploration of the determinants of overweight and obesity. Soc Sci Med. 2009;68(4):593–600.

40. Haute autorité de santé. Recommandations professionnelles. Préparation à la naissance et à la périnatalité. 2005. Available from: http://www.has-sante.fr/portail/upload/docs/application/pdf/preparation_naissance_recos.pdf. Accessed 17 Apr 2017.

41. Raleigh VS, Hussey D, Seccombe I, Hallt K. Ethnic and social inequalities in women's experience of maternity care in England: results of a national survey. J R Soc Med. 2010;103(5):188–98.

42. Baron R, Manniën J, te Velde SJ, Klomp T, Hutton EK, Brug J. Socio-demographic inequalities across a range of health status indicators and health behaviours among pregnant women in prenatal primary care: a cross-sectional study. BMC Pregnancy Childbirth. 2015;15:261.

43. Vilain A, Gonzalez L. Surveillance de la grossesse en 2010: des inégalités socio-démographiques. Etudes et Résultats (Drees). Drees. 2013. Available from: http://drees.social-sante.gouv.fr/IMG/pdf/er848.pdf. Accessed 17 Apr 2017.

44. Garner CD, McKenzie SA, Devine CM, Thornburg LL, Rasmussen KM. Obese women experience multiple challenges with breastfeeding that are either unique or exacerbated by their obesity: discoveries from a longitudinal, qualitative study: obese women's breastfeeding challenges. Matern Child Nutr. 2016. doi:10.1111/mcn.12344. Epub ahead of print.

45. Nohr EA, Vaeth M, Baker JL, Sørensen TIA, Olsen J, Rasmussen KM. Pregnancy outcomes related to gestational weight gain in women defined by their body mass index, parity, height, and smoking status. Am J Clin Nutr. 2009;90(5):1288–94.

46. Lan-Pidhainy X, Nohr EA, Rasmussen KM. Comparison of gestational weight gain-related pregnancy outcomes in American primiparous and multiparous women. Am J Clin Nutr. 2013;97(5):1100–6.

47. Henriksen T. The macrosomic fetus: a challenge in current obstetrics. Acta Obstet Gynecol Scand. 2008;87(2):134–45.

48. Hermann M, Le Ray C, Blondel B, Goffinet F, Zeitlin J. The risk of prelabor and intrapartum cesarean delivery among overweight and obese women: possible preventive actions. Am J Obstet Gynecol. 2015;212(2):241.e1–9.

49. Landon MB, Leindecker S, Spong CY, Hauth JC, Bloom S, Varner MW, et al. The MFMU cesarean registry: factors affecting the success of trial of labor after previous cesarean delivery. Am J Obstet Gynecol. 2005;193(3 Pt 2): 1016–23.

50. Chu SY, Callaghan WM, Kim SY, Schmid CH, Lau J, England LJ, et al. Maternal obesity and risk of gestational diabetes mellitus. Diabetes Care. 2007;30(8):2070–6.

51. Roberts JM, Bodnar LM, Patrick TE, Powers RW. The role of obesity in preeclampsia. Pregnancy Hypertens. 2011;1(1):6–16.

52. Diouf I, Charles MA, Blondel B, Heude B, Kaminski M. Discordant time trends in maternal body size and offspring birthweight of term deliveries in France between 1972 and 2003: data from the French National Perinatal Surveys. Paediatr Perinat Epidemiol. 2011;25(3):210–7.

53. Villamor E, Cnattingius S. Interpregnancy weight change and risk of adverse pregnancy outcomes: a population-based study. Lancet. 2006;368(9542): 1164–70.

54. Cnattingius S, Villamor E. Weight change between successive pregnancies and risks of stillbirth and infant mortality: a nationwide cohort study. Lancet. 2016;387(10018):558–65.

Examining the provisional guidelines for weight gain in twin pregnancies

Olha Lutsiv[1*†] [ID], Adam Hulman[1†], Christy Woolcott[2], Joseph Beyene[3], Lucy Giglia[4], B. Anthony Armson[5], Linda Dodds[2], Binod Neupane[3] and Sarah D. McDonald[6]

Abstract

Background: Weight gain during pregnancy has an important impact on maternal and neonatal health. Unlike the Institute of Medicine (IOM) recommendations for weight gain in singleton pregnancies, those for twin gestations are termed "provisional", as they are based on limited data. The objectives of this study were to determine the neonatal and maternal outcomes associated with gaining weight below, within and above the IOM provisional guidelines on gestational weight gain in twin pregnancies, and additionally, to explore ranges of gestational weight gain among women who delivered twins at the recommended gestational age and birth weight, and those who did not.

Methods: A retrospective cohort study of women who gave birth to twins at ≥20 weeks gestation, with a birth weight ≥ 500 g was conducted in Nova Scotia, Canada (2003–2014). Our primary outcome of interest was small for gestational age (<10th percentile). In order to account for gestational age at delivery, weekly rates of 2nd and 3rd trimester weight gain were used to categorize women as gaining below, within, or above guidelines. We performed traditional regression analyses for maternal outcomes, and to account for the correlated nature of the neonatal outcomes in twins, we used generalized estimating equations (GEE).

Results: A total of 1482 twins and 741 mothers were included, of whom 27%, 43%, and 30% gained below, within, and above guidelines, respectively. The incidence of small for gestational age in these three groups was 30%, 21%, and 20%, respectively, and relative to gaining within guidelines, the adjusted odds ratios were 1.44 (95% CI 1.01–2.06) for gaining below and 0.92 (95% CI 0.62–1.36) for gaining above. The gestational weight gain in women who delivered twins at 37–42 weeks with average birth weight ≥ 2500 g and those who delivered twins outside of the recommend ranges were comparable to each other and the IOM recommendations.

Conclusions: While gestational weight gain below guidelines for twins was associated with some adverse neonatal outcomes, additional research exploring alternate ranges of gestational weight gain in twin pregnancies is warranted, in order to optimize neonatal and maternal outcomes.

Keywords: Guidelines, Pregnancy, Small for gestational age, Twins, Weight gain

* Correspondence: olha.lutsiv@mail.mcgill.ca
†Equal contributors
[1]Department of Obstetrics and Gynecology, McMaster University, 1280 Main Street West, Room 3N52B, Hamilton, ON L8S 4K1, Canada
Full list of author information is available at the end of the article

Background

Weight gain during pregnancy is increasingly recognized as being a key, modifiable perinatal factor with an important impact on a number of maternal and infant outcomes [1]. Recognizing the importance of gestational weight gain (GWG), in 2009 the US Institute of Medicine (IOM) released a guideline specifying the recommended amounts of weight that women with singleton gestations should gain during their pregnancy, depending on their pre-pregnancy body mass index (BMI) [2]. Since the research on GWG in multiple gestations was limited, only "provisional" recommendations regarding the optimal GWG in twin pregnancies were released at the time.

Despite accounting for only 3% of births [3], disproportionately more twins than singletons experience morbidity and mortality, occupying 28% of neonatal intensive care unit (NICU) days [4–6]. Small for gestational age (SGA; defined as birth weight < 10th percentile according to singleton cut-offs) affects more twins (14–20% of twin births), as does low birth weight (LBW) [5]. Due to the morbidity and mortality associated with small infant size, the current IOM guidelines on GWG are designed to reduce the risk of small infant size as well as preterm birth (PTB). Since the incidence of twin pregnancies is likely to continue to increase due to delayed child bearing and assisted reproductive technologies [7], determining the optimal GWG range for this population is of great importance.

While some raise caution at the fact that excessive weight gain during pregnancy may be detrimental to the mother and her baby [8], others have speculated that the provisional GWG recommendations for twin gestations may not be high enough to prevent LBW [9]. GWG above the IOM guidelines for singleton pregnancies is associated with significant adverse maternal outcomes, including pre-eclampsia and overweight/obesity later in life [10–12], and neonatal outcomes, such as high birth weight, which in turn predisposes them to overweight/ obesity in adolescence [8, 13, 14]. Therefore, the benefits of higher GWG for reducing small infant size in twins need to be offset against the possible adverse effects associated with excessive gain [15].

Although several studies have since attempted to explore the adequacy of the provisional IOM GWG guidelines for twins, no consensus has yet been reached. Due to this, more current, robust research to guide optimal GWG in twin pregnancies has been called for [16].

The objectives of this study were two-fold: 1) to examine the association between the existing provisional IOM GWG guidelines for twin pregnancies and SGA (and other secondary maternal and neonatal outcomes), and 2) to determine the GWG in women who delivered twins at the recommended gestational age and birth weight, using a large cohort separate from that in which the provisional

guidelines were estimated, in order to explore similarities and/ or differences in optimal GWG.

Methods
Study design and data source

A retrospective cohort study was conducted of all women who gave birth to twins between January 1, 2003 and December 31, 2014 in Nova Scotia, which is an eastern province of Canada. Data for this study were obtained from the Nova Scotia Atlee Perinatal Database (NSAPD), a validated population–based database that captures information on all births within the province [17–19].

The NSAPD contains maternal and neonatal information on demographics, procedures/ interventions, diagnoses, morbidities and mortality for all pregnancies and births, which is extracted from antenatal and medical charts by trained personnel, using standardized forms. The NSAPD is a valid and reliable database, as confirmed by an ongoing quality assurance program, which carries out periodic abstraction studies.

Inclusion and exclusion criteria

Women who were between 18 and 45 years of age and gave birth to twins at ≥20 weeks were eligible for study inclusion. Women were excluded if one or both of their infants had a birth weight < 500 g, major congenital anomalies, twin-to-twin transfusion syndrome, or if they were conjoined or monoamniotic. Additionally, mothers of single infants with a co-twin loss, mothers of co-twins of infants lost presumably from pregnancies that started with >2 fetuses, and mothers of infants with undetermined, unknown, or missing chorionicity were also excluded. Records with missing data on gestational age at delivery, BMI, or maternal weight at the time of delivery were excluded. Women who were underweight (BMI < 18.5 kg/m^2) were excluded since the current IOM guidelines do not provide GWG recommendations for underweight women with twin pregnancies [2].

Exposure, outcome and other variables of interest

The primary exposure was maternal GWG, categorized as below, within, or above the IOM provisional guidelines for twin pregnancies, according to the woman's pre-pregnancy BMI group (normal weight BMI 18.5–24.9 kg/ m^2, overweight 25.0–29.9 kg/m^2 or obese ≥30.0 kg/m^2). Women's total GWG was calculated by subtracting their self-reported pre-pregnancy weight, or if unavailable, their first measured weight, from their last measured weight closest to delivery. The measure of pre-pregnancy weight as reported in the NSAPD is based on the value that is written by the physician on the Nova Scotia Prenatal Record (field: "Pre-Pregnancy Weight"). The NSAPD does not record the specific source of this information, however it is known that the physician can use a pre-pregnancy weight as reported by the mother or a weight at the first prenatal visit (which for most women will occur in the first trimester; the NSAPD does not capture the date of this visit).

Gestational age at delivery was based on the last menstrual period or ultrasound. The majority of the women (84.5%) in the NSAPD have an early-pregnancy ultrasound. In women with both gestational age estimates, 87.2% of the last menstrual period-based estimates are within the ultrasound-based estimates by +/– 1 completed week. The total GWG recommendations for twin pregnancies for normal weight, overweight and obese women are: 16.8–24.5 kg, 14.1–22.7 kg and 11.4–19.1 kg, respectively. According to the IOM, the average cumulative weight gains for the first trimester (up to 13 weeks of gestation) in women who deliver twins at the recommended gestational age and birth weight (i.e., gestational ages 37–42 weeks and an average twin birth weight > 2500 g) are: 3.6 kg, 2.1 kg and 2.0 kg, respectively, for the three BMI categories. The optimal length of gestation was not defined by the IOM, although they considered a gestational age of 37–42 weeks in their recommendations of total GWG. Since that time practice has shifted to twin delivery during the earlier portion of that range in most instances [20, 21]. For this reason, we assumed that a term twin pregnancy is 38 weeks, and thus the recommended 2nd and 3rd trimester weekly rates of weight gain were calculated for each BMI group according to the formula: (IOM recommended total GWG – IOM average cumulative GWG up to 13 weeks)/ (38 weeks – 13 weeks). A similar formula was applied to estimate each woman's actual 2nd and 3rd trimester weekly rate of GWG for her BMI group. The women's actual 2nd and 3rd trimester weekly rates of GWG were compared with the calculated IOM recommended rates of gain for their BMI group, and accordingly, women were categorized as gaining below, within, or above the guidelines.

Our primary outcome was SGA, defined as birth weight < 10th percentile for gestational age and sex based on singleton growth curves [22]. Singleton growth curves currently provide the best predictors of adverse outcomes in twins, and are thus recommended by obstetrical associations as the preferred method for evaluating growth abnormalities in twins [23]. According to the National Institute for Health and Care Excellence, no evidence-based growth charts specific to twin and triplet pregnancies are available for use [20].

Secondary neonatal outcomes included: birth weight (continuous outcome), LBW <2500 g, SGA more strictly defined as birth weight < 5th percentile for gestational age and sex, large for gestational age (LGA) defined as birth weight > 90th percentile for gestational age and sex, Apgar score < 7 at 5 min, umbilical cord pH <7.10, respiratory distress, hypoglycaemia, NICU admission, and NICU length of stay.

Secondary maternal outcomes included: gestational age at delivery (continuous outcome), PTB <37 weeks (overall and broken down into spontaneous and indicated), labour induction, mode of delivery (unassisted birth, instrumental birth, and Caesarean section), postpartum haemorrhage, and length of postpartum hospital stay.

Important covariates included: maternal age, ethnicity, marital status, smoking status and drug use during pregnancy, pre-existing diabetes mellitus, pre-existing hypertension, other physical health problems, mental health problems, prenatal class attendance, chorionicity, and babies' sex. In addition to a woman's level of education, a neighborhood-level measure of socioeconomic status was also included – the Quintile of Adjusted Income Per Person Equivalent (QAIPPE), where 1 corresponds to the lowest and 5 corresponds to the highest income quintiles [24]. Obstetrical history was also included: parity and past history of gestational diabetes, gestational hypertension, LBW, and neonatal death.

Statistical analyses

Baseline characteristics were compared across the three GWG groups – women who gained below, within, or above the IOM GWG guidelines. Continuous variables were compared with the analysis of variance (ANOVA) or Kruskal-Wallis test. Categorical data were compared with a χ^2 or Fisher's exact test. To address our primary objective, to determine the effects of gaining below, within, or above the IOM GWG guidelines on each of the individual outcomes, linear regression was used for continuous outcomes and logistic regression was used for binary outcomes, with generalized estimating equations (GEE) used for the neonatal outcomes in order to adjust for the correlation between twins in a set. In order to assess the independent effect of GWG on neonatal and maternal outcomes, multivariable analyses were performed, adjusting for baseline maternal and pregnancy characteristics that may confound the associations of interest. The multivariable analyses adjusted for relevant a priori determined variables, which included maternal age, maternal pre-pregnancy BMI, smoking, socioeconomic status, parity, and chorionicity, as well as any additional baseline characteristics significant with a p-value <0.2 in the univariate analyses. All effect estimates from the models using GEE for the neonatal outcomes and the regression models for the maternal outcomes were reported as mean differences (MD; for continuous outcomes) or odds ratios (OR; for binary outcomes), with their accompanying 95% confidence intervals (CI).

Additionally, in order to explore potential GWG effect measure modification by parity or chorionicity, the multivariable models for all maternal and neonatal outcomes were also reanalyzed with an additional interaction term between parity and GWG, and separately chorionicity and GWG. The Wald test was used to test the significance of the interaction terms.

In order to address our second objective and determine the GWG in women who delivered twins at the recommended gestational age and birth weight, we followed the calculations outlined in the IOM guidelines in our study population. The recommended gestational age was defined as birth at 37–42 weeks of gestation. The recommended birth weight was defined as an average twin birth weight ≥ 2500 g. The interquartile range (IQR: 25th and 75th percentiles of the 2nd and 3rd trimester weekly rates of GWG) was determined. To reflect more recent clinical practice, we repeated the calculations after replacing 42 with 38 [6/7] weeks as the upper limit of gestational age at birth, and further amending the definition of the recommended birth weight, such that both twins individually weighed ≥2500 g. We also determined ranges of GWG in women who delivered twins outside of the recommended gestational age and birth weight, based on both definitions for comparison.

Prior to study commencement, a sample size calculation was performed. Analyses were performed using SAS (version 9.1; SAS Institute Inc., Cary, NC). We followed the *Strengthening the Reporting of Observational Studies in Epidemiology* (STROBE) guideline [25]. Institutional review board approval was obtained from the Faculty of Health Sciences/ McMaster University Research Ethics Board (#12-140C), the Reproductive Care Program of Nova Scotia Data Access Committee and the IWK Health Centre Research Ethics Board (#1012023) prior to study commencement.

Results

There were 3294 twin hospital births to 1647 women between January 1, 2003 and December 31, 2014 in Nova Scotia (Fig. 1). After excluding records of women who did not meet our study criteria (N = 445), and those who had missing information on gestational age, maternal pre-pregnancy height or weight, or maternal weight at delivery (N = 461), 741 women and 1482 infants were included.

Baseline characteristics

The majority of the women did not gain the IOM recommended amount of weight during pregnancy; 27.1% gained below, 29.7% gained above, and only 43.2% gained within the guidelines according to the 2nd and 3rd trimester weekly rates of weight gain. The median

maternal age was 31 years (IQR 27, 34), with the majority of women being married or common-law (77.8%), overweight or obese according to their pre-pregnancy BMI classification (26.5% and 26.3%, respectively), multiparous (52.5%), and residing in the top two highest neighborhood-level income quintiles (4th and 5th quintile, 23.0% and 21.0%, respectively). Approximately one-fifth of the infants were monochorionic (19.4%), and 47.2% were male (with the sex of one baby being ambiguous). Additional baseline characteristics of all study participants are reported in Table 1, according to their IOM classification of GWG.

Women who were excluded from our analyses due to missing information (N = 461) had similar baseline characteristics as those included (Additional file 1: Table S1).

Objective 1: Neonatal and maternal outcomes according to IOM classification of GWG

Our primary outcome, SGA <10th percentile, occurred in 30.1% of neonates exposed to inadequate maternal weight gain, which was significantly higher than in neonates exposed to appropriate (21.1%) or excess maternal weight gain (19.8%, Table 2). After controlling for potential confounders, neonates of women who gained below recommendations had a 44% higher odds of SGA <10th percentile (95% CI 1.01 to 2.06) than neonates of women who gained within the guidelines (Table 3). They also had higher odds of LBW (adjusted OR 1.55, 95% CI 1.07 to 2.23), and a longer NICU stay (mean + 4.4 days, 95% CI 0.7 to 8.2 days). The adjusted odds of SGA or any secondary neonatal outcome was not significantly different in women who gained above the guidelines compared to those who gained within. Women who gained weight above the provisional guidelines had higher odds of labour induction (adjusted OR 1.65 [95% CI 1.08, 2.53], Tables 4 and 5).

Gestational age, PTB <37 weeks, instrumental delivery, or postpartum hemorrhage did not differ by groups of GWG. The low incidence of LGA >90th percentile, Apgar score < 7 at 5 min, and umbilical cord pH <7.10, prohibited their exploration with multivariable regression. We did not find evidence of interaction between the classification of GWG and either parity or chorionicity (i.e., all $p > 0.05$ for interaction terms).

Objective 2: GWG in women who delivered twins within and outside the recommended gestational age and birth weight

Forty-four percent of the women in our study population delivered twins between 37 and 42 weeks, with an *average* twin birth weight ≥ 2500 g, while 31% of the women delivered twins between 37 and 38 [6/7] weeks, with *each* twin individually having a birth weight ≥ 2500 g. The rates of 2nd and 3rd trimester weight gain appeared to be fairly

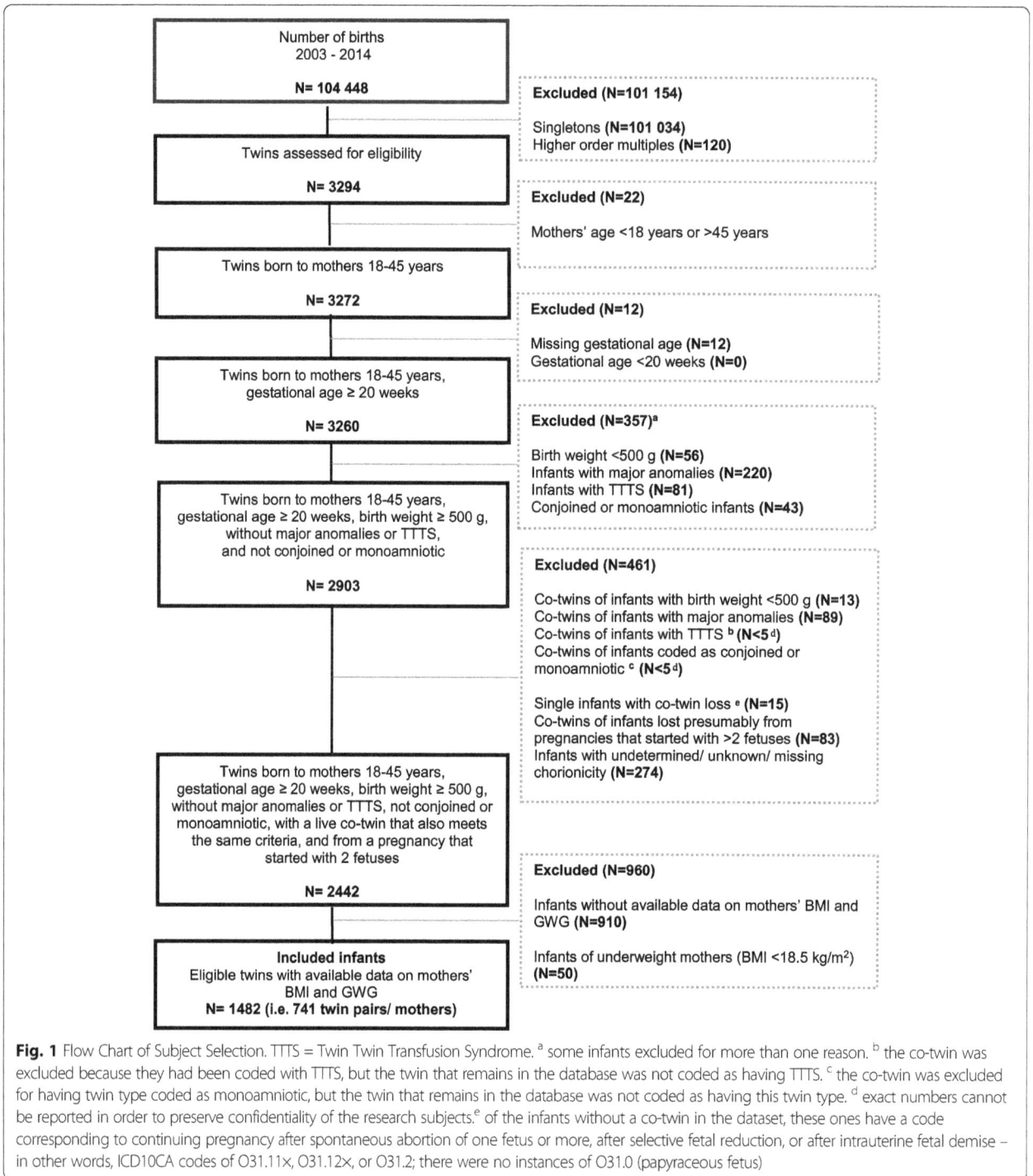

Fig. 1 Flow Chart of Subject Selection. TTTS = Twin Twin Transfusion Syndrome. [a] some infants excluded for more than one reason. [b] the co-twin was excluded because they had been coded with TTTS, but the twin that remains in the database was not coded as having TTTS. [c] the co-twin was excluded for having twin type coded as monoamniotic, but the twin that remains in the database was not coded as having this twin type. [d] exact numbers cannot be reported in order to preserve confidentiality of the research subjects. [e] of the infants without a co-twin in the dataset, these ones have a code corresponding to continuing pregnancy after spontaneous abortion of one fetus or more, after selective fetal reduction, or after intrauterine fetal demise – in other words, ICD10CA codes of O31.11x, O31.12x, or O31.2; there were no instances of O31.0 (papyraceous fetus)

comparable between women who delivered within the recommend gestational age and birth weight ranges and those who did not, regardless of which definition was used, and were also similar to the provisional recommendations from the IOM, regardless of pre-pregnancy BMI (Table 6). Examining the total GWG in women who delivered at the recommended gestational age and birth weight reveals a trend towards higher optimal GWG in normal

weight and overweight women compared to the IOM recommendations, but a lower optimal GWG in obese women (Fig. 2).

Discussion

In this large retrospective cohort study, we determined that relative to gaining within the provisional IOM guidelines for twins, gaining above the guidelines was

Table 1 Baseline characteristics of women with twin pregnancies according to gestational weight gain

Baseline Characteristic	All Participants (N = 741) N (%) [b]	Below IOM [a] GWG (N = 201) N (%) [b]	Within IOM [a] GWG (N = 320) N (%) [b]	Above IOM [a] GWG (N = 220) N (%) [b]	P value [c]
Maternal age, years, median (IQR)	31 (27, 34)	29 (25, 34)	32 (28, 35)	30 (26, 34)	<0.001
Caucasian	318 (82.8)	91 (82.0)	134 (84.3)	93 (81.6)	0.81
Married or common-law	556 (77.8)	145 (74.7)	255 (82.5)	156 (73.6)	0.03
Post-secondary education or higher	131 (50.4)	33 (47.1)	66 (56.4)	32 (43.8)	0.20
Neighborhood-level income quintile					0.36
1st quintile	139 (19.9)	46 (23.7)	51 (17.1)	42 (20.4)	
2nd quintile	109 (15.6)	33 (17.0)	46 (15.4)	30 (14.6)	
3rd quintile	143 (20.5)	38 (19.6)	57 (19.1)	48 (23.3)	
4th quintile	161 (23.0)	45 (23.2)	70 (23.4)	46 (22.3)	
5th quintile	147 (21.0)	32 (16.5)	75 (25.1)	40 (19.4)	
Pre-pregnancy BMI, kg/m^2, median (IQR)	25.5 (22.5, 30.3)	26.0 (22.6, 32.7)	25.0 (22.1, 29.5)	25.7 (23.0, 30.1)	0.07
Pre-pregnancy BMI classification					0.15
Normal weight (BMI 18.5 to 24.9 kg/m^2)	350 (47.2)	93 (46.3)	161 (50.3)	96 (43.6)	
Overweight (BMI 25.0 to 29.9 kg/m^2)	196 (26.5)	45 (22.4)	84 (26.3)	67 (30.5)	
Obese (BMI ≥ 30.0 kg/m^2)	195 (26.3)	63 (31.3)	75 (23.4)	57 (25.9)	
Parity ≥1	390 (52.6)	119 (59.2)	172 (53.8)	99 (45.0)	0.01
Previous gestational diabetes [d]	15 (2.0)	NA	NA	NA	0.76
Previous gestational hypertension	29 (3.9)	8 (4.0)	14 (4.4)	7 (3.2)	0.78
Previous Caesarean section	86 (11.7)	20 (10.1)	40 (12.6)	26 (12.0)	0.68
Previous LBW [d]	20 (2.8)	NA	NA	NA	0.31
Previous neonatal death	7 (1.0)	NA	NA	NA	0.31
Smoking during pregnancy	68 (10.3)	30 (17.2)	23 (7.8)	15 (7.9)	0.002
Drug use during pregnancy [d]	15 (2.0)	NA	NA	NA	0.64
Pre-existing diabetes mellitus [d]	9 (1.2)	NA	NA	NA	0.002
Pre-existing hypertension [d]	15 (2.0)	NA	NA	NA	0.32
Other physical health problems	194 (26.2)	57 (28.4)	84 (26.3)	53 (24.1)	0.61
Mental health problems	69 (9.3)	17 (8.5)	29 (9.1)	23 (10.5)	0.76
Attended prenatal classes	143 (41.9)	42 (43.3)	50 (35.2)	51 (50.0)	0.07
Twin type					0.52
Monochorionic – diamniotic	144 (19.4)	42 (20.9)	52 (16.3)	50 (22.7)	
Dichorionic (dissimilar sexes or blood groups)	294 (39.7)	77 (38.3)	128 (40.0)	89 (40.5)	
Dichorionic (similar sexes and blood groups)	135 (18.2)	34 (16.9)	64 (20.0)	37 (16.8)	
Dichorionic (similar sexes but blood groups undetermined)	168 (22.7)	48 (23.9)	76 (23.7)	44 (20.0)	
Sex of the baby [e]					0.40
Male	699 (47.2)	203 (50.5)	294 (45.9)	202 (46.0)	
Female	782 (52.8)	199 (49.5)	346 (54.1)	237 (54.0)	

Abbreviations: BMI, body mass index; GWG, gestational weight gain; IOM, Institute of Medicine; IQR, inter-quartile range; N, number; NA, not available
[a] GWG categories (below, within, and above IOM GWG) are based on the 2nd and 3rd trimester weekly rates of GWG
[b] Baseline characteristics are mostly reported as N (%), unless otherwise specified (i.e., median (IQR))
[c] P values were calculated with the Kruskal-Wallis test for continuous variables and with the χ^2 test or Fisher's exact test for categorical variables
[d] The proportions of previous gestational diabetes, previous LBW, previous neonatal death, drug use during pregnancy, pre-existing diabetes mellitus, and pre-existing hypertension could not be reported by GWG category in order to preserve the confidentiality of the research subjects, since some cells had <5 events
[e] Sex of the baby is reported at the neonatal level and not the maternal level, thus total N = 1482; the sex of one baby was ambiguous; the p-value is based on the analysis of generalized estimating equations parameter estimates

Table 2 Outcomes of twins according to mothers' gestational weight gain

Neonatal Outcome	All Participants (N = 1482)	Below IOM [a] GWG (N = 402)	Within IOM [a] GWG (N = 640)	Above IOM [a] GWG (N = 440)	
	N (%) [b]	N (%) [b]	N (%) [b]	N (%) [b]	P value [c]
SGA <10th percentile	343 (23.2)	121 (30.1)	135 (21.1)	87 (19.8)	0.004
SGA <5th percentile	193 (13.0)	69 (17.2)	85 (13.3)	39 (8.9)	0.005
LBW <2500 g	603 (40.7)	204 (50.8)	244 (38.1)	155 (35.2)	<0.001
LGA >90th percentile	31 (2.1)	5 (1.2)	11 (1.7)	15 (3.4)	0.22
Birth weight, g, median (IQR)	2603 (2260, 2885)	2475 (2100, 2765)	2653 (2290, 2905)	2637 (2356, 2910)	<0.001
Apgar score < 7 at 5 min	39 (2.6)	13 (3.3)	10 (1.6)	16 (3.7)	0.16
Umbilical cord pH <7.10	33 (2.7)	10 (2.9)	15 (2.8)	8 (2.2)	0.84
Respiratory distress	148 (10.0)	46 (11.4)	53 (8.3)	49 (11.1)	0.27
Hypoglycemia	160 (10.8)	43 (10.7)	71 (11.1)	46 (10.5)	0.96
NICU admission	555 (37.5)	170 (42.3)	230 (35.9)	155 (35.2)	0.21
NICU length of stay, days, median (IQR)	11 (2, 20)	13 (2, 23)	10 (2, 19)	11 (1, 20)	0.10

Abbreviations: BMI, body mass index; GWG, gestational weight gain; IOM, Institute of Medicine; IQR, inter-quartile range; LBW, low birth weight; LGA, large for gestational age (and sex); N, number; NICU, neonatal intensive care unit; SGA, small for gestational age (and sex)
[a] Gestational weight gain categories (below, within, and above IOM GWG) are based on the 2nd and 3rd trimester weekly rates of GWG
[b] Outcomes are mostly reported as N (%), unless otherwise specified (i.e., median (IQR))
[c] P values are based on the analysis of generalized estimating equations parameter estimates

associated with higher odds of labour induction, while gaining below was associated with higher odds of SGA, LBW, and longer NICU stay. Additionally, we determined that the rates of 2nd and 3rd trimester weight gain for women who delivered twins *within* the recommended gestational age and birth weight ranges, of all pre-pregnancy BMI classes, were fairly comparable to the rates computed based on current recommendations by the IOM, but they were not very different from the rates in women who delivered *outside* of the recommended gestational age and birth weight ranges.

The original 1990 IOM guidelines recommended 6–20 kg of GWG for women carrying twins, regardless of their BMI [26]. Given the concerns of small infant size that are associated with low GWG, the IOM revised their guidelines in 2009 to recommend significantly higher GWG (17–25 kg for normal weight women, 14–23 kg for overweight women, and 11–19 kg for obese women) [2]. These guidelines were "provisional", a seemingly reasonable term given that they were based on: a single study; historical in nature (1979 to 1999); with potential for selection bias (four teaching hospitals); and inclusion of

Table 3 Unadjusted and adjusted associations between gestational weight gain and neonatal outcomes

Neonatal Outcome	Below IOM GWG [a]		Above IOM GWG [a]	
	Unadjusted Analyses OR (95% CI)	Adjusted Analyses [b] OR (95% CI)	Unadjusted Analyses OR (95% CI)	Adjusted Analyses [b] OR (95% CI)
SGA <10th percentile	1.61 (1.18, 2.21)	1.44 (1.01, 2.06)	0.92 (0.66, 1.29)	0.92 (0.62, 1.36)
SGA <5th percentile	1.35 (0.93, 1.98)	1.07 (0.69, 1.65)	0.64 (0.40, 1.00)	0.67 (0.39, 1.14)
LBW <2500 g	1.67 (1.23, 2.28)	1.55 (1.07, 2.23)	0.88 (0.65, 1.20)	0.81 (0.58, 1.14)
Birth weight, g [c]	−1523 (−235, −71)	−145 (−233, −57)	18 (−64, 100)	39 (−48, 126)
Respiratory distress	1.43 (0.87, 2.36)	1.14 (0.65, 2.01)	1.39 (0.85, 2.27)	1.09 (0.63, 1.87)
Hypoglycemia	0.96 (0.60, 1.53)	0.73 (0.41, 1.28)	0.94 (0.60, 1.46)	1.13 (0.69, 1.84)
NICU admission	1.31 (0.94, 1.82)	1.29 (0.87, 1.91)	0.97 (0.70, 1.35)	0.92 (0.63, 1.35)
NICU length of stay, days [c]	3.76 (0.32, 7.21)	4.45 (0.69, 8.20)	0.92 (−2.38, 4.22)	1.59 (−2.04, 5.22)

Abbreviations: BMI, body mass index; CI; confidence interval; GWG, gestational weight gain; IOM, Institute of Medicine; IQR, inter-quartile range; LBW, low birth weight; N, number; NICU, neonatal intensive care unit; OR, odds ratio; PTB, preterm birth; SGA, small for gestational age (and sex)
[a] Gestational weight gain categories (below, within, and above IOM GWG) are based on the 2nd and 3rd trimester weekly rates of GWG; GWG within the IOM GWG is the referent group for all analyses
[b] All outcomes were adjusted for the a priori defined confounders, including maternal age, neighborhood-level income, maternal pre-pregnancy BMI, parity, smoking status, and chorionicity. Analyses were also adjusted for the baseline characteristics significant with a *p-value* < 0.2, including marital status. Despite having a *p-value* <0.2, pre-existing diabetes mellitus and attending prenatal classes were not included in the adjusted models, due to low frequency of occurrence in the three categories of GWG (pre-existing diabetes mellitus), or collinearity with other variables in the model (attending prenatal classes)
[c] The corresponding effect estimates are a mean difference (95% CI), instead of OR (95% CI)

Table 4 Outcomes of women with twin pregnancies by gestational weight gain

Maternal Outcome	All Participants (N = 741)	Below IOM [a] GWG (N = 201)	Within IOM [a] GWG (N = 320)	Above IOM [a] GWG (N = 220)	
	N (%) [b]	N (%) [b]	N (%) [b]	N (%) [b]	P value [c]
Gestational age at delivery, weeks, median (IQR)	37.0 (35.7, 38.0)	36.9 (35.6, 38.0)	37.1 (35.7, 38.0)	37.0 (35.7, 37.9)	0.49
PTB <37 weeks					
Overall	353 (47.6)	104 (51.7)	142 (44.4)	107 (48.6)	0.25
Spontaneous	155 (20.9)	49 (24.4)	67 (20.9)	39 (17.7)	0.25
Indicated	198 (26.7)	55 (27.4)	75 (23.4)	68 (30.9)	0.15
Labour induction	235 (31.7)	67 (33.3)	86 (26.9)	82 (37.3)	0.03
Mode of delivery					
Vaginal birth (unassisted)	304 (41.0)	98 (48.8)	125 (39.1)	81 (36.8)	0.03
Forceps/ vacuum	50 (6.8)	12 (6.0)	25 (7.8)	13 (5.9)	0.60
Caesarean section	387 (52.2)	91 (45.3)	170 (53.1)	126 (57.3)	0.04
Postpartum haemorrhage	148 (20.0)	42 (20.9)	63 (19.7)	43 (19.6)	0.93
Length of stay, days, median (IQR)	3.4 (2.7, 4.3)	3.2 (2.5, 4.1)	3.5 (2.8, 4.3)	3.6 (2.8, 4.6)	0.02

Abbreviations: BMI, body mass index; GWG, gestational weight gain; IOM, Institute of Medicine; IQR, inter-quartile range; N, number; PTB, preterm birth
[a] Gestational weight gain categories (below, within, and above IOM GWG) are based on the 2nd and 3rd trimester weekly rates of GWG
[b] Outcomes are mostly reported as N (%), unless otherwise specified (i.e., median (IQR))
[c] P values were calculated with the Kruskal-Wallis test for continuous variables and with the χ^2 test or Fisher's exact test for categorical variables

women who delivered between 37 and 42 weeks of gestation, despite the fact that delivery of twins is now recommended between 38 and 39 weeks, to reduce mortality and morbidity [27]; and a focus on twins *averaging* ≥ 2500 g, thereby precluding the ability to truly examine the association between GWG and individual small infant size [28]. The guidelines did not report on GWG among women with "suboptimal" outcomes (i.e., women who deliver outside of the recommended gestational age and birth weight), even though it is also important to consider

Table 5 Unadjusted and adjusted associations between gestational weight gain and maternal outcomes

Maternal Outcome	Below IOM GWG [a]		Above IOM GWG [a]	
	Unadjusted Analyses OR (95% CI)	Adjusted Analyses [b] OR (95% CI)	Unadjusted Analyses OR (95% CI)	Adjusted Analyses [b] OR (95% CI)
Gestational age at delivery, weeks [c]	−0.28 (−0.66, 0.10)	−0.34 (−0.76, 0.07)	−0.10 (−0.47, 0.27)	0.01 (−0.39, 0.41)
PTB <37 weeks				
Overall	1.34 (0.94, 1.91)	1.28 (0.86, 1.93)	1.19 (0.84, 1.68)	1.09 (0.73, 1.62)
Spontaneous	1.22 (0.80, 1.85)	1.16 (0.71, 1.90)	0.81 (0.53, 1.26)	0.78 (0.47, 1.30)
Indicated	1.23 (0.82, 1.84)	1.20 (0.76, 1.91)	1.46 (0.99, 2.15)	1.34 (0.86, 2.09)
Labour induction	1.36 (0.93, 2.00)	1.54 (0.99, 2.39)	1.62 (1.12, 2.34)	1.65 (1.08, 2.53)
Mode of delivery				
Vaginal birth (unassisted)	1.48 (1.04, 2.12)	1.47 (0.96, 2.25)	0.91 (0.64, 1.30)	1.03 (0.67, 1.56)
Forceps/ vacuum	0.75 (0.37, 1.53)	0.91 (0.40, 2.09)	0.74 (0.37, 1.48)	0.73 (0.32, 1.67)
Caesarean section	0.73 (0.51, 1.04)	0.71 (0.46, 1.08)	1.18 (0.84, 1.67)	1.07 (0.71, 1.61)
Postpartum haemorrhage	1.08 (0.70, 1.67)	1.10 (0.67, 1.81)	0.99 (0.64, 1.53)	1.01 (0.62, 1.63)
Length of stay, days [c]	−0.30 (−0.60, −0.01)	−0.35 (−0.68, −0.02)	0.03 (−0.25, 0.32)	−0.04 (−0.36, 0.28)

Abbreviations: BMI, body mass index; CI; confidence interval; GWG, gestational weight gain; IOM, Institute of Medicine; IQR, inter-quartile range; N, number; OR, odds ratio; PTB, preterm birth
[a] Gestational weight gain categories (below, within, and above IOM GWG) are based on the 2nd and 3rd trimester weekly rates of GWG; GWG within the IOM GWG is the referent group for all analyses
[b] All outcomes were adjusted for the a priori defined confounders, including maternal age, neighborhood-level income, maternal pre-pregnancy BMI, parity, smoking status, and chorionicity. Analyses were also adjusted for the baseline characteristics significant with a p-value < 0.2, including marital status. Despite having a p-value <0.2, pre-existing diabetes mellitus and attending prenatal classes were not included in the adjusted models, due to low frequency of occurrence in the three categories of GWG (pre-existing diabetes mellitus), or collinearity with other variables in the model (attending prenatal classes)
[c] The corresponding effect estimates are a mean difference (95% CI), instead of OR (95% CI)

Table 6 The 2nd-3rd trimester weekly GWG in women with twin pregnancies with optimal and suboptimal outcomes

	Normal weight BMI 18.5–24.9 kg/m^2	Overweight BMI 25.0–29.9 kg/m^2	Obese BMI ≥ 30 kg/m^2
	25th – 75th percentiles of 2nd + 3rd trimester weekly GWG (kg/week)[a]		
IOM provisional guideline	0.53–0.84	0.48–0.82	0.38–0.68
IOM definition in NSAPD			
Optimal outcome [b]	0.58–0.87	0.49–0.85	0.30–0.77
Sub-optimal outcome	0.45–0.85	0.52–0.87	0.34–0.72
New definition in NSAPD			
Optimal outcome [c]	0.61–0.86	0.48–0.88	0.29–0.80
Sub-optimal outcome	0.45–0.85	0.52–0.86	0.33–0.72

Abbreviations: BMI, body mass index; GWG, gestational weight gain; IOM, Institute of Medicine; NSAPD, Nova Scotia Atlee Perinatal Database
[a] 2nd and 3rd trimester weekly GWG were calculated according to the formula: (Total GWG – IOM Average Cumulative GWG up to 13 weeks) / (Gestational Age – 13). The IOM Average Cumulative GWGs up to 13 weeks were 3.6 kg, 2.1 kg and 2.0 kg in normal weight, overweight and obese women
[b] Optimal outcome defined as birth at 37–42 weeks and average twin birth weight ≥ 2500 g
[c] Optimal outcome defined as birth at 37–38 $^{6/7}$ weeks and birth weight of both twins individually ≥2500 g

the difference in GWG between women with "optimal" and "suboptimal" outcomes.

Several studies have attempted to examine the 2009 recommendations for twin gestations, with conflicting results. Only a few studies considered SGA <10th percentile specifically, and of those that did, one did not find a significant difference between women [29], while another found a lower incidence in normal weight women who gained within or above guidelines, but no differences in overweight or obese women [9]. A number of studies called into question the provisional recommendations as they found that weight gain in accordance with or in excess of the guidelines was associated with larger birth weight and decreased incidence of prematurity [30–32]. Other studies corroborated these results, as excessive GWG was associated with a larger birth

weight, without any significant increases in other adverse pregnancy outcomes [33]. Conversely, another study found both inadequate and excess weight gain were associated with lower birth weight and prematurity [29].

Strengths of this study include the methodology used to classify GWG as below, within, or above guidelines which took into account the length of gestation as recommended by the IOM. Unlike numerous previous studies that restricted their study population to 37 weeks or more, excluding up to 50% of the population of interest [30, 34] and making it impossible to examine "optimal" and "suboptimal" outcomes, or those that assumed a uniform rate of weight gain throughout the pregnancy, our classifications were based on the estimated weekly rates of weight gain for the 2nd and 3rd trimesters, reflective of the slower trajectory of weight gain during the

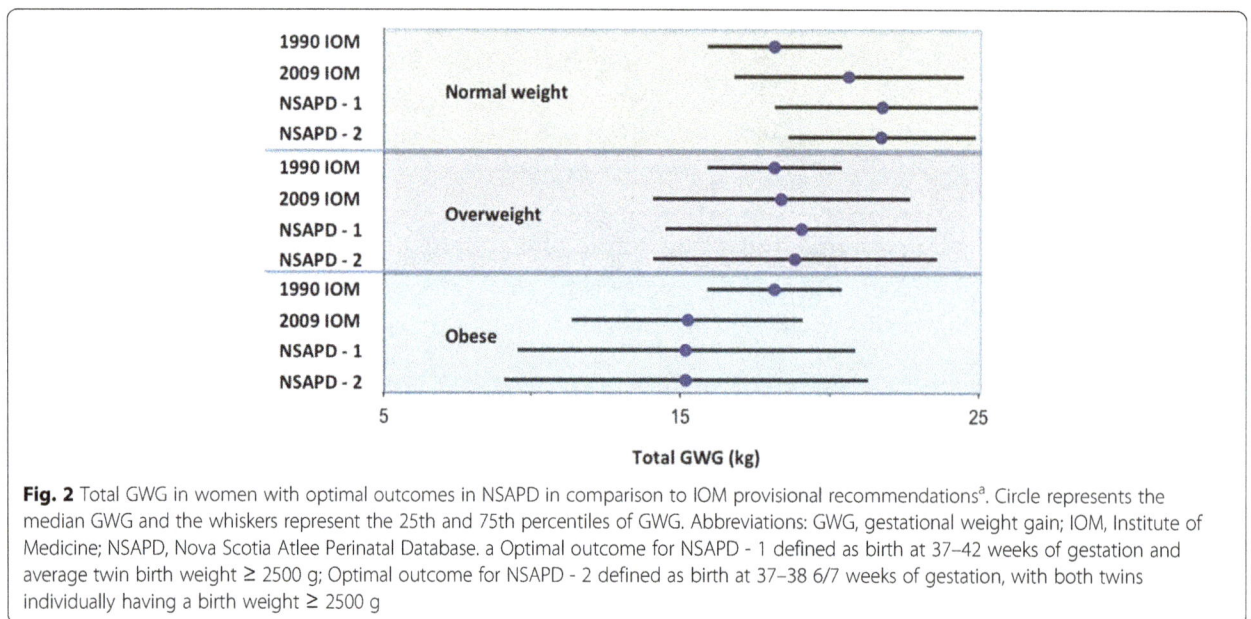

Fig. 2 Total GWG in women with optimal outcomes in NSAPD in comparison to IOM provisional recommendations[a]. Circle represents the median GWG and the whiskers represent the 25th and 75th percentiles of GWG. Abbreviations: GWG, gestational weight gain; IOM, Institute of Medicine; NSAPD, Nova Scotia Atlee Perinatal Database. a Optimal outcome for NSAPD - 1 defined as birth at 37–42 weeks of gestation and average twin birth weight ≥ 2500 g; Optimal outcome for NSAPD - 2 defined as birth at 37–38 6/7 weeks of gestation, with both twins individually having a birth weight ≥ 2500 g

first trimester. This allowed us not only to include a larger sample of women, but much more importantly, did not eliminate women with adverse outcomes, such as PTB. Using a weekly rate of GWG further overcomes some of the bias that can affect results based on total GWG, given its inherent correlation with gestational age. It should be noted, however, that this method may not fully remove the effects of gestational length, as it assumes a certain amount of weight gain in the first trimester; if this assumption is incorrect for some women, it will misclassify them as having inadequate, adequate or excessive weight gain as defined by the IOM provisional guidelines [35, 36].

We maintained three BMI groups, rather than grouping together women gaining within and above the guidelines to compare them to women gaining below, which dismisses differences in the incidence of adverse outcomes between the first two groups, and could therefore result in biased effect estimates [30–32]. The large sample size is another notable strength, as it ensured adequate statistical power to control for a number of key confounding variables. Finally, a strength of this study is the use of GEE in order to account for correlation between twins, resulting in robust and valid effect estimates and CIs. Thus we overcame limitations of the majority of previous studies which analyzed all outcomes at the maternal level (instead of the individual neonate level) or which did not account for correlation between twins altogether [29, 31, 33], which could result in seemingly significant differences between groups even when there are none.

Limitations of this study include some missing data as sometimes occurs with large databases, for some variables of interest, including GWG. However, a comparison of the baseline characteristics of the women who were included in the study and those who were excluded due to missing information did not reveal any significant differences. Furthermore, missing data does not necessarily bias our associations, although our study findings should not be over-generalized to be representative of all pregnant women. Additionally, while our sample size was large enough for us to control for a number of key confounding variables, we were unable to perform analyses stratified by pre-pregnancy BMI, as such analyses would have been underpowered.

Limitations of the method used to develop the provisional guidelines [2] should also be noted. First of all, a comparison of GWG between the women who deliver twins within and outside of the recommended gestational age and birth weight, is an important one, however it is lacking in the IOM guidelines. The smaller the difference between these two groups, the less robust the recommendation. Furthermore, the width of the IOM recommended range of GWG was based on data from a arbitrarily chosen percentiles (25th and 75th) from data from a single study as noted above [28] and not on outcomes. In addition to gestational age and birth weight, other maternal and neonatal outcomes should have also been considered when determining the recommended ranges. Since the currently published studies have mostly aimed to evaluate the provisional guidelines, more attention should be focused on developing new methodologies for defining recommendations, determining whether alternate ranges of GWG correspond with better outcomes, and examining optimal and suboptimal outcomes according to GWG. This is especially critical at this time because if the provisional recommendations are interpreted to be the gold standard, then it will be more difficult to prove that an alternate recommendation may lead to better outcomes, and to change practice.

Future research is required to examine different patterns of GWG throughout pregnancy on maternal and neonatal outcomes, using a longitudinal approach with serial antenatal weight measurements. Determining the optimal GWG for underweight women, and further refining and narrowing the recommended ranges of GWG for normal weight, overweight and obese women is also key. Studying the effects of GWG on SGA defined according to twin growth charts will also be important, if standardized, validated twin growth charts that are based on rigorous data are developed and recommended in clinical practice guidelines.

Conclusions

In summary, while GWG below the provisional guidelines for twins was associated with SGA and other adverse neonatal outcomes, GWG above the guidelines did not reduce the odds of SGA, and was further associated with adverse maternal outcomes, such as labour induction. As such, GWG recommendations outside of the provisional IOM guidelines may not be advisable, and further research is required to confirm the robustness of the provisional guidelines.

Abbreviations
ANOVA: Analysis of Variance; BMI: Body Mass Index; CI: Confidence Interval; GEE: Generalized Estimating Equations; GWG: Gestational Weight Gain; IOM: Institute of Medicine; IQR: Inter-Quartile Range; LBW: Low Birth Weight; LGA: Large for Gestational Age; MD: Mean Difference; NICU: Neonatal Intensive Care Unit; NSAPD: Nova Scotia Atlee Perinatal Database; OR: Odds Ratio; PTB: Preterm Birth; QAIPPE: Quintile of Adjusted Income Per Person Equivalent; SGA: Small for Gestational Age; STROBE: Strengthening the Reporting of Observational Studies in Epidemiology

Acknowledgements

Not Applicable.

Funding

This work was supported by an operating grant from the Hamilton Academic Health Sciences Organization Academic Funding Plan (HAHSO AFP) Innovation Fund. Additionally, Dr. Sarah D McDonald is supported by a Tier II Canada Research Chair. The funding agencies had no role in the design of the study, collection, analysis and interpretation of the data, and in writing the manuscript.

Authors' contributions

Each of the bylined authors has made a substantial contribution to the study and has fulfilled the International Committee of Medical Journal Editors criteria for authorship. OL made substantial contributions to the study design, performed the statistical analyses, interpreted the data, and drafted the manuscript. AH, JB, and BN made substantial contributions to the study design, analysis and interpretation of data. CW, LG, BAA, and LD made substantial contributions to the study design and interpretation of data. SDM made substantial contributions to the study conception and design, acquisition of data, analysis and interpretation of data. All authors were involved in revising the manuscript critically for important intellectual content, approved the final version to be published, and agreed to be accountable for all aspects of the work in ensuring that questions related to the accuracy or integrity of any part of the work are appropriately investigated and resolved.

Competing interests

The authors declare that they have no competing interests.

Author details

[1]Department of Obstetrics and Gynecology, McMaster University, 1280 Main Street West, Room 3N52B, Hamilton, ON L8S 4K1, Canada. [2]Departments of Obstetrics and Gynaecology, and Pediatrics, Dalhousie University, Halifax, NS, Canada. [3]Department of Clinical Epidemiology & Biostatistics, McMaster University, Hamilton, ON, Canada. [4]Department of Pediatrics, McMaster University, Hamilton, ON, Canada. [5]Department of Obstetrics and Gynaecology, Dalhousie University, Halifax, NS, Canada. [6]Departments of Obstetrics and Gynecology, Radiology, and Clinical Epidemiology & Biostatistics, McMaster University, Hamilton, ON, Canada.

References

1. Dzakpasu S, Fahey J, Kirby RS, et al. Contribution of prepregnancy body mass index and gestational weight gain to adverse neonatal outcomes: population attributable fractions for Canada. BMC Pregnancy Childbirth. 2015;15:21.
2. Institute of Medicine (IOM). National Research Council. Weight Gain During Pregnancy: Reexamining the Guidelines. In: Rasmussen KM, Yaktine AL, editors. Committee to Reexamine IOM Pregnancy Weight Guidelines. Washington, DC: National Academy Press; 2009.
3. Public Health Agency of Canada. Canadian Perinatal Health Report. 2008. Ottawa.
4. Bassil KL, Shah PS, Barrington KJ, et al. The changing epidemiology of preterm twins and triplets admitted to neonatal intensive care units in Canada, 2003 to 2008. Am J Perinatol. 2012;29(4):237–44.
5. Kogan MD, Alexander GR, Kotelchuck M, et al. Trends in twin birth outcomes and prenatal care utilization in the United States, 1981-1997. JAMA. 2000;284(3):335–41.
6. Martin JA, Hamilton BE, Sutton PD, Ventura SJ, Menacker F, Kirmeyer S. Births: final data for 2004. Centers for Disease Control and Prevention, National Center for Health Statistics, National Vital Statistics System. 2006;55(1):1–101.
7. Johnson JA, Tough S. Society of O, Gynaecologists of C. Delayed child-bearing. J Obstet Gynaecol Can. 2012;34(1):80–93.
8. Nohr EA, Vaeth M, Baker JL, Sorensen T, Olsen J, Rasmussen KM. Combined associations of prepregnancy body mass index and gestational weight gain with the outcome of pregnancy. Am J Clin Nutr. 2008;87(6):1750–9.
9. Lal AK, Kominiarek MA. Weight gain in twin gestations: are the Institute of Medicine guidelines optimal for neonatal outcomes? J Perinatol. 2015;35(6):405–10.
10. Macdonald-Wallis C, Tilling K, Fraser A, Nelson SM, Lawlor DA. Gestational weight gain as a risk factor for hypertensive disorders of pregnancy. Am J Obstet Gynecol. 2013;209(4):327 e1–17.
11. Gunderson EP, Abrams B. Epidemiology of gestational weight gain and body weight changes after pregnancy. Epidemiol Rev. 2000;22(2):261–74.
12. Rooney BL, Schauberger CW, Mathiason MA. Impact of perinatal weight change on long-term obesity and obesity-related illnesses. Obstet Gynecol. 2005;106(6):1349–56.
13. Thorsdottir I, Torfadottir JE, Birgisdottir BE, Geirsson RT. Weight gain in women of normal weight before pregnancy: complications in pregnancy or delivery and birth outcome. Obstet Gynecol. 2002;99(5 Pt 1):799–806.
14. Yu ZB, Han SP, Zhu GZ, et al. Birth weight and subsequent risk of obesity: a systematic review and meta-analysis. Obes Rev. 2011;12(7):525–42.
15. McDonald SD, Han Z, Mulla S, et al. High gestational weight gain and the risk of preterm birth and low birth weight: a systematic review and meta-analysis. J Obstet Gynaecol Can. 2011;33(12):1223–33.
16. Leese B, Jomeen J, Denton J. Appropriate maternal weight gain in singleton and twin pregnancies: what is the evidence? Hum Fertil (Camb). 2012;15(4):194–9.
17. A Provincial Program of the Nova Scotia Department of Health and Wellness. The Nova Scotia Atlee Perinatal Database; 2014. (cited 2015 Sep 20). Available from: http://rcp.nshealth.ca/atlee-database.
18. Fair M, Cyr M, Allen AC, Wen SW, Guyon G, MacDonald RC. An assessment of the validity of a computer system for probabilistic record linkage of birth and infant death records in Canada. The Fetal and Infant Health Study Group. Chronic Dis Can. 2000;21(1):8–13.
19. Joseph KS, Fahey J. Canadian Perinatal Surveillance System - Validation of perinatal data in the Discharge Abstract Database of the Canadian Institute for Health Information. Chronic Dis Can. 2009;29(3):96–100.
20. National Institute for Health and Clinical Excellence (NICE). Multiple Pregnancy: The Management of Twin and Triplet Pregnancies in the Antenatal Period. 2011. Manchester, UK.
21. Royal College of Obstetricians and Gynaecologists (RCOG). Management of Monochorionic Twin Pregnancy. 2008. London.
22. Kramer MS, Platt RW, Wen SW, et al. A new and improved population-based Canadian reference for birth weight for gestational age. Pediatrics. 2001; 108(2):E35.
23. Morin L, Lim K. Ultrasound in twin pregnancies. J Obstet Gynaecol Can. 2011;33(6):643–56.
24. Wilkins R. PCCF + version 5F: User's guide. Ottawa: Statistics Canada; 2010 (cited 2015 July 25). Available from: http://publications.gc.ca/collections/ collection_2016/statcan/CS82-0086-2005-eng.pdf.
25. von Elm E, Altman DG, Egger M, et al. The Strengthening the Reporting of Observational Studies in Epidemiology (STROBE) statement: guidelines for reporting observational studies. Epidemiology. 2007;18(6):800–4.
26. Institute of Medicine (IOM). Subcommittee on Nutritional Status and Weight Gain During Pregnancy. Washington. DC: National Academy Press; 1990.
27. Hartley RS, Emanuel I, Hitti J. Perinatal mortality and neonatal morbidity rates among twin pairs at different gestational ages: optimal delivery timing at 37 to 38 weeks' gestation. Am J Obstet Gynecol. 2001;184(3):451–8.
28. Luke B, Hediger ML, Nugent C, et al. Body mass index–specific weight gains associated with optimal birth weights in twin pregnancies. J Reprod Med. 2003;48(4):217–24.
29. Shamshirsaz AA, Haeri S, Ravangard SF, et al. Perinatal outcomes based on the institute of medicine guidelines for weight gain in twin pregnancies. J Matern Fetal Neonatal Med. 2014;27(6):552–6.
30. Fox NS, Rebarber A, Roman AS, Klauser CK, Peress D, Saltzman DH. Weight gain in twin pregnancies and adverse outcomes: examining the 2009 Institute of Medicine guidelines. Obstet Gynecol. 2010;116(1):100–6.
31. González-Quintero VH, Kathiresan AS, Tudela FJ, Rhea D, Desch C, Istwan N. The association of gestational weight gain per institute of medicine

guidelines and prepregnancy body mass index on outcomes of twin pregnancies. Am J Perinatol. 2012;29(6):435–40.

32. Pettit KE, Lacoursiere DY, Schrimmer DB, Alblewi H, Moore TR, Ramos GA. The association of inadequate mid-pregnancy weight gain and preterm birth in twin pregnancies. J Perinatol. 2015;35(2):85–9.

33. Fox NS, Saltzman DH, Kurtz H, Rebarber A. Excessive weight gain in term twin pregnancies: examining the 2009 Institute of Medicine definitions. Obstet Gynecol. 2011;118(5):1000–4.

34. Gavard JA, Artal R. Gestational weight gain and maternal and neonatal outcomes in term twin pregnancies in obese women. Twin Res Hum Genet. 2014;17(2):127–33.

35. Hutcheon JA, Bodnar LM, Joseph KS, Abrams B, Simhan HN, Platt RW. The bias in current measures of gestational weight gain. Paediatr Perinat Epidemiol. 2012;26(2):109–16.

36. Bodnar LM, Hutcheon JA, Parisi SM, Pugh SJ, Abrams B. Comparison of gestational weight gain z-scores and traditional weight gain measures in relation to perinatal outcomes. Paediatr Perinat Epidemiol. 2015;29(1):11–21.

Correlates of poor mental health in early pregnancy in obese European women

Matteo C. Sattler[1], Judith G. M. Jelsma[2], Annick Bogaerts[3], David Simmons[4], Gernot Desoye[5], Rosa Corcoy[6,7], Juan M. Adelantado[6], Alexandra Kautzky-Willer[8], Jürgen Harreiter[8], Frans A. van Assche[9], Roland Devlieger[9], Goele Jans[9], Sander Galjaard[9,10], David Hill[11], Peter Damm[12], Elisabeth R. Mathiesen[12], Ewa Wender-Ozegowska[13], Agnieszka Zawiejska[13], Kinga Blumska[13], Annunziata Lapolla[14], Maria G. Dalfrà[14], Alessandra Bertolotto[15], Fidelma Dunne[16], Dorte M. Jensen[17], Lise Lotte T. Andersen[17], Frank J. Snoek[18,19] and Mireille N. M. van Poppel[1,2]*

Abstract

Background: Depression during pregnancy is associated with higher maternal morbidity and mortality, and subsequent possible adverse effects on the cognitive, emotional and behavioral development of the child. The aim of the study was to identify maternal characteristics associated with poor mental health, in a group of overweight/obese pregnant women in nine European countries, and thus, to contribute to better recognition and intervention for maternal depression.

Methods: In this cross-sectional observational study, baseline data from early pregnancy (< 20 weeks) of the DALI (Vitamin D and Lifestyle Intervention for gestational diabetes mellitus prevention) study were analyzed. Maternal mental health was assessed with the World Health Organization Well-Being Index (WHO–5). Women were classified as having a low (WHO–5 $\leq$ 50) or high wellbeing.

Results.: A total of 735 pregnant women were included. The prevalence of having a low wellbeing was 27.2%, 95% CI [24.0, 30.4]. Multivariate analysis showed independent associations between low wellbeing and European ethnicity, $OR = .44$, 95% CI [.25, .77], shift work, $OR = 1.81$, 95% CI [1.11, 2.93], insufficient sleep, $OR = 3.30$, 95% CI [1.96, 5.55], self-efficacy, $OR = .95$, 95% CI [.92, .98], social support, $OR = .94$, 95% CI [.90, .99], and pregnancy-related worries (socioeconomic: $OR = 1.08$, 95% CI [1.02, 1.15]; health: $OR = 1.06$, 95% CI [1.01, 1.11]; relationship: $OR = 1.17$, 95% CI [1.05, 1.31]).

Conclusions: Mental health problems are common in European overweight/obese pregnant women. The identified correlates might help in early recognition and subsequent treatment of poor mental health problems during pregnancy. This is important to reduce the unfavorable effects of poor mental health on pregnancy outcomes.

Keywords: Mental health, Depression, Pregnancy, Obesity

* Correspondence: mireille.van-poppel@uni-graz.at
[1]Institute of Sport Science, University of Graz, Mozartgasse 14, 8010, Graz, Austria
[2]Department of Public and Occupational Health, Amsterdam Public Health Research Institute, VU University Medical Centre, Amsterdam, the Netherlands
Full list of author information is available at the end of the article

Background

The statement of the World Health Organization (WHO) that there can be no "health without mental health" [1] emphasizes the importance of mental health. Almost 30% of all people experience serious mental health problems, such as mood or anxiety disorders, across their lifetime [2]. Depression alone has a cross-cultural lifetime prevalence from 1 to 17% [3] and has a substantial influence both on disability and mortality [4]. It is associated with various adverse health conditions such as unexplained somatic symptoms [5], cardiovascular disease [6, 7], type 2 diabetes [8], HIV/AIDS [9] and tuberculosis [10]. In addition, depression is associated with obesity (body mass index (BMI) ≥ 30 kg/m^2) [11] and this association becomes stronger at an older age [12].

Moreover, depression is one of the more common complications during pregnancy [13] with a prevalence of up to 11% [14]. Pregnancy-related maternal depression has been found to be associated with obesity [15], poor socioeconomic status (including occupation, education and income), lack of social support, history of domestic violence or abuse, personal history of mental illness, unplanned pregnancy, adverse life events and high perceived stress, smoking, single status, past or present pregnancy complications and pregnancy loss [16, 17]. Furthermore, maternal depression appears to be inversely related with physical activity (PA) [18] and there is evidence to suggest that PA can help to reduce antenatal depression [19] as well as improve maternal physical health [20].

Depression in pregnancy not only affects the health of the woman, but also, potentially, the unborn child. The fetal period is a sensitive and challenging period, where changes and harm could have short- and long-term consequences for the development of the offspring. In contrast to parental genetic factors, fetal programming (e.g., programming of the child's stress response system) supposes *intra uterine* developmental origins of future health and disease, mainly through epigenetic mechanism [21]. Thus, a stressful in utero environment (e.g., poor maternal mental health) could lead to detrimental consequences for the offspring's physical and mental health [22, 23].

Indeed, there is substantial evidence that pregnancy-related depression is associated with higher risks for negative child outcomes, potentially lasting until late adolescence [24]. For instance, depression in pregnancy represents a risk factor for adverse birth outcomes such as preterm birth (< 37 weeks of gestation), low birth weight (< 2500 g), small-for-gestational age [25, 26] and poorer behavioral, neurophysiological and cognitive development (e.g., emotional and immune functioning) of the child [27, 28]. Consequently, there is no other period

in life where the statement "there is no health without mental health" is more true than during pregnancy [29].

Since obesity and depression are often comorbid [11], it is important to investigate mental health in obese pregnant women. The increasing prevalence of overweight (BMI ≥ 25 kg/m^2) and obese (BMI ≥ 30 kg/m^2) pregnant women is by itself already a growing public health concern worldwide [30, 31]. Maternal obesity increases the risk for pregnancy-related complications such as neonatal intensive care requirement, infection and haemorrhage [32] and may even affect future health of the offspring [33]. Although extensive research on the impact of obesity on maternal physical health has been carried out, less attention has been paid to relationship of obesity and maternal mental health. In particular, a better understanding of factors associated with poor mental health in obese pregnant women, and opportunities for early recognition and management is most important.

However, studies concerning mental health in pregnancy were often performed in low-risk populations such as women without serious health conditions and European-wide studies on a broad range of maternal mental health correlates are sadly lacking. This study combines these two aspects with the objective to explore the role of correlates, including lifestyle, socioeconomic, biological, and pregnancy-specific factors, associated with poor mental health in early pregnancy in a large group of overweight/obese European women.

Methods

Study design and setting

This cross-sectional observational study was part of the DALI (Vitamin D and Lifestyle Intervention for gestational diabetes mellitus prevention) project (ISRCTN70595832), which aimed to identify the best available preventive intervention (healthy eating (HE), PA, vitamin D) for gestational diabetes mellitus in a European cohort of obese pregnant women. Therefore, following a pilot study [34], a randomized controlled trial was implemented in nine European countries: Austria, Belgium, Denmark, Italy, Ireland, the Netherlands, Poland, Spain and the United Kingdom. Detailed study design and data collection of the DALI project were published previously [35]. Participants were recruited from January 2012 to April 2015 by participating hospitals, obstetrician, midwifes and general practices and randomly allocated to one of the eight intervention arms (HE, PA, HE & PA, HE & PA & vitamin D, HE & PA & placebo, vitamin D alone, placebo alone, control). Measurements took place at baseline (< 20 weeks of gestation), 24–28 weeks, 35–37 weeks and after delivery. Participants receiving the lifestyle interventions were assigned a lifestyle coach and those receiving the vitamin D interventions were asked to take four vitamin D tablets per day (each containing on average 400 IU vitamin D) from randomization until delivery. The lifestyle coaching was based on principles of patient empowerment and cognitive behavioral techniques inspired by motivational interviewing and included five face-to-face sessions, up to four telephone sessions, handbooks and educational materials in order to increase PA, HE or both.

For the purpose of the present study, cross-sectional data from early pregnancy (< 20 weeks; baseline) of the pilot study, Lifestyle trial and Vitamin D trial were used. The study received ethical approval in all nine countries. All participants provided written informed consent.

Participants

Inclusion criteria were defined as singleton pregnancy, less than 20 weeks of gestation, pre-pregnancy BMI ≥ 29 kg/m^2 (based on self-reported weight and measured height) or BMI ≥ 29 kg/m^2 at baseline measurement and age ≥ 18 years. The BMI cut off was based on data on the European obesity prevalence to ensure sufficiency in the recruiting process for countries with lower rates of maternal obesity [36]. Other exclusion criteria were pre-existing diabetes, inability to walk ≥100 m safely, multiple pregnancy, requiring a complex diet, significant chronic medical condition or psychiatric disease, unable to speak the major language of the country of recruitment fluently or unable to converse with the lifestyle coach in another language for which translated materials existed.

Of the 3544 women approached, 1069 (30.2%) consented to participate. Of those, a total of 738 women between 18.7 and 47.1 years (M = 32.0, SD = 5.4) fulfilled all inclusion criteria and were randomized and included at baseline. Seventy-six (10.3%) were overweight at baseline (BMI < 30). Please note that from now on we refer to the whole sample as *obese*, including this percentage of overweight pregnant women. Three of 738 women did not complete mental health measurements, and therefore, were excluded from the present study. Sociodemographic characteristics are presented in Table 1 in detail. Number of missing data was below 5% for all variables (see Table 1), except for heart rate data (5.6%). Differences between missing and non-missing data were assessed if there were more than 5% missing values for one variable.

Measures
Mental health
Assessment of maternal mental health was based on the World Health Organization Well-Being Index (WHO-5), a widely-used, unidimensional instrument measuring subjective wellbeing [37]. It has shown to be a valid screening instrument for clinical depression with high sensitivity and specificity, and has been validated for all languages required in the present multi-national study [38, 39].The scale consists of five items, each rated on a 6-point Likert scale (0: at no time, 5: all of the time), and following total scores, standardized scores (0–100) are calculated. Based on current literature on sensitivity and specificity for clinical depression, values ≤50 were

Table 1 Maternal socio-demographic characteristics

Characteristic	Total (N = 735)	Low wellbeing[a] (n = 200)	High wellbeing[a] (n = 535)
Age, *years* ($M \pm SD$)	32.0 ± 5.4	31.3 ± 5.9	32.3 ± 5.2
BMI, *kg/m^2* (median (IQR))	33.4 (31.4–36.6)	33.4 (31.7–36.9)	33.4 (31.3–36.6)
Pre-pregnancy BMI, *kg/m^2* (median (IQR))	32.7 (30.5–35.8)	33.0 (30.9–35.7)	32.5 (30.2–35.8)
Ethnicity, *European descent* (n (%))	638 (86.8)	160 (80.0)	478 (89.3)
Education (n (%), total = 734)			
Low (no qualification/intermediate)	89 (12.1)	28 (14.0)	61 (11.4)
Medium (higher school/apprenticeship)	233 (31.7)	75 (37.5)	158 (29.5)
High (diploma/university)	412 (56.1)	96 (48.0)	316 (59.1)
Occupational status (n (%), total = 733)			
Home duties	63 (8.6)	21 (10.5)	42 (7.9)
Unemployed/not able to work	109 (14.8)	37 (18.5)	72 (13.5)
Working (fulltime/part-time/student)	561 (76.3)	141 (70.5)	420 (78.5)
Household composition, *living with partner* (n (%))	672 (91.4)	177 (88.5)	495 (92.5)
Marital status, *with partner* (n (%), total = 734)	690 (93.9)	179 (89.5)	511 (95.5)
Shift work, *yes* (n (%), total = 730)	149 (20.3)	52 (26.0)	97 (18.1)

[a]Based on the World Health Organization Well-Being Index (WHO-5). Values ≤50 were considered as low wellbeing (poor maternal mental health), values >50 as high wellbeing

considered as low wellbeing (poor maternal mental health), values above 50 as high wellbeing [38]. Cronbach Alpha (α) was 0.82 for the whole scale.

Potential correlates

The selection of variables collected at baseline was based on current literature [7, 16, 17] and then clustered into 4 groups: a) socio-demographic (age, pre-pregnancy BMI, BMI at baseline, ethnicity, education, household composition, occupational status, shift work, marital status), b) lifestyle (smoking, alcohol consumption, hours of sleep per day (24 h), days of insufficient sleep per month, snoring, PA), c) biological (polycystic ovary syndrome, first degree relative with diabetes, fasting plasma glucose, fasting plasma insulin, Homeostasis Model Assessment of Insulin Resistance (HOMA-IR), systolic and diastolic blood pressure, chronic hypertension, resting heart rate) and d) pregnancy characteristics (weeks of gestation (at baseline), pregnant before, number of own children, previous stillbirths/miscarriages, previous fetal macrosomia, previous congenital malformation, previous gestational diabetes, pre-pregnancy to baseline weight gain, attitude/importance of current weight, social support, outcome expectancies, self-efficacy, pregnancy-related worries). Physiological parameters (plasma glucose, plasma insulin, blood pressure, heart rate) were quantified by standardized, commercially available devices, whereas all other variables were self-reported.

Hours of sleep per day (24 h), snoring and insufficient sleep were retrieved from single items (How many hours do you sleep per day on average; How many days in the last month have you had the feeling of insufficient sleep; How many days per week do you snore/are told you snore). Sleep hours per day were categorized into ≤6 h, 6–9 h and ≥9 h [40], ethnicity into European and non-European, education into low (no qualification/intermediate), medium (higher school/apprenticeship) and high (diploma/university), occupational status into working, not working and home duties, household composition into living with partner and not living with partner, marital status into with partner and without partner.

PA was based on the pregnancy physical activity questionnaire (PPAQ), which is a valid instrument for the assessment of PA during pregnancy [41]. In addition to 32 original activities, two more questions concerning *cycling to work* and *cycling for fun* have been added. Time spent in each activity was asked, and then multiplied by its intensity, resulting in an average weekly energy expenditure (MET hours/week) for each activity. After categorization of activities into sedentary, light, moderate or vigorous, total MET hours/week of moderate-to-vigorous physical activity (MVPA) and sedentary behavior (SB) were used for analysis.

Pregnancy-related worries have shown to be related to mood outcomes and were assessed by the Cambridge Worry Scale [42], a 13-item questionnaire (6-point Likert scale; 0: not a worry, 5: major worry) measuring worries across four domains: sociomedical (α = .71), socioeconomic (α = .59), health (α = .66) and relationship (α = .61). Cronbach Alpha for the whole scale was .77. Domain scores were used for analysis. Attitude (e.g., *It is important for me to manage my weight*), social support (e.g., *I am satisfied with the level of support I am receiving for eating healthily from my partner, family and friends*), outcome expectancies (e.g., *Staying physically active during this pregnancy, will help to reduce health risks for my baby*) and self-efficacy (e.g., *I am confident that I will succeed in managing my weight*) were based on the Health Action Process Approach (HAPA) model [43], referring to PA, nutrition and weight management during pregnancy, and collected with items on a 10-point Likert scale. Attitude to current weight as well as social support consisted of two items (α_a = .76, α_s = .87), outcome expectancies of six items (α = .93) and self-efficacy of five items (α = .88). Sum scores of each dimension were used for further analysis.

Statistical analysis

Statistical analyses were performed using SPSS Data Analysis version 22.0 (IBM Corp, Armonk, NY, USA). Descriptive statistics for all variables were calculated, including mean and standard deviation for continuous variables with normal distribution, median and interquartile range (IQR) for continuous variables without normal distribution, and frequencies and percentages for categorical variables. Normal distribution was assessed by Shapiro-Wilk, Q-Q-Plots and Histogram. Evaluation of missing and non-missing data was done by t test, Welch test and Chi square or Fisher's exact tests.

To evaluate the association between poor maternal mental health and potential correlates, logistic regression models were used, comprising a three-step procedure. In all analysis, the outcome was defined as the dichotomous variable derived from the WHO-5 index (low wellbeing vs. high wellbeing). Odds ratios (*OR*) with 95% confidence intervals (CI) were calculated for each association. In a first step, bivariate logistic regression models between outcome and each potential correlate were calculated. Significant correlates were included in the next step. In this second step, four multivariate logistic regression models were calculated, set up of blocks with related correlates (1) socioeconomic status (2) sleep (3) worries (4) perceptions and attitudes. All correlates of one block were entered at the same time and significant correlates were included in the next step. In this third and final step, remaining correlates were analyzed in one multivariate logistic regression model, entering all correlates at the same time.

Significance in step one and two was considered as $p < .10$ to allay beta error. In step 3 as well as in all other analyses, significance was considered as $p < .05$. BMI at baseline (based on measured weight and height) and pre-pregnancy BMI (based on self-reported weight and measured height) were both included in the first step, but if significant, BMI at baseline was used for step two and three. Linearity between outcome and each potential correlate was assessed by the interaction term between the potential correlate and its log transformation within the binary analysis, and if significant, tertiles of the predictor were calculated. To consider the possible clustering effect within countries, multilevel analysis with a random intercept was performed with Stata 12 (Stata-Corp, College Station, TX, USA). Multilevel analysis was carried out for the final model (step three), including a null model (random-intercept-only) and a random intercept model.

Results
Sample characteristics
Two hundred women (27.2%, 95% CI [24.0, 30.4]) had a "low wellbeing" and 535 women (72.8%) had a "high wellbeing" based on the pre-defined WHO-5 scores. In total, 561 women (76.5%) were working and 690 (94.0%) had a partner. 412 (56.1%) women were highly educated (diploma or university), whereas 89 (12.1%) had only a low education (no qualification or intermediate). Sample characteristics are displayed in Table 1 and Table 2 in detail.

Comparison of missing and non-missing data of resting heart rate showed no significant differences ($p \geq .05$) in age, education, ethnicity, household composition, shift work, marital status, BMI, gestational week, pregnancy-related worries, sleep hours, systolic and diastolic blood pressure. Nonetheless, significant differences were found between missing/non-missing data of resting heart rate and maternal mental health ($p < .01$) and occupational status ($p < .05$).

Bivariate analysis
Bivariate logistic regression models (first step) showed significant associations ($p < .10$, data not shown) between low wellbeing and age, BMI at baseline, weeks of gestation, ethnicity, household composition, education, occupational status, attitude to current weight, self-efficacy, social support, pregnancy-related worries (sociomedical, socioeconomic, health, relationship), marital status, pregnant before, shift work, hours of sleep per day, days of insufficient sleep per month, snoring, and systolic blood pressure.

No significant associations ($p \geq .10$, data not shown) were displayed between low wellbeing and smoking, alcohol consumption, outcome expectancies, number of own children, previous stillbirths/miscarriages, previous fetal macrosomia, previous congenital malformation, PA, previous gestational diabetes, chronic hypertension, polycystic ovary syndrome, pre to baseline weight gain, fasting plasma glucose, fasting plasma insulin, HOMA-IR, diastolic blood pressure, and resting heart rate.

Multivariate analysis
In a second step, four multivariate models (a-d) were developed. Remaining variables associated with socioeconomic status (ethnicity, household composition, education, occupational status, marital status, shift work) were analyzed in a first model (a). This model, χ^2 (8, N = 727) = 29.79, $p < .01$, $R^2 = .04$, showed significant associations between low wellbeing and ethnicity (European vs. not European: OR = .52, 95% CI [.33, .83], $p < .01$), occupational status (not working vs. working: OR = 1.51, 95% CI [.94, 2.41], $p = .09$), marital status (with vs. without partner: OR = .39, 95% CI [.18, .88], $p = .02$) and shift work (yes vs. no: OR = 1.79, 95% CI [1.19, 2.69], $p < .01$), but no longer with household composition ($p = .53$) and education (low: $p = .61$, medium: $p = .13$).

The second model (b), χ^2 (5, N = 704) = 53.44, $p < .01$, $R^2 = .07$, consisting of remaining variables related to sleeping quality (hours of sleep, days of insufficient sleep, snoring), showed significant associations of low wellbeing with hours of sleep per day (9 or more vs. normal: OR = 1.60, 95% CI [1.05, 2.45], $p = .03$) and days of insufficient sleep per month (moderate vs. low: OR = 1.73, 95% CI [1.08, 2.77], $p = .02$; high vs. low: OR = 4.13, 95% CI [2.63, 6.48], $p < .01$), but no longer with snoring ($p = .32$).

The third model (c), χ^2 (4, N = 720) = 72.94, $p < .01$, $R^2 = .10$, referring to remaining variables of the Cambridge Worry Scale, showed significant associations of low wellbeing with socioeconomic worries (OR = 1.11, 95% CI [1.05, 1.17], $p < .01$), health-related worries (OR = 1.06, 95% CI [1.02, 1.11], $p < .01$) and relationship-related worries (OR = 1.24, 95% CI [1.12, 1.37], $p < .01$), but no longer with sociomedical worries ($p = .90$).

The fourth model (d), χ^2 (3, N = 725) = 66.49, $p < .01$, $R^2 = .09$, referring to variables from the HAPA model, showed significant associations of low wellbeing and attitude to current weight (OR = 1.10, 95% CI [1.05, 1.16], $p < .01$), self-efficacy (OR = .96, 95% CI [.93, .98], $p < .01$) as well as social support (OR = .91, 95% CI [.87, .95], $p < .01$).

In the third and final step, all remaining variables of step two were analyzed within one multivariate logistic regression model. Results are displayed in Table 3, showing that low wellbeing was significantly associated with

Table 2 Specific maternal characteristics

Characteristic	Total (N = 735)	Low wellbeing[a] (n = 200)	High wellbeing[a] (n = 535)
Lifestyle			
Smoking behaviour, yes (n (%))	122 (16.6)	37 (18.5)	85 (15.9)
Any alcohol consumption, yes (n (%))	43 (5.9)	12 (6.0)	31 (5.8)
Sleep, hours per day (median (IQR), total = 734)	8.0 (7.0–8.5)	8.0 (7.0–9.0)	8.0 (7.0–8.0)
Insufficient sleep, days per month (median (IQR, total = 722)	7.0 (3.0–15.0)	15.0 (5.0–20.0)	5.0 (2.0–15.0)
Snoring, days per week (median (IQR, total = 714)	0.0 (0–2.0)	0.0 (0–3.0)	0.0 (0–2.0)
PPAQ, MET·h·wk.$^{-1}$ (median (IQR))			
MVPA	70.2 (34.7–127.8)	74.7 (32.3–128.2)	69.0 (35.5–127.8)
SB	42.0 (19.1–62.1)	36.8 (18.6–61.1)	43.2 (19.4–62.7)
Biological			
First degree relative with diabetes, yes (n (%))	168 (22.9)	48 (24.0)	120 (22.4)
Chronic hypertension, yes (n (%), total = 730)	98 (13.3)	30 (15.0)	68 (12.7)
Polycystic ovary syndrome, yes (n (%), total = 728)	73 (9.9)	24 (12.0)	49 (9.2)
Fasting plasma glucose, mmol/L (median (IQR), total = 727)	4.6 (4.3–4.8)	4.6 (4.3–4.8)	4.6 (4.3–4.8)
Fasting plasma insulin, mmol/L (median (IQR), total = 720)	12.7 (9.8–17.5)	13.1 (10.1–17.5)	12.5 (9.5–17.4)
HOMA-IR (median (IQR), total = 717)	2.6 (1.9–3.6)	2.7 (2.0–3.6)	2.6 (1.9–3.6)
Systolic blood pressure (median (IQR), total = 733)	116 (109–123)	114 (107–121)	116 (110–124)
Diastolic blood pressure (median (IQR), total = 733)	72 (67–79)	71 (67–77)	72 (67–79)
Resting heart rate (median (IQR), total = 694)	79 (72–86)	79 (71–87)	79 (73–85)
Pregnancy-specific			
Gestational week (median (IQR))	15.1 (13.4–16.7)	14.9 (13.3–16.2)	15.3 (13.6–17.0)
Number of own children (n (%), total = 734)			
Zero	366 (49.8)	93 (46.5)	273 (51.0)
One	256 (34.8)	73 (36.5)	183 (34.2)
Two or more	112 (15.2)	34 (17.0)	78 (14.6)
Pregnant before, yes (n (%))	460 (62.6)	136 (68.0)	324 (60.6)
Previous stillbirths/miscarriage, ≥ 1 (n (%), total = 445)	200 (27.2)	63 (31.5)	137 (25.6)
Previous fetal macrosomia, yes (n (%), total = 453)	81 (11.0)	22 (11.0)	59 (11.0)
Previous congenital malformation, yes (n (%), total = 454)	16 (2.2)	4 (2.0)	12 (2.2)
Previous gestational diabetes, yes (n (%), total = 455)	36 (4.9)	12 (6.0)	24 (4.5)
Pre to baseline weight gain, kg (median (IQR))	1.7 (−0.4–4.0)	1.6 (−0.6–4.2)	1.7 (−0.3–4.0)
Perceptions and attitude[b] (median (IQR))			
Attitude to current weight (total = 729)	16.0 (14.0–18.0)	17.0 (14.0–19.0)	16.0 (13.0–18.0)
Self-efficacy (total = 730)	35.0 (30.0–41.0)	31.0 (27.0–38.0)	37.0 (31.0–41.0)
Social support (total = 731)	16.0 (13.0–18.0)	14.0 (10.0–17.0)	16.0 (14.0–18.0)
Outcome expectancy (total = 723)	52.0 (46.0–58.0)	52.0 (46.0–58.0)	52.0 (46.0–58.0)
Cambridge worry scale (median (IQR))			
Total 13 items (total = 720)	18.0 (12.0–26.0)	24.0 (16.0–32.0)	17.0 (12.0–24.0)
Sociomedical (total = 731)	5.0 (2.0–8.0)	6.0 (2.0–10.0)	5.0 (2.0–8.0)
Socioeconomic (total = 733)	4.0 (2.0–7.0)	6.0 (3.0–9.0)	4.0 (1.0–6.0)
Health (total = 729)	8.0 (5.0–12.0)	10.0 (6.0–13.0)	8.0 (5.0–11.0)
Relationship (total = 729)	0.0 (0–2.0)	1.0 (0–3.0)	0.0 (0–1.0)

PPAQ = pregnancy physical activity questionnaire; MET = metabolic equivalents; MVPA = moderate-to-vigorous physical activity; SB = sedentary behavior
[a]Based on the World Health Organization Well-Being Index (WHO-5). Values ≤50 were considered as low wellbeing (poor maternal mental health), values >50 as high wellbeing. [b]Based on the Health Action Process Approach (HAPA) model [43]

Table 3 Multivariate logistic regression. Associations of low wellbeing and maternal characteristics

Maternal characteristic	Odds Ratio, 95% CI			
	OR	Lower	Upper	p
Ethnicity (European)	.44	.25	.77	< .01*
Marital status (with partner)	.45	.20	1.02	.06
Shift work (yes)	1.81	1.11	2.93	.02*
Occupational status (working = ref)				
Not working	1.39	.80	2.42	.24
Home duties	1.28	.59	2.78	.53
Sleep h/d (6–9 h = ref)[a]				
≤ 6 h	.90	.52	1.56	.70
≥ 9 h	1.11	.68	1.84	.67
Insufficient sleep d/m (low = ref)[b]				
Medium	1.26	.73	2.17	.41
High	3.30	1.96	5.55	< .01*
Perceptions and attitude[c]				
Attitude to current weight	1.05	.99	1.12	.11
Self-efficacy	.95	.92	.98	< .01*
Social support	.94	.90	.99	.03*
Cambridge worry scale				
Socioeconomic	1.08	1.02	1.15	.01*
Health	1.06	1.01	1.11	.03*
Relationship	1.17	1.05	1.31	< .01*
Age (young = ref)[d]				
middle	.81	.50	1.31	.39
old	.90	.54	1.49	.68
BMI at baseline	1.03	.98	1.08	.32
Weeks of gestation	.95	.87	1.03	.17
Pregnant before (yes)	1.11	.72	1.71	.64
Systolic blood pressure	.99	.97	1.01	.21

Only variables remaining after step two were included in the model (method = enter, outcome = WHO-5 index: low wellbeing), $\chi 2$ (21, N = 692) = 163.71, p < .001, R^2 = .21, Durbin Watson = 2.10
[a]sleep hours per day (24 h, self-reported); ≤ 6 h; 6–9 h; ≥ 9 h
[b]days per month (self-reported), based on tertiles
[c]Based on the Health Action Process Approach (HAPA) model [43]
[d]based on tertiles
*< .05

non-European ethnicity, shift work, insufficient sleep, low self-efficacy, low social support and pregnancy-related worries (socioeconomic, health, relationship), χ^2 (21, N = 692) = 163.71, p < .001, R^2 = .21.

Although multilevel analysis revealed significant level 2 variances for country, τ_{00} = .10, 95% CI [.02, .48], ρ = .03, p < .05, in the null model (random-intercept-only), there was no significant improvement of the final model in step 3, when adding a random intercept. Therefore, results of step 3 are presented without a random intercept (Table 3).

Discussion

In summary, this study showed independent associations between low wellbeing and non-European ethnicity, shift work, insufficient sleep, low self-efficacy, low social support and pregnancy-related worries (socioeconomic, health, relationship) in obese pregnant women.

A recent meta-analysis [15] on the prevalence of depressive symptoms in pregnancy showed higher rates for obese (33%) than normal-weight pregnant women (22.6%). Likewise, in the present study, 27.2% of all women with BMI ≥ 29 had a low wellbeing. There is a reciprocal relationship between poor mental health and obesity [11] and both have been linked with numerous adverse pregnancy outcomes such as neonatal intensive care requirement, preterm birth and gestational diabetes [24, 32, 33]. Thus, healthcare providers should be aware of the high prevalence of obese pregnant women experiencing mental health problems.

A number of studies reported a broad range of potential correlates of maternal mental health [16, 17], although some variability appears, largely based either on bivariate or multivariate analysis, sample composition and study design. For example, the present study demonstrated an association between maternal mental health and European ethnicity, which is in line with previous studies, showing both independent and mutual influences of ethnicity and variables of socioeconomic status (e.g., occupation, education, income) on maternal mental health [16, 44, 45]. Likewise, sleep quality is associated with depression in the general population [46] and during pregnancy, where poor sleep quality and sleep loss are linked with a greater risk of both maternal mood problems [47] and adverse birth outcomes [48]. This confirms our finding of the linkage between low wellbeing and insufficient sleep. In addition, previous studies confirm our findings of associations between low wellbeing and individual variables such as low self-efficacy, worrying and less perceived social support as well [16].

In contrast to other studies, we did not find associations (neither univariate nor multivariate) for previously described correlates of mental health in pregnancy such as age, alcohol consumption, smoking, number of own children or previous pregnancy complications [16, 17]. This may be due to the selection of women participating in the DALI study, small frequencies for some correlates (e.g., alcohol consumption, previous congenital malformation, previous gestational diabetes) or restriction of inclusion for BMI and gestational week.

Interestingly, no association between low wellbeing and PA was found, in contrast to previous research [18, 49, 50]. This may be related to the study context, where women were included in a lifestyle trial, partly focused on physically activity. Moreover, we studied women in early pregnancy, while the decrease in PA may be more pronounced later in pregnancy [18].

According to pregnancy-related worries, pregnancy is a sensitive period in a woman's life, and is likely to evoke heightened levels of anxiety and worrying [51] with unique influences on mood outcomes [42]. As shown in the present study, pregnancy-related worries should be considered as possible correlates of poor maternal mental health states. Furthermore, it may be possible that pregnancy-related worries play a crucial role in intervention strategies on improving maternal mental health. However, in pursuance of achieving the best outcomes when developing such intervention strategies, more insight into the relevance of a woman's current worries in pregnancy and how to deal with them is needed.

Under the terms of the health action process approach [43], social support and self-efficacy are important factors for forming intentions and maintaining changes in health behaviors (e.g., for PA or HE). Since many studies reported an inverse relationship between depression in pregnancy and PA [18], it could be possible that lack of social support and low self-efficacy deteriorate the unfavorable effects of an unhealthy lifestyle on mental and physical health. These effects might be even stronger in late pregnancy. Considering low social support and self-efficacy as correlates might help for an early recognition of poor maternal mental health states and the design of interventions. In particular, implementing intervention strategies, which include for instance, participation of family members and friends in order to increase social support or specific tasks to increase perceived self-efficacy are advisable. The inclusion of such individual characteristics into tailored intervention strategies would probably result in the best outcomes of maternal mental health.

Finally, the well-known association between poor mental health and shift work [52] was confirmed in pregnancy as well. In short, working in shifts (e.g., night work, rotating shifts) disturbs the circadian rhythm, a dynamic system which regulates most of our physiological processes based on the day-night cycle, and which is associated with pregnancy complications such as pre-term birth or low birth weight [53]. Together with sleep deprivation, the disruption of the circadian system could act as stressor with detrimental consequences on many body systems, including woman's reproductive function, while leading to a cumulative wear out of the whole system [54]. With this in view, integrating shift work as a correlate of poor maternal mental health is highly recommended.

During the last decade, researchers have shown an increased interest in mental health during pregnancy. However, the use of maternal mental health correlates for early recognition of poor mental health into clinical practice seems to be limited as yet. Clearly, some of the identified correlates would be difficult to routinely assess

in clinical practice but others (e.g., non-European ethnicity, worrying, insufficient sleep, shift work) could be easily assessed without the requirement of laboratory equipment or standardized questionnaires. Such an implementation (e.g., for screening) would be possible both in primary (e.g., general practitioners, midwifes) and secondary health care settings (obstetricians) and could help in early recognition of maternal mental health problems at a low threshold. In addition, identified correlates give direction to further intervention development for prevention or treatment of mental health problems in pregnancy. Finally, because of the reciprocal relationship between obesity and poor mental health, tackling mental health problems of obese pregnant women might help to mitigate part of the adverse effects of obesity on pregnancy outcomes.

Limitations and strengths

Our study has limitations and strengths that deserve to be mentioned. First, due to the cross-sectional design, no conclusions about causality can be drawn. To confirm whether the identified factors are indeed predictors for low mood in the course of pregnancy and to establish the consequences for both the woman and the child, longitudinal studies are warranted. In addition, the cross-sectional design and the chosen analysis strategy hinders the detection of causal pathways of variables associated with mental health in pregnancy. However, this study focused on the detection of correlates of poor mental health rather than causal pathways. Secondly, our data were derived from a large group of women from different European countries participating in the DALI study who might have a better mental health compared to others, possibly leading to a selection bias.

Yet, 27% reported low wellbeing, as defined by their WHO-5 score, which is in concert with previous research on other populations, and thus does not suggest an underestimation. Of course, we need to acknowledge that we used a relatively short measure of mental health (subjective wellbeing) rather than a diagnostic interview, which is the gold standard for establishing the true prevalence of major depression. Such a procedure was not feasible in the context of this large multi-national lifestyle study. Regardless, the WHO-5 scale has shown good screening properties for clinically relevant depressive symptoms, was used worldwide and tested in all languages required in the present study, as well as variations of the scale dependent on country of recruitment were statistically evaluated in the present study [38, 39]. Therefore, a bias is very unlikely and our data can be regarded as valid. Future studies should aim to thoroughly investigate the prevalence and course of minor and major depression in pregnancy.

Nonetheless, to our knowledge, this is the first study, which investigated a broad range of potential correlates of poor maternal mental health in a crucial period such as the early pregnancy in conjunction with a wide and representative European sample.

Conclusions

One of the great challenges is to recognize maternal mental health problems very early in pregnancy in order to prevent harmful health consequences. This study showed that mental health problems are common in European obese pregnant women (27.2%) and that non-European ethnicity, having shift work, insufficient sleep, low self-efficacy, low social support, and pregnancy-related worries have to be considered as correlates of poor maternal mental health in this population. Other factors such as smoking, alcohol consumption, marital status, occupational status and maternal age do not seem be associated with maternal mental health in this population. Some of these identified correlates may further help for an early recognition in clinical practice and the design of interventions. Especially insufficient sleep and non-European ethnicity seem to play a prominent role according to their effect sizes.

Abbreviations

BMI: body mass index; HAPA: health action process approach; HE: healthy eating; HOMA-IR: homeostasis model assessment of insulin resistance; IQR: interquartile range; MET: metabolic equivalent of task; MVPA: moderate-to-vigorous physical activity; PA: physical activity; PPAQ: pregnancy physical activity questionnaire; SB: sedentary behavior; WHO: world health organization

Acknowledgments

The authors thank Kenneth B. Smale for proofreading the manuscript.

Funding

The DALI project was registered as an RCT (ISRCTN70595832) and received funding from the European Community's 7th Framework Programme (FP7/2007–2013) under grant agreement no 242187. In the Netherlands, further funding was provided by the Netherlands Organisation for Health Research and Development (ZonMw; grant number: 200,310,013). The funders had no role in any aspect of the study beyond funding.

Authors' contributions

MS contributed to the data analysis and writing of the manuscript and took the lead in redrafting the script following editorial review. DS coordinated the study. DS GD RC JA AKW FAA RD DH PD EM EWO AZ AL MD AB FD DJ LLA FS MP contributed to the conception and design of the study. KB GJ JJ SG JH contributed to the acquisition of data. MS AB MP contributed to the analysis and interpretation of data. All authors read and corrected draft versions of the manuscript and approved the final manuscript.

Ethics approval and consent to participate

All procedures performed in studies involving human participants were in accordance with the ethical standards of the institutional and/or national research committee and with the 1964 Helsinki declaration and its later amendments or comparable ethical standards. For each country, the study design and procedures were approved by the local Medical Ethics committee (Amsterdam, the Netherlands: Ethical Committee of the VU University Medical Center; Barcelona, Spain: Comité Ético de Investigación Clínica de la Fundació de Gestió Sanitaria del Hospital de la Santa Creu i Sant Pau; Cambridge, United Kingdom: National Research Ethics Service, Norwich Research Ethics Committee; Copenhagen and Odense, Denmark: De Videnskabsetiske Komiteer D for Region Hovedstaden; Galway, Ireland: Clinical Research Ethics Committee, Galway University Hospitals; Leuven, Belgium: Commissie Medische Ethiek van de Universitaire Ziekenhuizen KU Leuven; Padua, Italy: Il Comitato Etico per la Sperimentazione Clinica della Provincia di Padova; Poznan, Poland: Komisja Bioetyczna Przy Uniwersytecie Medycznym im. Karola Marcinkowskiego W Poznaniu; Vienna, Austria: Ethik Kommission Medizinische Universität Wien). Written informed consent was obtained from all individual participants included in the study.

Consent for publication

Not applicable.

Competing interests

The authors declare that they have no competing interests.

Author details

[1]Institute of Sport Science, University of Graz, Mozartgasse 14, 8010, Graz, Austria. [2]Department of Public and Occupational Health, Amsterdam Public Health Research Institute, VU University Medical Centre, Amsterdam, the Netherlands. [3]Department of Development and Regeneration KULeuven, University of Leuven, Leuven, Belgium and Faculty of Medicine and Health Sciences, Centre for Research and Innovation in Care (CRIC), University of Antwerp, Belgium and Faculty of Health and Social Work, research unit Healthy Living, UC Leuven-Limburg, Leuven, Belgium. [4]Institute of Metabolic Science, Addenbrookes Hospital, Cambridge, England and Macarthur Clinical School, Western Sydney University, Sydney, Australia. [5]Department of Obstetrics and Gynecology, Medizinische Universität Graz, Graz, Austria. [6]Institut de Recerca de L'Hospital de la Santa Creu i Sant Pau, Barcelona, Spain. [7]CIBER Bioengineering, Biomaterials and Nanotechnology, Instituto de Salud Carlos III, Zaragaza, Spain. [8]Division of Endocrinology and Metabolism, Department of Medicine III, Medical University of Vienna, Vienna, Austria. [9]KU Leuven Department of Development and Regeneration: Pregnancy, Fetus and Neonate, Gynaecology and Obstetrics, University Hospitals, Leuven, Belgium. [10]Department of Obstetrics and Gynaecology Division of Obstetrics and Prenatal Medicine, Erasmus Medical Centre, Rotterdam, The Netherlands. [11]Recherche en Santé Lawson SA, Bronschhofen, Switzerland. [12]Center for Pregnant Women with Diabetes, Departments of Endocrinology and Obstetrics, Rigshospitalet, University of Copenhagen, Copenhagen, Denmark. [13]Division of Reproduction, Poznan University of Medical Sciences, Poznan, Poland. [14]Universita Degli Studi di Padova, Padova, Italy. [15]Università di Pisa, Pisa, Italy. [16]National University of Ireland, Galway, Ireland. [17]Odense University Hospital, Odense, Denmark. [18]Department of Medical Psychology, VU University Medical Centre, Amsterdam, the Netherlands. [19]Department of Medical Psychology, Academic Medical Centre, Amsterdam, the Netherlands.

References

1. World Health Organization Mental health-facing the challenges, building solutions: report from the WHO European ministerial conference: World Health Organization; 2005.
2. Steel Z, Marnane C, Iranpour C, Chey T, Jackson JW, Patel V, Silove D. The global prevalence of common mental disorders: a systematic review and meta-analysis 1980-2013. Int J Epidemiol. 2014;43:476–93. doi:10.1093/ije/dyu038.
3. Kessler RC, Bromet EJ. The epidemiology of depression across cultures. Annu Rev Public Health. 2013;34:119–38. doi:10.1146/annurev-publhealth-031912-114409 .
4. Prince M, Patel V, Saxena S, Maj M, Maselko J, Phillips MR, Rahman A. No health without mental health. Lancet. 2007;370:859–77. doi:10.1016/S0140-6736(07)61238-0 .

5. Russo J, Katon W, Sullivan M, Clark M, Buchwald D. Severity of somatization and its relationship to psychiatric disorders and personality. Psychosomatics. 1994;35:546–56.

6. Compare A, Zarbo C, Manzoni GM, Castelnuovo G, Baldassari E, Bonardi A, et al. Social support, depression, and heart disease: a ten year literature review. Front Psychol. 2013; doi:10.3389/fpsyg.2013.00384 .

7. Cohen BE, Edmondson D, Kronish IM. State of the art review: depression, stress, anxiety, and cardiovascular disease. Am J Hypertens. 2015;28:1295–302. doi:10.1093/ajh/hpv047 .

8. Holt RIG, de Groot M, Golden SH. Diabetes and depression. Curr Diab Rep. 2014; doi: 10.1007/s11892-014-0491-3.

9. Ciesla JA, Roberts JE. Meta-analysis of the relationship between HIV infection and risk for depressive disorders. AJP. 2001;158:725–30. doi:10.1176/appi.ajp.158.5.725 .

10. Sweetland A, Oquendo M, Wickramaratne P, Weissman M, Wainberg M. Depression: a silent driver of the global tuberculosis epidemic. World Psychiatry. 2014;13:325–6. doi:10.1002/wps.20134 .

11. Luppino FS, de Wit LM, Bouvy PF, Stijnen T, Cuijpers P, Penninx BWJH, Zitman FG. Overweight, obesity, and depression. Arch Gen Psychiatry. 2010; 67:220. doi:10.1001/archgenpsychiatry.2010.2.

12. Kivimaki M, Batty GD, Singh-Manoux A, Nabi H, Sabia S, Tabak AG, et al. Association between common mental disorder and obesity over the adult life course. Br J Psychiatry. 2009;195:149–55. doi:10.1192/bjp.bp.108.057299 .

13. Gavin NI, Gaynes BN, Lohr KN, Meltzer-Brody S, Gartlehner G, Swinson T. Perinatal depression: a systematic review of prevalence and incidence. Obstet Gynecol. 2005;106:1071–83.

14. Howard LM, Molyneaux E, Dennis C-L, Rochat T, Stein A, Milgrom J. Non-psychotic mental disorders in the perinatal period. Lancet. 2014;384:1775–88. doi:10.1016/S0140-6736(14)61276-9 .

15. Molyneaux E, Poston L, Ashurst-Williams S, Howard LM. Obesity and mental disorders during pregnancy and postpartum: a systematic review and meta-analysis. Obstet Gynecol. 2014;123:857–67. doi:10.1097/AOG.0000000000000170 .

16. Biaggi A, Conroy S, Pawlby S, Pariante CM. Identifying the women at risk of antenatal anxiety and depression: a systematic review. J Affect Disord. 2016; 191:62–77. doi:10.1016/j.jad.2015.11.014 .

17. Lancaster CA, Gold KJ, Flynn HA, Yoo H, Marcus SM, Davis MM. Risk factors for depressive symptoms during pregnancy: a systematic review. Am J Obstet Gynecol. 2010;202:5–14. doi:10.1016/j.ajog.2009.09.007 .

18. Poudevigne MS, O'Connor PJA. Review of physical activity patterns in pregnant women and their relationship to psychological health. Sports Med. 2006;36:19–38.

19. Daley AJ, Foster L, Long G, Palmer C, Robinson O, Walmsley H, Ward R. The effectiveness of exercise for the prevention and treatment of antenatal depression: systematic review with meta-analysis. BJOG. 2015;122:57–62. doi:10.1111/1471-0528.12909 .

20. Downs DS, Chasan-Taber L, Evenson KR, Leiferman J, Yeo S. Physical activity and pregnancy. Res Q Exerc Sport. 2012;83:485–502. doi:10.1080/02701367.2012.10599138 .

21. Barker DJP. The origins of the developmental origins theory. J Intern Med. 2007;261:412–7. doi:10.1111/j.1365-2796.2007.01809.x .

22. Bale TL, Baram TZ, Brown AS, Goldstein JM, Insel TR, McCarthy MM, et al. Early life programming and neurodevelopmental disorders. Biol Psychiatry. 2010;68:314–9. doi:10.1016/j.biopsych.2010.05.028 .

23. Kim DR, Bale TL, Epperson CN. Prenatal programming of mental illness: current understanding of relationship and mechanisms. Curr Psychiatry Rep. 2015; doi:10.1007/s11920-014-0546-9 .

24. Stein A, Pearson RM, Goodman SH, Rapa E, Rahman A, McCallum M, et al. Effects of perinatal mental disorders on the fetus and child. Lancet. 2014; 384:1800–19. doi:10.1016/S0140-6736(14)61277-0 .

25. Accortt EE, Cheadle ACD, Dunkel Schetter C. Prenatal depression and adverse birth outcomes: an updated systematic review. Matern Child Health J. 2015;19:1306–37. doi:10.1007/s10995-014-1637-2 .

26. Szegda K, Markenson G, Bertone-Johnson ER, Chasan-Taber L. Depression during pregnancy: a risk factor for adverse neonatal outcomes? A critical review of the literature. J Matern Fetal Neonatal Med. 2013;27:960–7. doi:10.3109/14767058.2013.845157 .

27. O'Connor TG, Monk C, Fitelson EM. Practitioner review: maternal mood in pregnancy and child development–implications for child psychology and psychiatry. J Child Psychol Psychiatry. 2014;55:99–111. doi:10.1111/jcpp.12153 .

28. Kingston D, McDonald S, Austin M-P, Tough S. Association between prenatal and postnatal psychological distress and toddler cognitive development: a systematic review. PLoS One. 2015;10:e0126929. doi:10.1371/journal.pone.0126929 .

29. Howard LM, Piot P, Stein A. No health without perinatal mental health. Lancet. 2014;384:1723–4. doi:10.1016/S0140-6736(14)62040-7 .

30. Fisher SC, Kim SY, Sharma AJ, Rochat R, Morrow B. Is obesity still increasing among pregnant women? Prepregnancy obesity trends in 20 states, 2003-2009. Prev Med. 2013;56:372–8. doi:10.1016/j.ypmed.2013.02.015 .

31. Heslehurst N, Ells LJ, Simpson H, Batterham A, Wilkinson J, Summerbell CD. Trends in maternal obesity incidence rates, demographic predictors, and health inequalities in 36,821 women over a 15-year period. BJOG. 2007;114: 187–94. doi:10.1111/j.1471-0528.2006.01199.x.

32. Heslehurst N, Simpson H, Ells LJ, Rankin J, Wilkinson J, Lang R, et al. The impact of maternal BMI status on pregnancy outcomes with immediate short-term obstetric resource implications: a meta-analysis. Obes Rev. 2008; 9:635–83. doi:10.1111/j.1467-789X.2008.00511.x .

33. O'Reilly JR, Reynolds RM. The risk of maternal obesity to the long-term health of the offspring. Clin Endocrinol. 2013;78:9–16. doi:10.1111/cen.12055 .

34. Simmons D, Jelsma JGM, Galjaard S, Devlieger R, van Assche A, Jans G, et al. Results from a European multicenter randomized trial of physical activity and/or healthy eating to reduce the risk of gestational diabetes mellitus: the DALI lifestyle pilot. Diabetes Care. 2015;38:1650–6. doi:10.2337/dc15-0360 .

35. Jelsma JGM, van Poppel MNM, Galjaard S, Desoye G, Corcoy R, Devlieger R, et al. DALI: vitamin D and lifestyle intervention for gestational diabetes mellitus (GDM) prevention: an European multicentre, randomised trial – study protocol. BMC Pregnancy Childbirth. 2013;13:142. doi:10.1186/1471-2393-13-142 .

36. Vellinga A, Zawiejska A, Harreiter J, Buckley B, Di Cianni G, Lapolla A, et al. Associations of body mass index (maternal BMI) and gestational diabetes mellitus with neonatal and maternal pregnancy outcomes in a multicentre European database (diabetes and pregnancy vitamin D and lifestyle intervention for gestational diabetes mellitus prevention). ISRN Obes. 2012; 2012:424010. doi:10.5402/2012/424010 .

37. World Health Organization. Wellbeing measures in primary health care: the DepCare project: report on a WHO meeting Stockholm, Sweden 12-13 February 1998: WHO Regional Office for Europe; 1998.

38. Topp CW, Østergaard SD, Søndergaard S, Bech P. The WHO-5 well-being index: a systematic review of the literature. Psychother Psychosom. 2015;84: 167–76. doi:10.1159/000376585.

39. Krieger T, Zimmermann J, Huffziger S, Ubl B, Diener C, Kuehner C, Grosse Holtforth M. Measuring depression with a well-being index: further evidence for the validity of the WHO well-being index (WHO-5) as a measure of the severity of depression. J Affect Disord. 2014;156:240–4. doi:10.1016/j.jad.2013.12.015 .

40. Grandner MA, Patel NP, Gehrman PR, Perlis ML, Pack AI. Problems associated with short sleep: bridging the gap between laboratory and epidemiological studies. Sleep Med Rev. 2010;14:239–47. doi:10.1016/j.smrv.2009.08.001 .

41. Chasan-Taber L, Schmidt MD, Roberts DE, Hosmer D, Markenson G, Freedson PS. Development and validation of a pregnancy physical activity questionnaire. Med Sci Sports Exerc. 2004;36:1750–60. doi:10.1249/01.MSS.0000142303.49306.0D .

42. Green JM, Kafetsios K, Statham HE, Snowdon CM. Factor structure, validity and reliability of the Cambridge worry scale in a pregnant population. J Health Psychol. 2003;8:753–64. doi:10.1177/13591053030086008 .

43. Schwarzer R. Modeling health behavior change: how to predict and modify the adoption and maintenance of health behaviors. Appl Psychol. 2008;57: 1–29. doi:10.1111/j.1464-0597.2007.00325.x.

44. Prady SL, Pickett KE, Croudace T, Fairley L, Bloor K, Gilbody S, et al. Psychological distress during pregnancy in a multi-ethnic community: findings from the born in Bradford cohort study. PLoS One. 2013;8:e60693. doi:10.1371/journal.pone.0060693 .

45. Fellenzer JL, Cibula DA. Intendedness of pregnancy and other predictive factors for symptoms of prenatal depression in a population-based study. Matern Child Health J. 2014;18:2426–36. doi:10.1007/s10995-014-1481-4 .

46. Murphy MJ, Peterson MJ. Sleep disturbances in depression. Sleep Medicine Clinics. 2015;10:17–23. doi:10.1016/j.jsmc.2014.11.009 .

47. Bei B, Coo S, Trinder J. Sleep and mood during pregnancy and the postpartum period. Sleep Medicine Clinics. 2015;10:25–33. doi:10.1016/j.jsmc.2014.11.011 .

48.   Palagini L, Gemignani A, Banti S, Manconi M, Mauri M, Riemann D. Chronic sleep loss during pregnancy as a determinant of stress: impact on pregnancy outcome. Sleep Med. 2014;15:853–9. doi:10.1016/j.sleep.2014.02.013 .

49.   Gaston A, Prapavessis H. Tired, moody and pregnant? Exercise may be the answer. Psychol Health. 2013;28:1353–69. doi:10.1080/08870446.2013.809084 .

50.   de Wit L, Jelsma JGM, van Poppel MNM, Bogaerts A, Simmons D, Desoye G, et al. Physical activity, depressed mood and pregnancy worries in European obese pregnant women: results from the DALI study. BMC Pregnancy Childbirth. 2015;15:158. doi:10.1186/s12884-015-0595-z.

51.   Gourounti K, Anagnostopoulos F, Lykeridou K, Griva F, Vaslamatzis G. Prevalence of women's worries, anxiety, and depression during pregnancy in a public hospital setting in Greece. Clinical and experimental obstetrics & gynecology. 2012;40:581–3.

52.   Foster RG, Wulff K. The rhythm of rest and excess. Nat Rev Neurosci. 2005;6: 407–14. doi:10.1038/nrn1670.

53.   Gamble KL, Resuehr D, Johnson CH. Shift work and circadian dysregulation of reproduction. Front Endocrinol (Lausanne). 2013;4:92. doi:10.3389/fendo. 2013.00092 .

54.   McEwen BS, Karatsoreos IN. Sleep deprivation and circadian disruption: stress, Allostasis, and allostatic load. Sleep Medicine Clinics. 2015;10:1–10. doi:10.1016/j.jsmc.2014.11.007.

Exercise training during pregnancy reduces circulating insulin levels in overweight/obese women postpartum

Kirsti K. Garnæs[1], Siv Mørkved[2,3], Kjell Å. Salvesen[4,5], Øyvind Salvesen[2] and Trine Moholdt[1,5]*

Abstract

Background: The primary aim was to investigate if supervised exercise training during pregnancy could reduce postpartum weight retention (PPWR) three months after delivery in overweight and obese women. We also measured circulating markers of cardiometabolic health, body composition, blood pressure, and physical activity level.

Methods: This was a secondary analysis of a randomised controlled trial in which 91 women with BMI $\geq$ 28 kg/m^2 were allocated 1:1 to an exercise program or a control group. Women in the exercise group were prescribed three weekly, supervised sessions of 35 min of moderate intensity walking/running followed by 25 min of resistance training. The control group received standard maternal care. Assessments were undertaken in early pregnancy, late pregnancy, and three months postpartum. PPWR was defined as postpartum body weight minus early pregnancy weight.

Results: Seventy women participated three months after delivery, and PPWR was −0.8 kg in the exercise group ($n = 36$) and −1.6 in the control group ($n = 34$) (95% CI, −1.83, 3.84, $p = 0.54$). Women in the exercise group had significantly lower circulating insulin concentration; 106.3 pmol/l compared to the control group; 141.4 pmol/l (95% CI, −62.78, −7.15, $p = 0.01$), and showed a tendency towards lower homeostatic measurement of insulin resistance (HOMA2-IR) (3.5 vs. 5.0, 95% CI, −2.89, 0.01, $p = 0.05$). No women in the exercise group compared to three women in the control group were diagnosed with type 2 diabetes postpartum ($p = 0.19$). Of the women in the exercise group, 46.4% reported of exercising regularly, compared to 25.0% in the control group ($p = 0.16$).

Conclusions: Offering supervised exercise training during pregnancy among overweight/obese women did not affect PPWR three months after delivery, but reduced circulating insulin levels. This was probably due to a higher proportion of women being active postpartum in the exercise group.

Keywords: Pregnant, Physical activity, Maternal risks, Diabetes, High BMI

* Correspondence: trine.moholdt@ntnu.no
[1]Department of Circulation and Medical Imaging, NTNU, Norwegian
University of Science and Technology, Box 8905, 7491 Trondheim, Norway
[5]Department of Obstetrics and Gynaecology, St. Olavs Hospital, Trondheim
University Hospital, Trondheim, Norway
Full list of author information is available at the end of the article

Background

Overweight and obesity among women in fertile age are associated with adverse health outcomes for mother and child, both during pregnancy and postpartum [1–11]. Overweight is defined as body mass index (BMI) ≥ 25 kg/m^2, and obesity as BMI ≥ 30 kg/m^2 (according to the WHO classification system) [12]. Pre-pregnancy overweight and obese women are at increased risk for high postpartum weight retention (PPWR) [10, 11]. Obese women are two times more likely than normal weight women to exceed the Institute of Medicine's (IOM) recommendations for gestational weight gain [13], and half of the PPWR can be explained by excessive gestational weight gain [14]. High PPWR is associated with reduced insulin sensitivity, hypertension, and later development of type 2 diabetes mellitus and cardiovascular disorders [7, 8, 15, 16]. High PPWR also predisposes for high pre-pregnancy BMI [7, 8] and further reduced maternal metabolic function in future pregnancies [17].

Finding lifestyle interventions to limit gestational weight gain and PPWR among overweight and obese women is important. Previous research investigating the effect of lifestyle programs during pregnancy targeting this group of women have demonstrated conflicting results on PPWR, glucose tolerance, and other cardiometabolic health variables [18–21]. Further, few trials have investigated the effect of regular exercise during pregnancy as the only intervention.

The primary aim of the Exercise Training in Pregnancy (ETIP) trial was to assess if offering supervised exercise training during pregnancy would reduce gestational weight gain in women with pre-pregnancy BMI of ≥ 28.0 kg/m^2 [22, 23]. At delivery we found no difference in gestational weight gain between the groups, but we observed a lower incidence of gestational diabetes mellitus (GDM) and lower blood pressure in the exercise group [22].

This is a secondary analysis of data from the ETIP trial where we assessed if providing a supervised exercise program during pregnancy could reduce PPWR three months after delivery. Our a priori hypothesis was that the women in the exercise group would have a lower PPWR. We also investigated effects of the intervention during pregnancy on body composition, blood pressure, physical activity level, and various circulating markers of cardiometabolic health three months postpartum.

Methods
Trial design

The ETIP trial was a single-centre, parallel-group randomised controlled trial (RCT) investigating effects of offering supervised regular exercise training during pregnancy compared to standard maternal care only, in overweight and obese women. The primary outcome measure in ETIP was gestational weight gain. The trial

was conducted between September 2010 and March 2015 at the Norwegian University of Science and Technology (NTNU) and St. Olavs Hospital, Trondheim University Hospital, Norway. The study was approved by the Regional Committee for Medical and Health Research Ethics (REK-midt 2010/1522), registered in ClinicalTrials.gov (NCT01243554) and was in accordance with the Helsinki Declaration of 1975. The ETIP study protocol and primary findings of the trial have been published previously [22, 23].

We experienced slow recruitment in the trial and made changes to the study protocol after commencement of the trial to accommodate the need for more participants [22]. We experienced eligible women making contact for participation too late for randomisation within gestational week 16, therefore the originally criterion for maximum inclusion time in gestational week 16 was changed to gestational week 18 in November 2012. The inclusion criterion pre-pregnancy BMI was changed from ≥ 30 kg/m^2 to ≥ 28 kg/m^2 in March 2013, in attempt to increase the number of women eligible for participation [22]. The changes were approved by the Regional Committee for Medical and Health Research Ethics.

Participants

Women were eligible if they had a pre-pregnancy BMI ≥ 28, age ≥ 18 years, gestational week < 18, carrying one singleton live foetus at the 11–14-week ultrasound scan, and were able to attend assessments and exercise sessions at St. Olavs Hospital. Exclusion criteria were; habitual exercise training (twice or more weekly) in the period before pregnancy, high risk for preterm delivery, diseases that could interfere with participation, and contraindications in accordance to The American College of Obstetricians and Gynecologists (ACOG) recommendations for physical activity and exercise during pregnancy [24, 25]. The women received written information and signed informed consent on behalf of themselves and their foetus before participation and randomisation.

Intervention

All participants received standard maternal care. In addition, women in the exercise group were offered supervised exercise sessions three times per week at the hospital from time of inclusion (at gestational week 12–18) until delivery [22]. The exercise program provided was in accordance with the recommendations from ACOG [26]. Women in the exercise group walked or ran on treadmills for 35 min at moderate intensity (65–80% of maximal capacity, estimated using a rate of perceived exertion of 12–15 on the Borg 6–20 scale [27]), followed by 25 min of resistance exercises for large muscle groups and a strength training program for the pelvic floor muscles. The strength training consisted of weight-bearing exercises such as squats, push-ups, diagonal lifts on all fours, oblique abdominal crunches, and pelvic floor muscle exercises, with three sets of ten repetitions of each exercise separated by one minute rest between sets. In addition, the women also performed three sets of the "plank exercise" for 30 s. A physical therapist supervised all sessions and registered each woman's adherence to the program. We also advised women in the exercise group to do 35 min of endurance exercise and 15 min of resistance exercise at home at least once weekly, as well as daily pelvic floor muscle strengthening exercises. The participants' exercise sessions at the hospital, including duration, intensity and possible adjustments, were registered by study personnel. The participants' registered their home-based exercise and general physical activities in a training diary. The women in the exercise group were informed of recommended weight gain during pregnancy, based on the guidelines of the Institute of Medicine (IOM) [28]. They received an individually adjusted weight gain curve, where they weekly registered their weight measured at the hospital. The supervised exercise sessions were terminated at delivery. Women in the control group were informed about the recommended level of physical activity during pregnancy and were not discouraged from exercising on their own.

Outcomes

The principal outcome of this secondary analysis was PPWR, defined as body weight (kg) at the postpartum visit minus body weight (kg) at early pregnancy. Weight was measured using a calibrated electronic scale (SECA 770, Medema, Norway). We also assessed the difference between postpartum weight and self-reported weight before pregnancy.

All participants underwent the same test protocol at early pregnancy (gestational week 12–18), in late pregnancy (gestational week 34–37), and three months postpartum. The participants fasted overnight for ≥ 10 h before undergoing an oral glucose tolerance test where they drank 75 g of glucose dissolved in 2.5 dl of water. We report the number of women who fulfilled the WHO definition of type 2 diabetes; fasting plasma glucose ≥ 7.0 mmol/l, and/or 2 h concentration ≥ 11.1 mmol/l. [29] We measured plasma insulin by enzyme immunoassay (ELISA, IBL-International, Germany), using a DS2 ELISA processing system (Dynex Technologies, USA), according to the manufacturer's procedures. As a measure of insulin resistance, we used the homeostatic assessment of insulin resistance (HOMA2-IR), calculated as [glucose*insulin]/22.5 [30]. All other blood measurements were analysed by Roche Modular P-system (Roche, Switzerland).

Blood pressure measurements were taken three times at two-minute intervals, and the average was used in the

analysis. Hypertension was defined as a systolic blood pressure ≥ 140 mmHg and/or a diastolic blood pressure ≥ 90 mmHg. We used a Harpenden Caliper (Holtain Ltd., UK) to measure subscapular-, biceps-, and triceps skinfold thickness. Body composition was additionally measured with air displacement plethysmography (BOD POD, COSMED The Metabolic Company, Italy). We measured waist circumference at the postpartum visit, using measuring tape at the level of the umbilicus at normal expiration. Assessments were undertaken by principal investigators (KKG and TM), trained nurses and biomechanical laboratory personnel. For a more detailed description of outcome measures, see Garnæs et al. [22]

At the three months postpartum visit, as well as in early and late pregnancy, the participants answered questionnaires about their physical activity and exercise training. They were asked if they adhered to the recommendations of ≥ 150 min of moderate intensity physical activity per week, and about their amount and intensity of exercise training. Women were also asked about breastfeeding at the time of the postpartum visit; whether they were exclusively breastfeeding and the number of meals per 24 h.

Sample size

The sample size calculation in the ETIP-trial was based on a primary outcome of gestational weight gain from baseline to delivery [22, 23]. To detect a 6 kg clinically significant difference in weight gain between the groups, we needed a minimum of 118 participants (with alpha 0.05, beta 0.90). We did not do a separate power calculation for the analyses presented in this report.

Randomisation and blinding

After early pregnancy assessments were undertaken, we allocated participants 1:1 to the exercise or the control group, using a computer random number generator. The participants allocated to the intervention were invited to exercises sessions immediately after randomisation. For details about the randomisation procedure, see Garnæs et al. [22] The personnel measuring weight at birth and undertaking blood analyses and the statistician were blinded for group allocation. All other measurements were unmasked. To limit bias were blinding was not possible, detailed test-protocols were used, and a low number of- and the same study personnel performed the assessments in the trial.

Statistical methods

Analyses were done according to the "intention to treat" principle. All available data was used at all time points. Baseline data (early pregnancy) was tested for normality and compared between groups by independent samples t-tests and Fisher's Exact Tests. The effect of treatment on the continuous postpartum outcomes was assessed with mixed linear models. The effect of time and treatment was specified as a fixed effect having the levels 'baseline', 'training late pregnancy', 'control late pregnancy', 'training postpartum' and 'control postpartum'. No systematic differences between groups at baseline were assumed due to randomisation. Participant ID was included as a random effect to account for repeated measurements. To account for apparent variance heterogeneity across time, the covariance structure for the error term was specified as diagonal. The effect of treatment on dichotomous postpartum outcomes was analysed using exact logistic regression adjusted for the baseline (early pregnancy) outcome when available, with the exercise group as the reference group.

Analyses were performed using IBM SPSS Statistics 22 for baseline values, R version 2.13.1 for continuous outcome data, and Stata version 13.1 for dichotomous outcome data. All results are given as mean values with 95% confidence intervals and p-values < 0.05 were considered as significant.

We did supplementary mixed model analyses of PPWR where we adjusted for the number of days since delivery, lactation and physical activity. We also investigated association between PPWR and gestational weight gain, lactation and physical activity. We performed, as described in the protocol [23], per protocol analyses of women in the exercise group adhering to the exercise protocol. In these analyses we included women in the exercise group who undertook one of the following: 1) attending ≥ 42 organized exercise sessions, 2) attending ≥ 28 exercise sessions + performing ≥ 28 home exercise sessions, 3) performing ≥ 60 home exercise sessions. The exercise had to be ≥ 50 min of aerobic and/or strength training to count as a home session.

Results

The trial was conducted between September 2010 and March 2015, and enrolment was ended due to prolonged time for inclusion and fewer eligible participants than expected. Figure 1 outlines the flow of participants during the trial. Seventy (77%) of 91 women included in the ETIP trial were assessed at three months postpartum and two women in each group dropped out from late pregnancy/delivery until the postpartum visit (Figure 1). Table 1 shows participants' demographic characteristics at baseline. Additional baseline characteristics of the whole sample in the ETIP trial has been published previously [22]. Apart from a lower fasting glucose in the exercise group ($p = 0.02$), baseline (early pregnancy) characteristics did not differ between groups. Of the women in the exercise group included in the postpartum analyses, 54.3% adhered to the training protocol. The

mean time for postpartum testing was 99.8 ± 10.2 days after delivery in the exercise group and 95.7 ± 10.4 days in the control group. The women in the exercise group performed 31.7 ± 15.3 (range 0–53) supervised sessions at the hospital, and 19.2 ± 16.5 (range 0–72) exercise sessions at home. Mean gestational weight gain during pregnancy was 10.5 ± 4.6 kg in the exercise group and 9.7 ± 6.9 kg in the control group ($p = 0.55$). Among women in the exercise group, 58% gained more weight during pregnancy than recommended by the IOM guidelines compared with 44% in the control group [22]. Table 2 presents model-based outcomes at baseline (means for all participants) and at the postpartum visit.

Postpartum weight retention

PPWR was not significantly different between groups, with –0.8 kg in the exercise group and –1.6 kg in the control group ($p = 0.54$) (Table 2). Women in both groups had returned to their early pregnancy body weight three months postpartum. We observed no association between PPWR and gestational weight gain ($p = 0.79$), PPWR and lactation ($p = 0.63$), or between PPWR and fulfilling recommendations of 30 min of physical activity per day ($p = 0.20$).

Other outcome measures

Fasting glucose was equal between groups at the postpartum visit (Fig. 2a), but we observed a tendency towards lower 120 min glucose in the exercise group compared to the control group (5.2 mmol/l vs 5.8 mmol/l, $p = 0.10$) (Fig. 2b). The insulin concentration was significantly lower in the exercise group compared to the control group ($p = 0.01$) (Table 1). Figure 2c outlines the insulin levels at baseline, in late pregnancy, and postpartum. HOMA2-IR (insulin resistance) was lower in the exercise group, but the group difference was not statistically significant (Fig. 2d). No women in the exercise group compared to three women in the control group fulfilled the diagnostic criteria for type 2 diabetes postpartum ($p = 0.19$, Table 2). All three women were diagnosed with GDM in late pregnancy, and none had diabetes before pregnancy. We also observed a trend towards lower systolic and diastolic blood pressure in the exercise group (Table 1). Approximately 75% of the total study population fulfilled the recommended amount of weekly general physical activity three months postpartum (Table 3). Twice as many women in the exercise group reported regular exercise (defined as $\geq$ 90 min with moderate intensity and/or ≥ 45 min with high intensity per week) postpartum, but the between-group difference was not statistically significant. The number of women exclusively breastfeeding at the postpartum visit was not significantly different between groups (Table 3).

CONSORT Flow Diagram

Enrollment

Assessed for eligibility (n=136)

Excluded (n=45)
- Not meeting inclusion criteria (n=25)
- Declined to participate (n=12)
- Abortion (n=8)

Randomized (n=91)

Allocation

Allocated to exercise (n=46)
- Received allocated intervention (n=46)

Allocated to control (n=45)
- Received allocated intervention (n=45)

Follow-up Late pregnancy

Lost to follow-up (n=8)
Discontinued intervention
- Abortion (between gestational week 12 and 22) (n=3)
- Not meeting inclusion criteria (moved from Trondheim) (n=1)
- Other reasons (n=4)

Lost to follow-up (n=9)
Discontinued intervention
- Abortion (between gestational week 12 and 22) (n=3)
- Not meeting inclusion criteria (diagnosed with twins at late ultrasound) (n =2)
- Other reasons (n=4)

Follow-up Postpartum

Lost to follow-up (n=2)

Lost to follow-up (n=2)

Analysis

Analysed (n=36)
Excluded from analysis (n=0)

Analysed (n=34)
Excluded from analysis (n=0)

Fig. 1 Flow chart of the ETIP trial

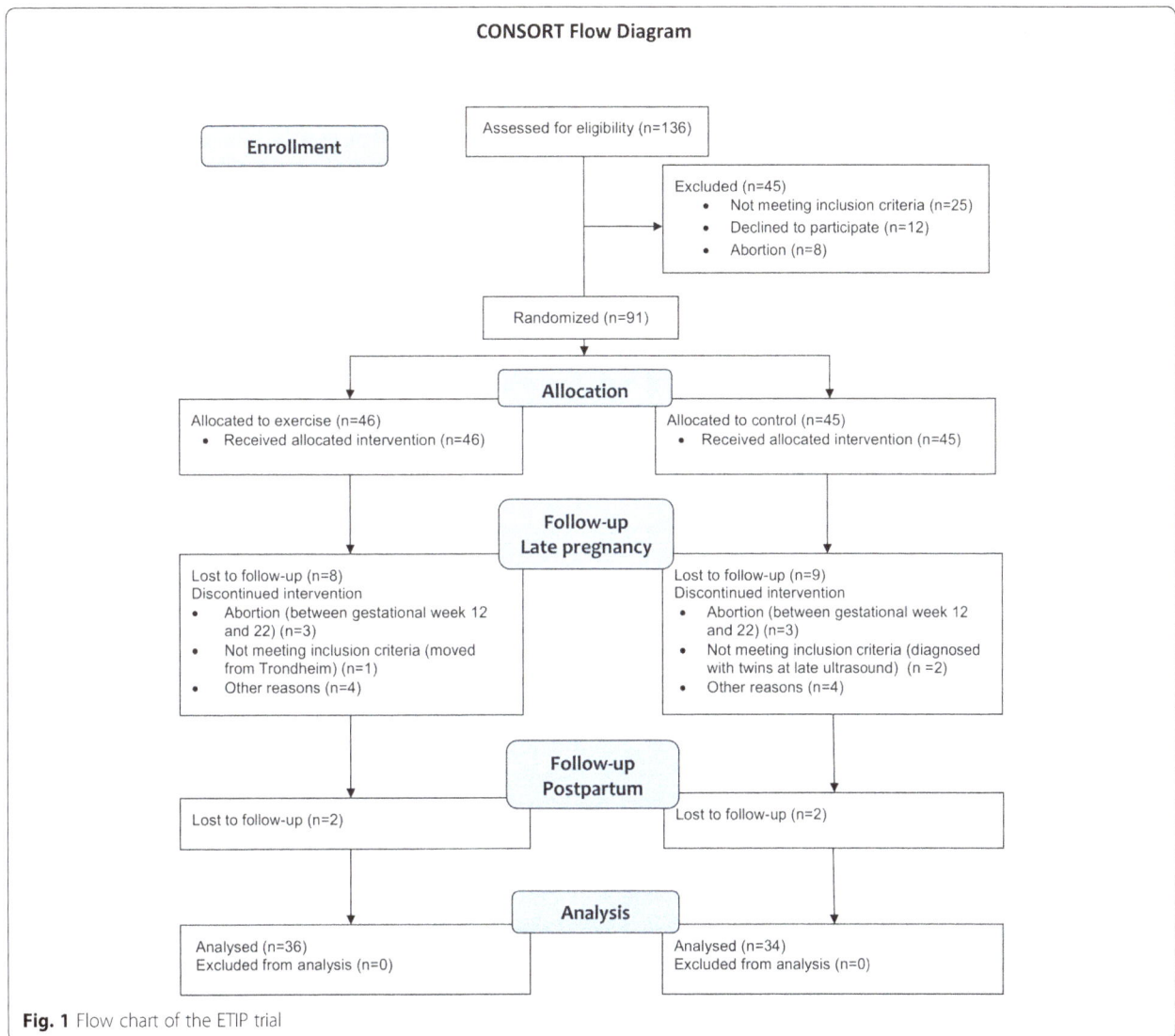

Additional analyses

We analysed PPWR in both groups adjusted for number of days from birth to postpartum test and observed no significant effect on postpartum weight ($p = 0.76$) or PPWR ($p = 0.32$). The effect estimate of weight loss per day was –0.016 kg. We found no effect of adjusting for lactation and physical activity. Half of the exercising women included in the postpartum analysis ($n = 19$) fulfilled the training intervention during pregnancy as described in the study protocol [23]. Detailed data are presented in Additional file 1 and Additional file 2. We found no difference in PPWR (postpartum minus early pregnancy) between the per protocol exercise group (–0.1 kg, 95% CI, –2.7, 1.1) and the control group (–1.7 kg, 95% CI, –3.5, 0.3) ($p = 0.35$), and no difference in PPWR when using self-reported pre-pregnancy weight between the per protocol exercise group (2.5 kg, 95% CI,

–0.7, 3.8) and the control group (0.2 kg, 95% CI, –1.8, 2.9) ($p = 0.28$). At postpartum, there was no difference in mean weight between the exercise group (95.9 kg) and the control group (94.8 kg) ($p = 0.47$) (Additional file 1). Women in the per protocol exercise group had significantly lower resting systolic and diastolic blood pressure compared to the control group, (117.0/73.1 mmHg vs. 124.0/78.4 mmHg) (systolic BP, $p = 0.01$, diastolic BP, $p < 0.01$), and they had lower insulin levels (14.1 mmol/l vs 19.7 mmol/l, $p = 0.04$) (Additional file 1). No harmful, unintended or adverse events were reported.

Discussion

Offering supervised regular exercise during pregnancy for overweight and obese women did not lower PPWR compared to women receiving standard maternal care. Both groups regained the pre-pregnancy weight three

Table 1 Participants' demographic characteristics at baseline (early pregnancy). Observed data presented as mean ± standard deviation or number of participants (percent)

Participant characteristics at baseline	Exercise Group ($n = 36$)	Control Group ($n = 34$)	
	Mean ± SD	Mean ± SD	p-value
Age (years)	31.6 ± 3.6	31.3 ± 4.6	0.73
Weight (kg)	94.7 ± 12.4	99.3 ± 14.4	0.16
Height (cm)	167.0 ± 5.7	167.8 ± 6.3	0.59
BMI (kg/m^2)	33.9 ± 3.8	35.2 ± 4.5	0.20
	n (%)	n (%)	
Weight classification			0.35
Overweight, BMI 28.0–29.9 kg/m^2	2 (5.6%)	3 (8.8%)	
Class 1 obesity, BMI 30.0–34.9 kg/m^2	23 (63.9%)	15 (44.1%)	
Class 2 obesity, BMI 35.0–39.9 kg/m^2	9 (25.0%)	11 (32.4%)	
Class 3 obesity, BMI ≥ 40.0 kg/m^2	2 (5.6%)	5 (14.7%)	
Parity			0.71
0	18 (50.0%)	15 (44.1%)	
1	15 (41.7%)	14 (41.2%)	
2	3 (8.3%)	4 (11.8%)	
≥ 3	0 (0.0%)	1 (2.9%)	
Current smoking	2 (5.6%)	4 (11.8%)	
Education			0.85
Primary/secondary school	0 (0.0%)	0 (0.0%)	
High school	9 (25.0%)	6 (18.2%)	
University ≤ 4 y	13 (36.1%)	10 (29.4%)	
University > 4 y	14 (38.9%)	17 (50.0%)	
Currently employed	32 (88.9%)	26 (76.5%)	0.21

Missing: Education: Control group: 1
Statistics: Current Smoking and Currently employed were analysed by Fisher's Exact Test. Weight classification, Parity and Education were analysed by Pearson Chi-Square Test
Abbreviations: *BMI* Body Mass Index

months after delivery. However, we found a significantly lower blood insulin concentration and a tendency towards lower HOMA2-IR in the exercise group compared to the control group. These findings may indicate a reduced risk for developing type 2 diabetes among the exercising women, however, studies with higher power is needed to confirm this. Among women who adhered to the training protocol during pregnancy, we also found significantly lower systolic and diastolic blood pressure three months postpartum.

Pre-pregnancy BMI is a strong predictor of PPWR with higher weight retention in overweight and obese women [31, 32]. We have found no RCTs assessing the isolated effects of exercise training in pregnancy on PPWR in exclusively overweight and obese women. Previous studies have combined different types of intervention, such as diet and exercise, and/or included participants of all BMI categories. Those RCTs have shown divergent results; some have found no effect [33–36], whereas others have found lower

PPWR in the intervention group [32, 37]. Phelan and colleagues [32], found lower PPWR in normal weight and overweight women after a lifestyle intervention program, but not among obese women. According to a meta-analysis by Nascimento and colleagues, trials reporting positive effects on PPWR are characterised by including women in all BMI categories and have combined supervised exercise training and intensive dietary interventions [21]. Among studies providing ancillary analyses, some have suggested positive effects of exercise on PPWR among women adhering to the intervention protocol [32–35]. We did not show any differences in PPWR between groups using early pregnancy weight measurement, self-reported weight prepregnancy, or analysing women who exercised per protocol. However, women in both groups had almost regained their pre-pregnancy and early pregnancy weight at the postpartum visit. Our trial included supervised exercise training from early pregnancy and throughout the pregnancy, but the results indicate that the amount or intensity of the

Table 2 Outcomes at three months postpartum. "Intention to treat" model based analyses with early pregnancy (baseline) mean for all participants, and comparisons between groups at postpartum presented as mean, 95% confidence interval (CI) and p-value. Weight retention was estimated based both on the difference between postpartum weight and early pregnancy (baseline) weight, and between postpartum weight and self-reported pre-pregnancy weight

Outcomes at postpartum	Baseline	Exercise Group (n = 36)		Control Group (n = 34)		Between-Group Comparison		
		Mean	95% CI	Mean	95% CI	Mean Diff	95% CI	p-value
Weight (kg)	96.8	96.0	92.7, 99.3	95.2	91.9, 98.5	0.82	−1.83, 3.46	0.54
PPWR[1] (kg)[a]		- 0.8	−2.7, 1.1	−1.6	−3.5, 0.3	0.82	−1.83, 3.84	0.54
PPWR[2] (kg)[b]		1.52	−0.73, 3.78	0.52	−1.82, 2.86	1.0	−2.15, 4.16	0.53
BMI (kg/m[2])	34.5	34.2	33.2, 35.3	33.9	32.9, 35.0	0.29	−0.67, 1.25	0.55
Waist circumference (cm)	107.5	105.0	101.7, 108.2	102.9	99.6, 106.2	2.06	−1.34, 5.47	0.24
Body composition[c]								
Fat mass (kg)	43.1	42.1	39.6, 44.6	42.0	39.5, 44.5	0.11	−2.05, 0.92	0.92
Fat mass (%)	44.6	44.2	43.0, 45.5	43.9	42.7, 45.2	0.28	−0.83, 1.38	0.62
Fat-free mass (kg)	52.7	52.1	50.4, 53.7	53.0	51.4, 54.7	−0.96	−2.83, 0.92	0.32
Fat-free mass (%)	55.4	55.7	54.4, 57.1	56.4	55.1, 57.7	−0.65	−1.97, 0.67	0.33
Skinfold thickness								
Biceps area (mm)	21.1	16.7	14.7, 18.7	17.5	15.5, 19.6	−0.85	−3.15, 1.44	0.47
Triceps area (mm)	30.0	26.4	24.4, 28.4	26.8	24.8, 28.8	−0.43	−2.67, 1.82	0.71
Subscapular area (mm)	31.8	28.5	26.3, 30.8	30.0	27.7–32.3	−1.44	−4.03, 1.16	0.28
Blood pressure								
Systolic BP (mm/Hg)	124.5	120.6	117.5, 123.8	124.02	120.7, 127.4	−3.40	−7.70, −0.99	0.13
Diastolic BP (mm/Hg)	76.0	75.8	73.3, 78.4	78.4	75.7, 81.1	−2.61	−6.19, 0.96	0.15
Blood measurements								
Fasting glucose (mmol/l)	4.7	5.1	4.9, 5.3	5.1	4.8, 5.26	0.02	−0.24, 0.27	0.91
120-min glucose (mmol/l)	5.9	5.2	4.7, 5.8	5.8	5.3, 6.4	−0.60	−0.60, 1.31	0.10
Insulin (pmol/l)	139.6	106.3	83.3, 129.2	141.4	118.1, 164.6	−35.10	−62.78, −7.15	*0.01*
HbA1c (%)	5.2	5.3	5.2, 5.4	5.4	5.3, 5.5	−0.10	−0.25, 0.04	0.17
Insulin C-peptide (nmol/l)	0.6	0.7	0.6, 0.8	0.7	0.6, 0.8	−0.01	−0.14, 0.11	0.82
Triglycerides (mmol/l)	1.4	0.8	0.6, 1.0	1.0	0.8, 1.2	−0.21	−0.47, 0.05	0.12
Ferritin (pmol/l)	127.0	69.9	56.0, 83.6	64.5	49.7, 79.1	5.46	−14.81, 25.71	0.60
HDL cholesterol (mmol/l)	1.7	1.5	1.5, 1.6	1.5	1.4, 1.6	−0.02	−0.14, 0.11	0.81
LDL cholesterol (mmol/l)	2.8	3.1	2.8, 3.4	3.2	2.8, 3.5	−0.08	−0.51, 0.34	0.71
Total cholesterol (mmol/l)	5.0	4.9	4.5, 5.2	5.1	4.7, 5.4	−0.23	−0.71, 0.25	0.34
Haemoglobin (g/l)	126.7	128.4	125.4, 131.5	129.7	126.5, 132.9	−1.30	−5.50, 2.90	0.56
High-sensitive CRP (mg/l)	10.7	4.2	2.9, 5.6	4.8	3.4, 6.2	−0.58	−2.50, 1.34	0.55
HOMA2-IR	2.5	3.5	2.5, 4.6	5.0	3.9, 6.0	−1.44	−2.89, 0.01	0.05

Missing: The number of missing in the exercise group varied between 1and 5, in the control group between 1 and 3

Statistics: The effect of treatment was assessed with linear mixed models. For the primary and secondary outcomes, the effect of time and treatment was taken as a fixed effect. Due to randomisation, no systematic differences between groups at baseline were assumed. Insulin was significantly lower (p = 0.01) in th exercise group postpartum

Abbreviations: PPWR postpartum weight retention, BMI Body mass index, BP blood pressure, HbA1c Glycated Haemoglobin, HDL High-density lipoprotein, LDL Low-density lipoprotein, CRP C-reactive protein, HOMA2-IR homeostatic assessment of insulin resistance

[a]PPWR[1], postpartum weight minus weight at early pregnancy (baseline)

[b]PPWR[2], postpartum weight minus pre-pregnancy weight. Weight at pre-pregnancy was based on self-reported data. Mean pre-pregnancy weight for all participants were 94.4 kg

[c]Body composition was measured by air displacement plethysmography (BOD POD)

exercise ought to be higher or combined with dietary intervention to improve outcomes. Adherence to the training protocol was low, and may have reduced the difference between groups. Low adherence to the training protocol is a common challenge in trials including obese pregnant women.

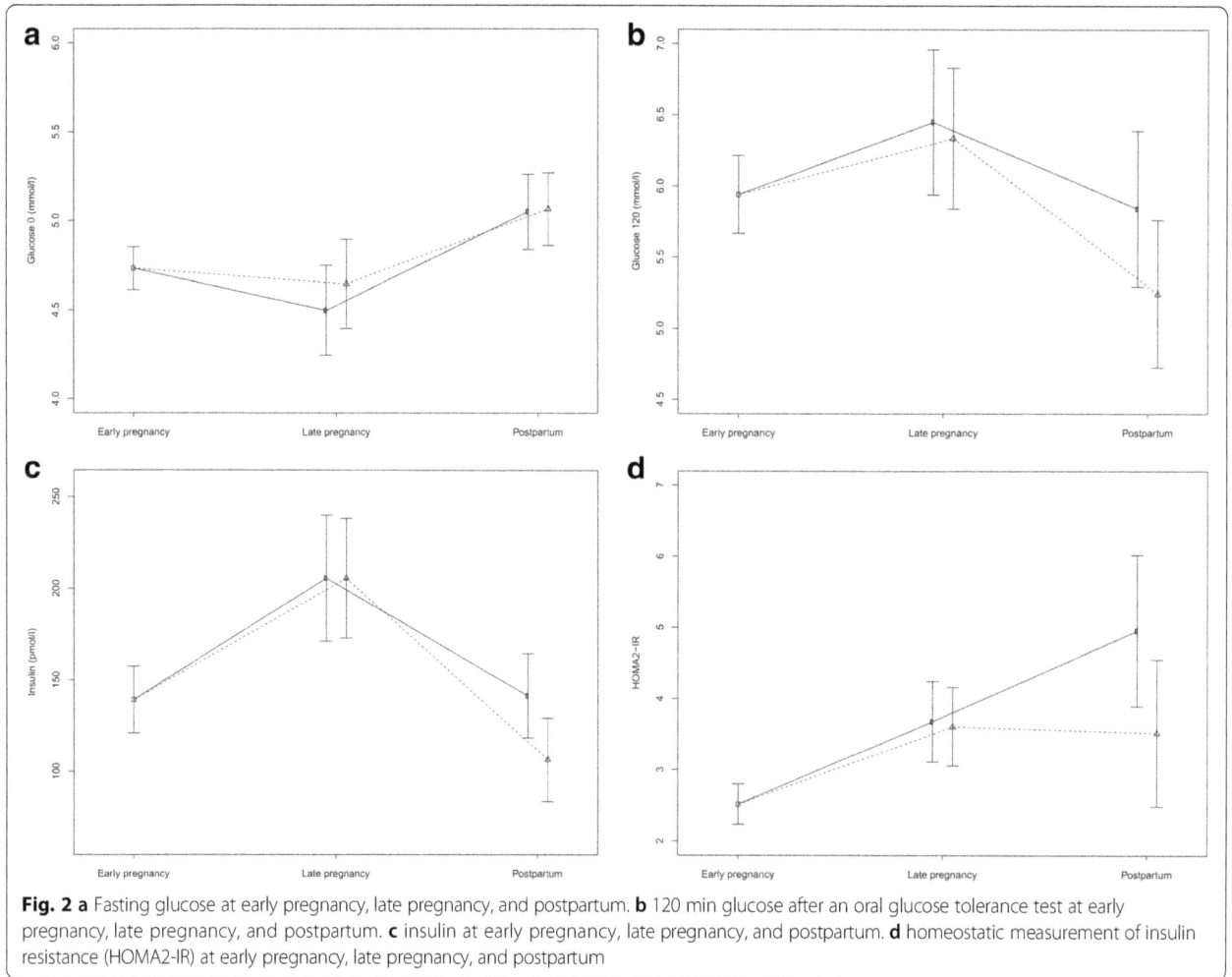

Fig. 2 a Fasting glucose at early pregnancy, late pregnancy, and postpartum. **b** 120 min glucose after an oral glucose tolerance test at early pregnancy, late pregnancy, and postpartum. **c** insulin at early pregnancy, late pregnancy, and postpartum. **d** homeostatic measurement of insulin resistance (HOMA2-IR) at early pregnancy, late pregnancy, and postpartum

Table 3 Outcomes at three months postpartum. "Intention to treat" analysis, observed data, for the exercise and the control group and comparison between groups are presented in number of participants (N), percentage (%), odds ratio (OR), 95% confidence interval (CI), and p-value

Outcomes at postpartum	Exercise group $n = 36$	Control group $n = 34$	Between-Group Comparison		
	n (%)	n (%)	Odds Ratio	95% CI	p-value
Type 2 diabetes	0 (0)	3 (9.1)	4.96	0.46, ∞	0.19
Hypertension	3 (8.8)	3 (10.0)	1.17	0.15, 9.30	1.00
Physical activity ≥ 150 min/week[a]	21 (72.4)	22 (78.6)	1.17	0.68, 2.02	0.76
Exercise training[b]	13 (46.4)	7 (25.0)	0.39	0.12, 1.19	0.16
Exclusively breastfeeding	18 (60.0)	21 (77.8)	1.44	0.90, 2.31	0.17
Breastfeeding 3–4 meals/24 h	4 (13.3)	1 (3.7)	0.63	0.37, 1.05	0.36

Missing: Type 2 diabetes: Exercise group 1 missing, control group 1 missing. Hypertension: Exercise group 1 missing, control group 4 missing. Physical activity questionnaire: Exercise group 7 missing, control group 6 missing. Lactating questionnaire: Exercise group 6 missing, control group 7 missing

Statistics: Type 2 diabetes and hypertension were analysed by exact logistic regression Model. Data on physical activity and breastfeeding are based on a self-reported questionnaire and were analysed by Fisher's Exact test

Definitions: Type 2 diabetes: Fasting plasma glucose ≥7.0 mmol/l or 2 h concentration ≥ 11.1 mmol/l, according to the definition of the World Health Organization (WHO). Hypertension: Systolic blood pressure ≥ 140, diastolic blood pressure ≥ 90

[a]Physical activity ≥150 min/week: 30 min of daily physical activity

[b]Exercise training ≥90 min with moderate intensity and/or ≥45 min with high intensity per week

Obese women have an increased risk for high insulin values and for developing diabetes mellitus type 2 postpartum [38]. We found significantly lower concentration of insulin in the exercise group compared to the control group. During pregnancy the insulin resistance increases, especially in obese women [39, 40]. To compensate, increased insulin secretion is needed [39]. Lower insulin, and trends towards lower 120 min glucose level and lower HOMA2-IR among women in the exercise group, may indicate lower risk of developing type 2 diabetes. The difference between groups in incidence of type 2 diabetes was not significant, but our results may have been affected by a small sample size.

Obese women are at increased risk for high blood pressure during pregnancy and postpartum [41–43]. We observed significantly lower systolic and diastolic blood pressure among women who adhered to the prescribed exercise, compared to the control group. We are not aware of any previous trial assessing the effect of exercise training during pregnancy on postpartum blood pressure. However, exercise has been shown to lower resting blood pressure among obese, non-pregnant subjects [44, 45].

Women are recommended to be physically active during pregnancy and postpartum to maintain a healthy weight and to prevent negative health outcomes [12, 46]. However, physical activity tends to decrease significantly during these periods, especially among women with BMI ≥ 25 kg/m^2 [47]. About 60% of the women in the ETIP trial (in both groups) reported to be physically active, whereas 77% in the exercise group versus 23% in the control group, reported to exercise regularly in late pregnancy [22]. At the postpartum visit, approximately 75% of all women in our study reported fulfilling the recommendations of minimum 150 min of weekly moderate intensity physical activity. A higher proportion of women in the exercise group (46% vs 25%) reported regular exercise postpartum. These results show that the amount of general physical activity is equal between groups both during the pregnancy and after delivery, but with a tendency of more structured exercise training in the exercise group also postpartum. Concerning the inclusion criteria "not exercising regularly pre-pregnancy", these numbers show an increase in exercise training for both groups postpartum compared to before pregnancy. A low number of participants in each group likely hampers the statistical comparison between groups.

Gestational weight gain and lactation are important factors for PPWR [32, 48]. In the present study, we found no associations between gestational weight gain and PPWR or between lactation and PPWR.

Study strength and limitations
The ETIP trial had a randomised, controlled study design. The exercise program was described in detail and should be easy to reproduce. Previous research has found supervised exercise to be important for adherence to the exercise protocol, for motivation, and for the safety of the participant, and to be more effective than general guidance [18]. We measured weight objectively at study entry and at postpartum, and we only included sedentary overweight/obese women in the trial. We measured skinfold thickness and body composition in addition to weight, and provided information on potential confounding factors such as lactation and GWG. Our intervention included the exercise program only, and no diet. Thus, we could assess the effect of exercise alone in contrast to previous trials with mixed interventions.

The main limitation was a small study sample. We did not recruit as many participants as originally planned and experienced additional drop-outs during the intervention period. This affected the power of the study and decreased the possibility of detecting true effects of the intervention. The proportion of drop-outs was, however, equally distributed between groups, and we had only two drop-outs in each group after delivery. In addition, only 50% of women in the exercise program adhered to the protocol. We report exercise intensity only by the rate of perceived exertion in this trial, due to the lack of a precise estimate of maximum heart rate for each participant. Since pregnancy can influence the heart rate during exercise [49], we chose not to include data on heart rate during exercise. We prolonged the time limit for inclusion in the trial from gestational week 16 to 18, which reduced the mean number of weeks of exercise before delivery, and thus the effect of the intervention. Our change in inclusion criteria BMI from ≥ 30 to ≥ 28 kg/m^2, may have reduced the homogeneity of the trial population, but only five women in the postpartum analysis had a pre-pregnancy BMI below 30 kg/m^2.

The current trial did not provide any information on diet and possible changes in eating habits in the groups. The control group underwent comprehensive health assessments during pregnancy and after delivery and this may have motivated also the women in the control group to undertake lifestyle changes.

Generalisability
The participants were recruited from Google advertisement and through an information letter to all pregnant women in Trondheim. There is a risk for over-representation of highly motivated women in the trial. This may influence the external validity (generalizability) of the trial, but not the internal validity (comparisons between groups).

Clinical relevance
The exercise intervention in the current trial was based on the ACOG recommendations for physical activity and exercise during pregnancy. The program required

no equipment and consisted of exercises that could easily be implemented by women themselves at home. The findings are relevant for sedentary overweight and obese pregnant women. The finding of lower concentration of insulin in the exercise group is clinically important as this may reduce the risk of future type 2 diabetes [50]. The blood pressure was lower in the women who reported to exercise per protocol during pregnancy and imply a reduced risk for developing cardiovascular diseases. This highlights the need of increasing adherence to exercise training in pregnancy for this population. No adverse events related to exercise occurred, and the findings in the current trial support the recommendations for exercise training during pregnancy.

Conclusion

Offering supervised exercise during pregnancy among overweight and obese women did not affect PPWR three months after delivery compared to standard antenatal care. Both groups had regained their early pregnancy weight three months postpartum. We observed lower circulating insulin among the women in the exercise group, as well as lower blood pressure in those who adhered to the exercise protocol. These findings may decrease the risk for developing both type 2 diabetes and cardiovascular diseases later in life. Further studies are needed to assess if supervised exercise during pregnancy can reduce the risk for development of type 2 diabetes and hypertension postpartum.

Abbreviations

ACOG: American College of Obstetricians and Gynecologists; BMI: Body mass index (kg/m^2); ETIP: Exercise training in pregnancy; GDM: Gestational diabetes mellitus; IOM: Institute of Medicine; OGTT: Oral glucose tolerance test; PPWR: Postpartum weight retention; RCT: Randomised controlled trial; WHO: World Health Organization

Acknowledgements

We acknowledge the personnel at the Clinical Research Facility at NTNU; Nina Backlund, Gøril Bakken Rønning, Anne Risdal and Guro Almvik, for undertaking the blood sampling in the ETIP trial.

Funding

The presents study was supported by grants from The Norwegian Fund for Post-Graduate Training in Physiotherapy, The Liaison Committee between the Central Norway Regional Health Authority (RHA) and the Norwegian University of Science and Technology (NTNU).

Authors' contributions

KK has coordinated the trial, collected data, supervised the training sessions, analysed the data and has been the main contributor of the writing of the paper. SM initiated and had the major contribution in designing the trial, and has contributed in data collection and writing of the paper. KAS has contributed to the design of the trial, and writing of the paper. ØS provided the ETIP trial with statistical assistance in analysing the data. TM was the project manager, and provided major contribution to data collection, analyses and writing of the paper. All authors have read and approved the final version of this manuscript.

Competing interests

The authors declare that they have no competing interest.

Author details

[1]Department of Circulation and Medical Imaging, NTNU, Norwegian University of Science and Technology, Box 8905, 7491 Trondheim, Norway. [2]Department of Public Health and General Practice, NTNU, Norwegian University of Science and Technology, Trondheim, Norway. [3]Research Department, St. Olavs Hospital Trondheim University Hospital, Trondheim, Norway. [4]Institute of clinical and molecular medicine, Norwegian University of Science and Tecnology, Trondheim, Norway. [5]Department of Obstetrics and Gynaecology, St. Olavs Hospital, Trondheim University Hospital, Trondheim, Norway.

References

1. Brunner S, Stecher L, Ziebarth S, et al. Excessive gestational weight gain prior to glucose screening and the risk of gestational diabetes: a meta-analysis. Diabetologia. 2015;58(10):2229–37.
2. Lutsiv O, Math J, Beyene J, McDonald SD. The effects of morbid obesity on maternal and neonatal health outcomes: a systematic review and meta-analyses. Obes Rev. 2015;16(7):531–46.
3. Oken E, Kleinman KP, Belfort MB, Hammitt JK, Gillman MW. Associations of gestational weight gain with short- and longer-term maternal and child health outcomes. Am J Epidemiol. 2009;170(2):173–80.
4. Kim SS, Zhu Y, Grantz KL, et al. Obstetric and neonatal risks among obese women without chronic disease. Obstet Gynecol. 2016;128(1):104–12.
5. Weiss JL, Malone FD, Emig D, et al. Obesity, obstetric complications and cesarean delivery rate–a population-based screening study. Am J Obstet Gynecol. 2004;190(4):1091–7.
6. Gaudet L, Ferraro ZM, Wen SW, Walker M. Maternal obesity and occurrence of fetal macrosomia: a systematic review and meta-analysis. Biomed Res Int. 2014;2014:640291.
7. Schmitt NM, Nicholson WK, Schmitt J. The association of pregnancy and the development of obesity - results of a systematic review and meta-analysis on the natural history of postpartum weight retention. Int J Obes. 2007;31(11):1642–51.
8. Gavard JA, Artal R. Effect of exercise on pregnancy outcome. Clin Obstet Gynecol. 2008;51(2):467–80.
9. Rando OJ, Simmons RA. I'm eating for two: parental dietary effects on offspring metabolism. Cell. 2015;161(1):93–105.
10. Nehring I, Schmoll S, Beyerlein A, Hauner H, von Kries R. Gestational weight gain and long-term postpartum weight retention: a meta-analysis. Am J Clin Nutr. 2011;94(5):1225–31.
11. Siega-Riz AM, Viswanathan M, Moos MK, et al. A systematic review of outcomes of maternal weight gain according to the Institute of Medicine recommendations: birthweight, fetal growth, and postpartum weight retention. Am J Obstet Gynecol. 2009;201(4):339 e331–14.
12. World Health Organization, WHO. Obesity and overweight. 2016. http://www.who.int/mediacentre/factsheets/fs311/en/.
13. Cedergren M. Effects of gestational weight gain and body mass index on obstetric outcome in Sweden. Int J Gynaecol Obstet. 2006;93(3):269–74.
14. Ronnberg A, Hanson U, Ostlund I, Nilsson K. Effects on postpartum weight retention after antenatal lifestyle intervention - a secondary analysis of a randomized controlled trial. Acta Obstet Gynecol Scand. 2016;95(9):999-1007.
15. Geiss LS, Wang J, Cheng YJ, et al. Prevalence and incidence trends for diagnosed diabetes among adults aged 20 to 79 years, United States, 1980-2012. JAMA. 2014;312(12):1218–26.
16. Colditz GA, Willett WC, Rotnitzky A, Manson JE. Weight-gain as a risk factor for clinical diabetes-mellitus in women. Ann Intern Med. 1995;122(7):481–6.
17. Catalano PM, Shankar K. Obesity and pregnancy: mechanisms of short term and long term adverse consequences for mother and child. BMJ. 2017;356;j1.
18. Choi J, Fukuoka Y, Lee JH. The effects of physical activity and physical activity plus diet interventions on body weight in overweight or obese women who are pregnant or in postpartum: a systematic review and meta-analysis of randomized controlled trials. Prev Med. 2013;56(6):351–64.
19. Berger AA, Peragallo-Urrutia R, Nicholson WK. Systematic review of the

effect of individual and combined nutrition and exercise interventions on weight, adiposity and metabolic outcomes after delivery: evidence for developing behavioral guidelines for post-partum weight control. BMC Pregnancy Childbirth. 2014;14:319.

20. Ostbye T, Krause KM, Lovelady CA, et al. Active mothers postpartum: a randomized controlled weight-loss intervention trial. Am J Prev Med. 2009;37(3):173–80.

21. Nascimento SL, Pudwell J, Surita FG, Adamo KB, Smith GN. The effect of physical exercise strategies on weight loss in postpartum women: a systematic review and meta-analysis. Int J Obes. 2014;38(5):626–35.

22. Garnaes KK, Morkved S, Salvesen O, Moholdt T. Exercise training and weight gain in obese pregnant women: a randomized controlled trial (ETIP trial). PLoS Med. 2016;13(7):e1002079.

23. Moholdt TT, Salvesen K, Ingul CB, Vik T, Oken E, Morkved S. Exercise training in pregnancy for obese women (ETIP): study protocol for a randomised controlled trial. Trials. 2011;12:154.

24. Exercise during pregnancy and the postpartum period. Clin Obstet Gynecol. 2003;46(2):496–9.

25. ACOG Committee Opinion No. 650. Physical activity and exercise during pregnancy and the postpartum period. Obstet Gynecol. 2015;126(6):e135–42.

26. ACOG Committee opinion. Number 267, January 2002: exercise during pregnancy and the postpartum period. Obstet Gynecol. 2002;99(1):171–3.

27. Borg GA. Psychophysical bases of perceived exertion. Med Sci Sports Exerc. 1982;14(5):377–81.

28. Rasmussen KM, Abrams B, Bodnar LM, Butte NF, Catalano PM, Maria S-RA. Recommendations for weight gain during pregnancy in the context of the obesity epidemic. Obstet Gynecol. 2010;116(5):1191–5.

29. World Health Organization, WHO. Definition and diagnosis of diabetes mellitus and intermediate hyperglycemia: report of a WHO/IDF consultation. 2006. 01.08.2016. http://www.who.int/diabetes/publications/diagnosis_diabetes2006/en/.

30. Matthews DR, Hosker JP, Rudenski AS, Naylor BA, Treacher DF, Turner RC. Homeostasis model assessment: insulin resistance and beta-cell function from fasting plasma glucose and insulin concentrations in man. Diabetologia. 1985;28(7):412–9.

31. Gore SA, Brown DM, West DS. The role of postpartum weight retention in obesity among women: a review of the evidence. Ann Behav Med. 2003;26(2):149–59.

32. Phelan S, Phipps MG, Abrams B, et al. Does behavioral intervention in pregnancy reduce postpartum weight retention? Twelve-month outcomes of the fit for delivery randomized trial. Am J Clin Nutr. 2014;99(2):302–11.

33. Price BB, Amini SB, Kappeler K. Exercise in pregnancy: effect on fitness and obstetric outcomes-a randomized trial. Med Sci Sports Exerc. 2012;44(12):2263–9.

34. Asci O, Rathfisch G. Effect of lifestyle interventions of pregnant women on their dietary habits, lifestyle behaviors, and weight gain: a randomized controlled trial. J Health Popul Nutr. 2016;35:7.

35. Sagedal LR, Sanda B, Overby NC, et al. The effect of prenatal lifestyle intervention on weight retention 12 months postpartum: results of the Norwegian fit for delivery randomised controlled trial. BJOG. 2016;124(1): 111-121. doi:10.1111/1471-0528.13863.

36. Vinter CA, Jensen DM, Ovesen P, et al. Postpartum weight retention and breastfeeding among obese women from the randomized controlled lifestyle in pregnancy (LiP) trial. Acta Obstet Gynecol Scand. 2014;93(8):794–801.

37. Ronnberg A, Hanson U, Ostlund I, Nilsson K. Effects on postpartum weight retention after antenatal lifestyle intervention - a secondary analysis of a randomized controlled trial. Acta Obstet Gynecol Scand. 2016;95(9):999–1007.

38. Leuridan L, Wens J, Devlieger R, Verhaeghe J, Mathieu C, Benhalima K. Glucose intolerance in early postpartum in women with gestational diabetes: who is at increased risk? Prim Care Diabetes. 2015;9(4):244–52.

39. Buchanan TA, Xiang A, Kjos SL, Watanabe R. What is gestational diabetes? Diabetes Care. 2007;30(Suppl 2):S105–11.

40. Catalano PM. Obesity, insulin resistance, and pregnancy outcome. Reproduction. 2010;140(3):365–71.

41. Ramakrishnan A, Lee LJ, Mitchell LE, Agopian AJ. Maternal hypertension during pregnancy and the risk of congenital heart defects in offspring: a systematic review and meta-analysis. Pediatr Cardiol. 2015;36(7):1442–51.

42. Gaudet L, Wen SW, Walker M. The combined effect of maternal obesity and fetal macrosomia on pregnancy outcomes. J Obstet Gynaecol Can. 2014;36(9):776–84.

43. Marchi J, Berg M, Dencker A, Olander EK, Begley C. Risks associated with obesity in pregnancy, for the mother and baby: a systematic review of reviews. Obes Rev. 2015;16(8):621–38.

44. Whelton SP, Chin A, Xin X, He J. Effect of aerobic exercise on blood pressure: a meta-analysis of randomized, controlled trials. Ann Intern Med. 2002;136(7):493–503.

45. Schwingshackl L, Dias S, Hoffmann G. Impact of long-term lifestyle programmes on weight loss and cardiovascular risk factors in overweight/obese participants: a systematic review and network meta-analysis. Syst Rev. 2014;3:130.

46. American College of O, Gynecologists. Exercise during pregnancy and the postpartum period. Clin Obstet Gynecol. 2003;46(2):496–9.

47. Sui Z, Moran LJ, Dodd JM. Physical activity levels during pregnancy and gestational weight gain among women who are overweight or obese. Health Promot J Austr. 2013;24(3):206–13.

48. Straub H, Simon C, Plunkett BA, et al. Evidence for a complex relationship among weight retention, Cortisol and breastfeeding in postpartum women. Matern Child Health J. 2016;20(7):1375–83.

49. Avery ND, Wolfe LA, Amara CE, Davies GA, McGrath MJ. Effects of human pregnancy on cardiac autonomic function above and below the ventilatory threshold. J Appl Physiol (1985). 2001;90(1):321–8.

50. Kim C, Newton KM, Knopp RH. Gestational diabetes and the incidence of type 2 diabetes: a systematic review. Diabetes Care. 2002;25(10):1862–8.

Enablers and barriers to physical activity in overweight and obese pregnant women: an analysis informed by the theoretical domains framework and COM-B model

C. Flannery[1*], S. McHugh[2], A. E. Anaba[2], E. Clifford[3], M. O'Riordan[4], L. C. Kenny[5], F. M. McAuliffe[6], P. M. Kearney[2] and M. Byrne[1]

Abstract

Background: Obesity during pregnancy is associated with increased risk of gestational diabetes mellitus (GDM) and other complications. Physical activity is a modifiable lifestyle factor that may help to prevent these complications but many women reduce their physical activity levels during pregnancy. Interventions targeting physical activity in pregnancy are on-going but few identify the underlying behaviour change mechanisms by which the intervention is expected to work. To enhance intervention effectiveness, recent tools in behavioural science such as the Theoretical Domains Framework (TDF) and COM-B model (capability, opportunity, motivation and behaviour) have been employed to understand behaviours for intervention development. Using these behaviour change methods, this study aimed to identify the enablers and barriers to physical activity in overweight and obese pregnant women.

Methods: Semi-structured interviews were conducted with a purposive sample of overweight and obese women at different stages of pregnancy attending a public antenatal clinic in a large academic maternity hospital in Cork, Ireland. Interviews were recorded and transcribed into NVivo V.10 software. Data analysis followed the framework approach, drawing on the TDF and the COM-B model.

Results: Twenty one themes were identified and these mapped directly on to the COM-B model of behaviour change and ten of the TDF domains. Having the social opportunity to engage in physical activity was identified as an enabler; pregnant women suggested being active was easier when supported by their partners. Knowledge was a commonly reported barrier with women lacking information on safe activities during pregnancy and describing the information received from their midwife as 'limited'. Having the physical capability and physical opportunity to carry out physical activity were also identified as barriers; experiencing pain, a lack of time, having other children, and working prevented women from being active.

Conclusion: A wide range of barriers and enablers were identified which influenced women's capability, motivation and opportunity to engage in physical activity with "knowledge" as the most commonly reported barrier. This study is a theoretical starting point in making a 'behavioural diagnoses' and the results will be used to inform the development of an intervention to increase physical activity levels among overweight and obese pregnant women.

Keywords: Overweight, Obesity, Pregnant women, Maternal health, Physical activity, Theoretical domains framework, COM-B model, Behaviour change wheel

* Correspondence: cflannery@ucc.ie
[1]Health Behaviour Change Research Group, School of Psychology, National University of Ireland, Galway, Ireland
Full list of author information is available at the end of the article

Background

Recent studies identify increasing trends in maternal obesity worldwide and associated complications such as gestational diabetes mellitus (GDM) [1–3]. Maternal obesity also has adverse neonatal outcomes, such as macrosomia [4] and offspring born to obese women are more likely to develop obesity, type 2 diabetes, cardiovascular disease and cancer in later life [5]. A recent systematic review identified maternal pre-pregnancy overweight as a significant risk factor for childhood overweight [6]. Children of mothers who were overweight before pregnancy were 1.37 times more likely to be overweight at 3 years of age than children of normal weight parents [7]. These trends and risks have increased interest in antenatal interventions which focus on women's eating, physical activity, their impact on gestational weight gain and GDM [8–10]. Strong evidence exists on the benefits associated with physical activity during pregnancy including an increase in functional mobility and a reduction in nausea and vomiting [11, 12]. Higher levels of physical activity before pregnancy or in early pregnancy also significantly lowers the risk of developing GDM [13]. A recent meta-analysis reported that antenatal physical activity in women of any body mass index led to a small reduction in offspring birth weight [14]. It is possible that this modest reduction in birth weight in offspring of overweight and obese women may be beneficial in reducing the long-term obesity risk [14, 15]. Furthermore, behavioural changes made during pregnancy may continue after childbirth and possibly throughout the woman's life [16] which in turn may have positive effects on child physical activity levels [17].

Despite these benefits, women's physical activity levels often reduce or cease during pregnancy [18]. Similar to Health Service Executive (HSE) recommendations in Ireland, the American Congress of Obstetricians and Gynaecologists (ACOG) and the Royal College of Obstetricians and Gynaecologists (RCOG), UK, recommend 30 min of daily moderate intensity physical activity for pregnant women [19–22]. Previous studies, carried out in different countries, reported low rates of physical activity during pregnancy. In the United States, only 15.8% of pregnant women vs. 26.1% of non-pregnant women reported engaging in the recommended physical activity guidelines [7]. This figure was even lower in a study from Brazil, where only 4.7% of pregnant women were physically active [8]. Only one-fifth of pregnant women in Ireland met the recommended guidelines and over 10% reported no physical activity [23]. Furthermore, a study examining lifestyle changes using the Pregnancy Risk Assessment Monitoring system (PRAMS), Ireland found that adherence to physical activity guidelines of moderate intensity activity was low (12.3%) but was particularly low for pregnant women with a body mass index > 25 kg/m^2 (6.4%) [24]. A cross-sectional study carried out in Danish women who wore a pedometer for at least 5 days, found that mean footsteps were higher among normal-weight women compared to obese women [25]. Furthermore, a decline in physical activity in pregnancy was found in a study carried out in 305 overweight or obese women [26]. These low rates of physical activity during pregnancy, particularly for overweight and obese women, are concerning given the significant health benefits for both mother and baby [12].

Previous research on clinical effects of lifestyle interventions in overweight and obese pregnant women has shown conflicting results [27–31]. These results have been attributed to poor study design, lack of power, lack of consistency in terms of the target behaviour, and failing to identify the psychological determinants and behavioural mechanisms by which the intervention is expected to have an effect [32, 33]. These complex lifestyle interventions have consisted of interacting components including dietary and physical activity counselling, monitoring of weight and group exercise sessions or have been designed to prevent excessive gestational weight gain (GWG) and reduce the risk of GDM [34]. Other interventions include individual counselling sessions on weight control and motivational interviewing [35, 36]. Most of these studies have examined the combined effect of physical activity and dietary advice and guidance. Three randomized controlled trials (RCTs) [31, 37, 38] that assessed the isolated effects of exercise in pregnancy on GWG and clinical outcomes in overweight and obese women found no significant difference in GWG between exercise and control groups. However, a recent meta-analysis [39], found that structured physical exercise programs during pregnancy do decrease the risk of GDM. Future research needs to address these conflicting results, hence, there is a need to establish the potential effects of physical activity on clinical indicators, especially in overweight and obese pregnant women.

Using theory to identify the determinants of behaviour can increase the likelihood that an intervention will be effective [40, 41]. A systematic review [42] examining the determinants of physical activity during pregnancy found that intention to exercise, self-efficacy and barriers such as lack of time and tiredness were strong predictors of exercise. Moreover, a systematic review that evaluated the content of physical activity interventions in pregnancy found theoretically developed interventions were more likely to help reduce the decline of physical activity throughout pregnancy [43]. Therefore, more attention should be placed on using theory to identify perceived determinants of behaviour and barriers to physical activity behaviour in pregnancy in order to develop effective interventions.

Health psychology offers theories of behaviour that can be used in maternity care interventions to help women make changes to lifestyle behaviours [34, 43, 44].

Michie and colleagues developed a framework derived from 33 commonly used behavioural theories and 128 psychological constructs called The Theoretical Domains Framework (TDF). The TDF has been identified as a useful tool for identifying determinants of behaviour and barriers to behaviour change. The TDF is an elaboration of the COM-B model which stands for "capability", "opportunity", "motivation" and "behaviour" [45, 46](Fig. 1). The COM-B model proposes that for any behaviour to occur a person must have the psychological and physical capability to perform the behaviour; the physical and social opportunity to engage in it and must be motivated to do so. Furthermore, when little is known about the population, qualitative research is useful to develop a theoretical understanding of the target behaviour [47–50]. To date, a number of empirical studies have used either the TDF or COM-B in order to develop behaviour change interventions in different contexts [51, 52] but to our knowledge this has not yet been done for physical activity in an overweight and obese pregnant population.

Therefore, the aim of this study was to use the TDF and corresponding COM-B model to identify enablers and barriers to physical activity in overweight and obese pregnant

women, and to use this information to inform the development of an antenatal lifestyle intervention to improve physical activity levels during pregnancy.

Method
Study design
A qualitative approach was used. Semi-structured interviews were conducted with a sample of overweight and obese pregnant women at risk of GDM. Ethical approval was obtained from the University College Cork Clinical Research Ethics Committee of the Cork Teaching Hospitals (ref: ECM 4 (y) 06/01/15).

Sampling and recruitment
Medical chart review identified a purposive sample of pregnant women with a body mass index (≥ 25 kg/m^2) recruited during pregnancy from a public antenatal clinic at Cork University Maternity Hospital (CUMH). CUMH is a large academic maternity hospital in the South of Ireland where approximately 6657 new obstetrics patients entered in 2015 [53]. Eligible participants were approached individually and informed about the study by the attending midwife and researcher on site at their antenatal appointment. They were

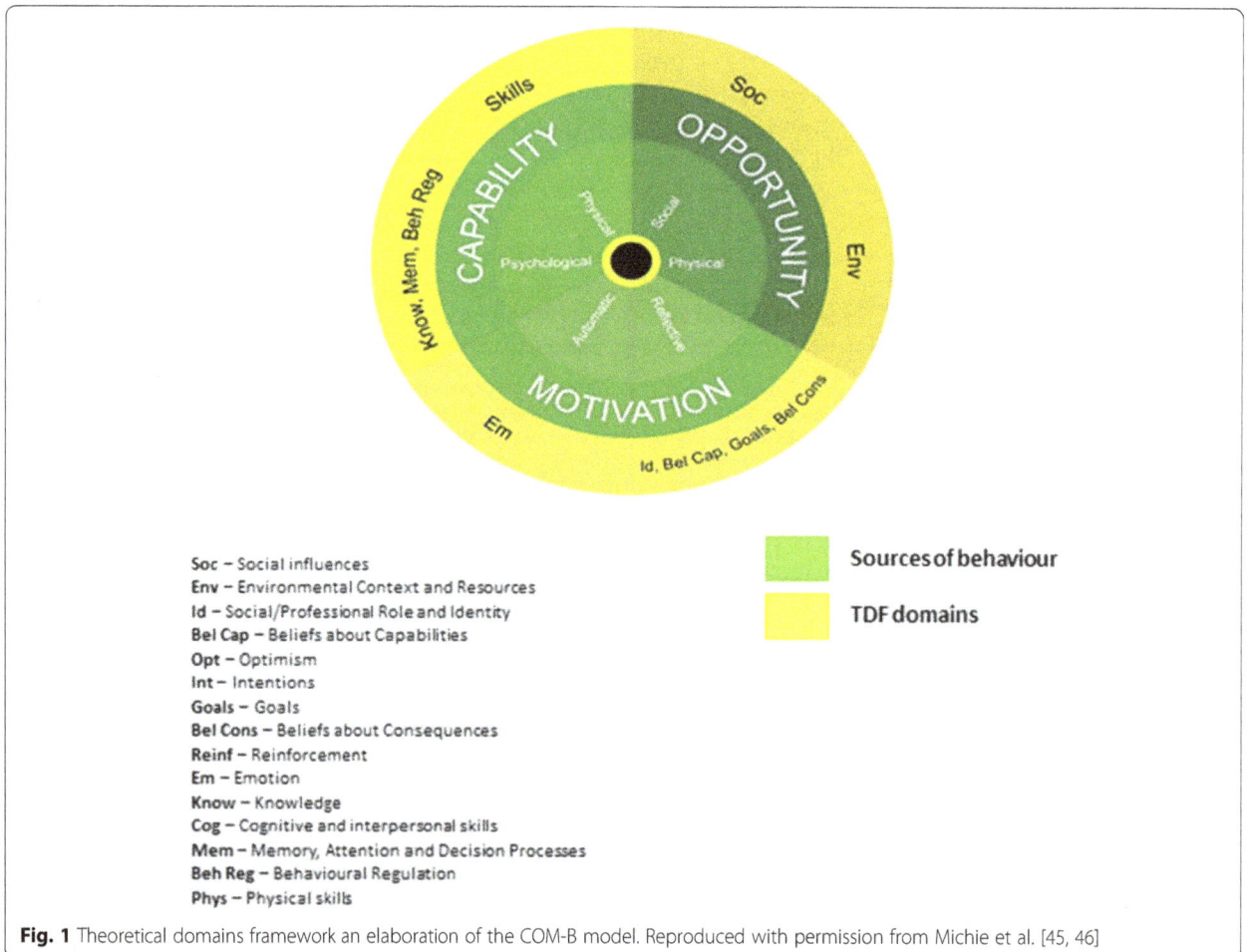

Soc – Social influences
Env – Environmental Context and Resources
Id – Social/Professional Role and Identity
Bel Cap – Beliefs about Capabilities
Opt – Optimism
Int – Intentions
Goals – Goals
Bel Cons – Beliefs about Consequences
Reinf – Reinforcement
Em – Emotion
Know – Knowledge
Cog – Cognitive and interpersonal skills
Mem – Memory, Attention and Decision Processes
Beh Reg – Behavioural Regulation
Phys – Physical skills

Sources of behaviour

TDF domains

Fig. 1 Theoretical domains framework an elaboration of the COM-B model. Reproduced with permission from Michie et al. [45, 46]

also provided with an information leaflet explaining the purpose of the study, how to participate and offered a small monetary compensation for participation. A €20 'One for All' voucher for a local shopping centre was posted to each woman who participated once the interview had been completed. Simultaneously, a sub-study examining diet and physical activity behaviours in pregnant African women led by researcher (AEA) was on-going. These women were recruited from the same antenatal clinic, during the same period using the same sampling criteria and interview guide. Therefore, interview data on physical activity for these women were included in this analysis. Data on age, nationality, body mass index (BMI) and gestational age were recorded from medical charts where possible. GDM, employment status and miscarriages were recorded only for those women who reported them spontaneously during the interview.

Interview process

Written informed consent was obtained from all participants at the start of the interviews. Face-to-face interviews were carried out in the antenatal clinic in CUMH on a day and time suitable for the participant by two researchers (CF) and (AEA) between June and September 2015. A semi-structured interview schedule was developed based on existing literature [34, 43, 54–56] and was used to facilitate the discussion (see Table 1). It consisted of open-ended questions and prompts about current lifestyle behaviours (physical activity and diet), challenges to engaging in healthy lifestyle and support mechanisms available. The interview schedule and process were piloted by interviewing two pregnant women at University College Cork. Following this pilot, additional probes and prompts were included to further explore women's experiences in terms of weight management and lifestyle changes. Pilot interviews were not included in the final sample as the women were not eligible for inclusion in the study.

Data analysis

Interviews were recorded and transcribed verbatim. NVivo software was used to facilitate data analysis. Data

Table 1 Interview schedule used to facilitate the interviews

	Questions	Prompts/Probes
Intro	Tell me a little about your home life?	• First pregnancy? • Married, single? • Other Children – how many? • Employed – how many hours you work?
	Tell me a bit about your lifestyle at the moment?	• Diet – cravings, nausea • **PA** – active before pregnancy, frequency, duration • Have diet/**PA** patterns changed since pregnancy? • In what way and why?
Health	Has a HCP made you aware of the risks surrounding your pregnancy	• Excessive weight gain • GDM • Potential difficulties during delivery • How does that make you feel?
PA and Diet	What **PA** do you/would you like doing?	• Walking, running, exercises tailored for pregnancy, sports, gym?
	How important do you feel exercise and **PA** is during pregnancy?	• Fitness level • Mobility • Give you more energy • Help sleep
	Tell me what you think would be the best way to encourage women to be watchful of diet and **PA** during pregnancy?	• Through friends, other pregnant women, GP, nurses, information sessions, individual or group, exercise and diet programmes
Behaviour Change	Have you been given advice about dietary habits and **PA** since you became pregnant?	• HCP, family, friend, book, internet? • When was this? • How did you feel about the advice?
	What to do think are the main challenges to **PA** and diet changes during pregnancy?	• Lack of information/ support/ time/ resources
	Would you be interested in using technology to help you track and improve you **PA** and diet	• Mobile phone apps, text message/phone, web based information forums, pedometer? • Would these support mechanisms be useful? • If it provided you with information as well • If it provided you HCP with your information
	How would you feel about participating in a study where technology would be used as encouragement to increase **PA**?	• Mobile phone apps, text message/phone, web based information forums, pedometer • Access to internet, mobile phone
	Is there anything I haven't asked you today you would like to mention?	

PA Physical activity, *HCP* Health care professional, *GDM* Gestational diabetes mellitus analysis followed a framework approach [57]. An inductive thematic analysis was conducted to identify new emerging themes and to investigate a priori objectives using the TDF and COM-B model. Each transcript was read and re-read numerous times by the researcher (CF). Transcripts were coded line by line and analysed to identify similarities and differences. Following open-coding, broader categories were mapped onto the domains of the TDF and then, directly onto the six components of the COM-B model identifying emerging themes relating to enablers and barriers to physical activity. See Table 3 for description of the TDF domains and components of the COM-B model. All transcripts were coded by the researcher (CF) and a subset of interviews were independently coded and analysed by a second researcher (SMH). Minor differences arose in relation to the mapping of codes to the TDF domains, particularly when codes mapped to more than one domain. Differences were resolved by consensus involving a third researcher with expertise in using the TDF and COM-B model (MB) on one occasion, as some themes were coded into multiple TDF domains. Specifically, the domain of "behavioural regulation" and "goals" were merged due to the overlapping theme of action planning. Recruitment continued until new issues ceased to emerge and saturation occurred across the theoretical domains. Two further pregnant women were interviewed to check if any new themes emerged.

Results

Participants' characteristics

In total twenty two overweight and obese pregnant women were interviewed. Data saturation occurred at interview twenty, as subsequent interviews did not contribute to the development of new themes. Eight interviews were included from the sub-study giving the overall sample of thirty overweight and obese pregnant women. Table 2 provides details of the participants' characteristics including age, nationality, BMI and gestational age. GDM, employment status and miscarriages were only recorded if mentioned by the woman during the interview.

Physical activity clusters identified in pregnancy

From the open coding of the interview data, pregnant women identified a number of factors surrounding physical activity in pregnancy. Given the importance of physical activity during pregnancy and in order to highlight pregnant women's perceptions, these different factors were categorised into four clusters that focus around friends and family, pregnancy, antenatal care and the community. These clusters are summarised in Fig. 2. Participants discussed different types of physical activity in pregnancy, the resources available and how family and friends could provide an important supportive role in physical activity participation. Participants also described the context in which these physical

Table 2 Profile characteristics of participants (N = 30)

Nationality	
Chinese	2
French	1
Hungarian	1
Lithuanian	1
Irish	16
Nigerian	5
Sudanese	2
Congolese (Democratic Republic of Congo)	1
Ghanaian	1
Age	
20–29	6
30–39	14
40+	1
Unknown[a]	9
Gestation	
First Trimester (0 to 13 Weeks)	1
Second Trimester (14 to 26 Weeks)	8
Third Trimester (27 to 40 Weeks)	20
Not stated	1
BMI (kg/m2\)[b]	
Overweight 25–29	12
Obese ≥30	12
Unknown[c]	6
Pregnancy	
Singleton	29
Twins	1
Employment	
Working full time	10
Working part time	2
Out sick from work	2
Not working	6
Not stated	10
Gestational Diabetes Mellitus[d]	
GDM	5
Not stated	25
Miscarriages[e]	
Miscarriages	8
Not stated	22

[a]Not recorded from medical chart
[b]BMI taken from medical chart (calculated at booking visit by midwife)
[c]Midwife identified women as overweight and obese from chart but did not record BMI
[d]Only 5 women mentioned having gestational diabetes
[e]Only 8 women discussed having one or more miscarriages

activity behaviours occur. Certain factors identified within these clusters are also present in the TDF and COM-B analysis, see results below. The main type of physical activity identified by the pregnant women includes walking, swimming, pilates, yoga and physical activity classes tailored for pregnancy.

Summary of the TDF and COM-B model: Barriers and enablers to physical activity

Twenty one themes were identified that mapped directly onto ten of the TDF domains and the six COM-B components. The ten TDF domains included "skills", "knowledge", "behavioural regulation", "goals"; "environmental context and resources", "social influences", "social/professional role and identity", "beliefs about capability", "intentions", and "emotion". The TDF domains not relevant to the context of physical activity in overweight and obese pregnant women were "optimism", "reinforcement" "memory" and "belief about consequences". These findings are described in greater detail below using the TDF and corresponding COM-B model (Table 3).

Capability
Physical skills

In terms of the domain "physical skills", pregnancy related symptoms were a common reason given by participants for undertaking little or no physical activity. These included muscle pain, pelvic or lower back pain, swelling and other conditions.

'The problems I had just stopped me [PA]. Like I got a polyp...which was heavy bleeding and the more I strained the body, even just a swim it was just like there was more pressure on it so I just said it was better to cut everything' (Participant 15; 32 weeks pregnant)

Furthermore, women who knew their pregnancy was high risk, decided themselves, that it was best not to engage in physical activity.

'I'm a high risk pregnancy so I couldn't do any of the exercise then on this pregnancy. And then I have factor 5 blood so really clotting and all that, I have to take it easy' (Participant 05; 28 weeks pregnant)

Another barrier was that of feeling too tired to engage in physical activity; finding it hard to move, lack of energy and being physically drained.

'It's harder to move faster now that I am pregnant. Like sometimes I have energy and some days I don't... It's

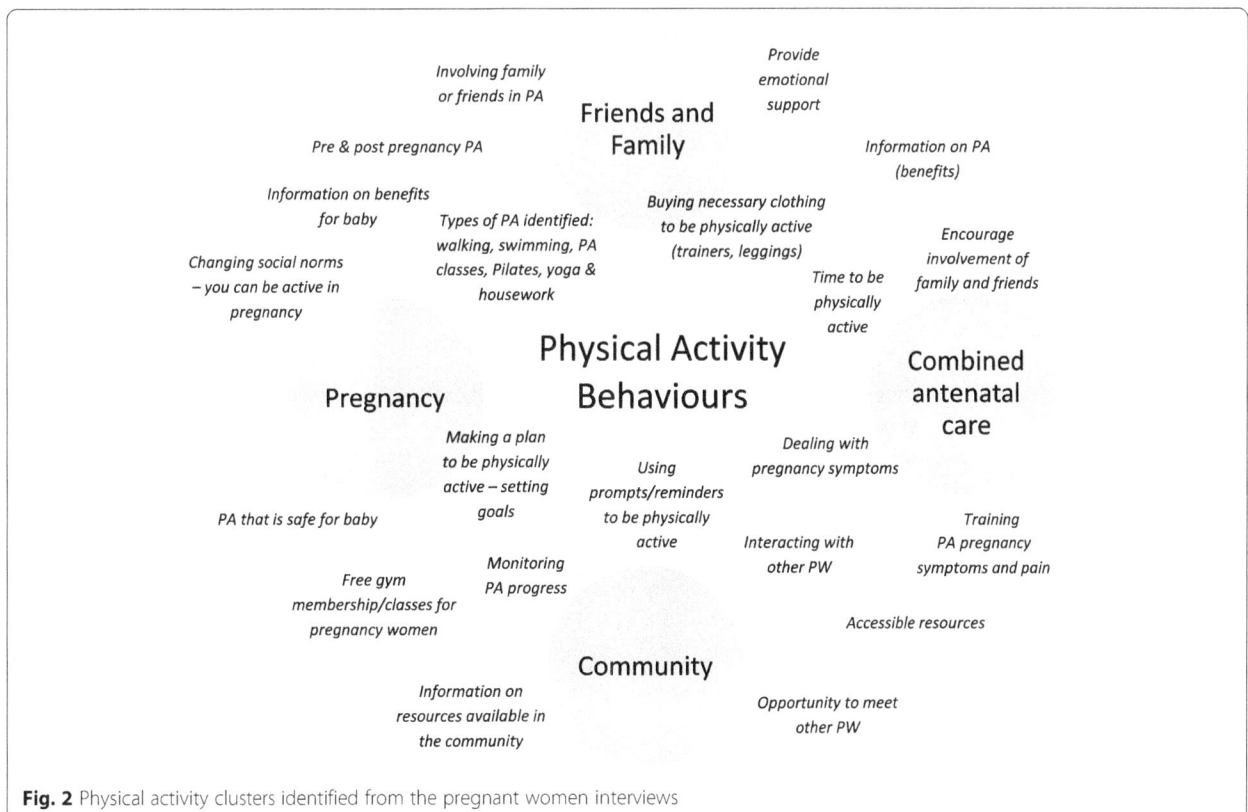

Fig. 2 Physical activity clusters identified from the pregnant women interviews

Table 3 Mapping of themes to the TDF domains and COM-B model

Themes	TDF	COM-B
- Fitness level prior to pregnancy - House work as a form of PA - Medical conditions and pregnancy symptoms (pain/energy/tiredness)	Knowledge (awareness of the existence of something: knowledge of condition)	Psychology capability Knowledge or psychological skills, strength or stamina to engage in the necessary mental process
- Limited knowledge surrounding PA benefits, types of PA in pregnancy and PA resources - Pregnant women discussed concerns around having that 'conversation'	Knowledge (awareness of the existence of something: knowledge of condition)	Psychology capability Knowledge or psychological skills, strength or stamina to engage in the necessary mental process
- Self- monitoring, use of pedometer/step count/phone apps	Behavioural regulation (managing or changes action – self monitoring)	
- Women expressed interest in goal setting	Goals[a] (mental representations of outcome or end states, that an individual wants to achieve)	
- Pregnant woman's situation (family life/children/work/pets) - Financial situation - Weather/ built environment and resources within the community	Environmental context and resources (persons situation or environment)	Physical Opportunity Opportunity afforded by the environment involving time, resources, location, cues physical affordance
- Acknowledged support from family members, partner and friends - Interaction with other pregnant women [PA classes] was mentioned	Social influences (Process that can change thoughts feelings or behaviours – social pressure)	Social opportunity Opportunity afforded by interpersonal influences, social cues and cultural norms that influence the way we think
- 'Every pregnant women is different' - Differences in pregnancies	Social role and identity (set of behaviours and displayed personal qualities in a social or work setting)	Reflective Motivation Reflective process involving plans (self-conscious intentions) and evaluations (beliefs about what is good and bad)
- Using pregnancy as an 'excuse' - Concern for health of the baby - Feeling responsible - Difficulty breaking habits/mind-set	Beliefs about capability (acceptance of the truth, reality or validity about an ability, perceived behavioural control,, self-esteem, confidence)	
- Post-partum intentions (planning weight loss/healthy lifestyle)	Intentions (A conscious decision to perform a behaviour)	Reflective Motivation Reflective process involving plans (self-conscious intentions) and evaluations (beliefs about what is good and bad)
- Feelings of worry, concern and guilt during pregnancy - Fear based on previous pregnancy outcome/miscarriage	Emotion (complex reactions - fear, anxiety, affect, stress, depression, positive and negative effect, burn out)	Automatic Motivation Automatic processes involving emotional reactions, desires(wants and needs) impulses inhibitions drive states and reflex responses

[a]Behavioural regulation and goals were merged due to the overlapping construct of 'action planning'
TDF domain not identified: optimism, reinforcement and belief about consequences

difficult, like you feel like you want to do stuff but you can't, your body is just tired and drained physically' (Participant 20; 28 weeks pregnant)

However, some women felt that physical activity during pregnancy did benefit them (e.g. helped them wake up, gave them energy and made them feel good). Likewise, being physically fit before pregnancy was identified as an enabler; if a woman was active before pregnancy she was more likely to keep it up.

'I don't know I think it depends on everyone's circumstances. Like a lot of women would be fit before they got pregnant and they would keep up their

walking or running' (Participant 01; gestation unknown)

House work emerged as an enabler particularly for women who did not like exercise. These women considered household activities as part of their daily activity.

'No I wouldn't get out and walk or anything like that... housework would be my activity during the day' (Participant 04; 28 weeks pregnant)

'Not really, there's nothing really, I'm not a big fan of exercise. I will do the house work, the cleaning and the cooking' (Participant 17; 36 weeks pregnant)

Knowledge

When considering the domain of "knowledge" there was concerns about safety and types of exercise appropriate in pregnancy.

'To be honest, I'm not good in what physical activities a pregnant woman should do because nobody really has told me about the kind of exercise you should be doing' (Participant 28; 32 weeks pregnant).

'I mean I don't know can you do certain exercises so I would be worried that I could pull a muscle so I would be extra cautious I suppose at the gym cause I'm afraid and I wouldn't really know' (Participant 13; 32 weeks pregnant)

These doubts were partly due to the limited information they reported receiving from their midwife or health care professional. This information was described as a *'limited', 'quick', 'automatic', 'like a checklist'* and women felt the benefits of physical activity was rarely discussed.

'It's very limited really, very limited. It's a quick one minute conversation really in relation to it [PA/ Diet]....I suppose nobody really sits you down to go through the implications of that or the benefits and stuff like that' (Participant 21; 26 weeks pregnant)

Furthermore when discussing 'the conversation' women felt more emphasis was placed on the clinical aspect of the visit rather than information and advice.

'They don't tend to offer any advice good or bad in terms of weight management and activity and stuff like that. It's more the blood pressure, checking the baby and stuff like that' (Participant 21; 26 weeks pregnant)

Some women felt that midwives assumed because they had other children they already had knowledge and information around being physically active in pregnancy.

'...what I found different was when they know that you have children already they kind of thinking that you know everything which is not true...you may forget, years apart, like between now and the last time I had a baby there is a three year gap so I can't remember everything but they seem to assume because you have had other children you know already what to do' (Participant 28; 32 weeks pregnant)

Women actually felt less confident in terms of what they knew about physical activity and would have preferred more advice from their midwife.

'there's no such thing as really showing you or describing it you know, or making sure that you are doing it [PA], I think that could be discussed or checked a little bit more' (Participant 14: 30 weeks pregnant)

Some women were active when they had "knowledge" of the health benefits (e.g. keeping muscles strong for labour). Furthermore, women expressed interest in attending pregnancy exercise classes; if they were provided with information on these classes in their area they would be more likely to attend.

'I think that would be a good idea [PA information & resources], like if you were given like numbers and sort of classes around that area at your clinic appointments for like types of yoga and stuff like that' (Participant 04; 28 weeks pregnant)

Behavioural regulation and goals

In terms of "behavioural regulation" women's comments on technology suggested that action planning and self-monitoring would be an enabler to physical activity. When discussing technology, women explained that a 'pedometer' or 'step count' might help in terms of motivation and to monitor current levels of physical activity.

'If there was definitely some sort of measurement like a pedometer or something like that, just something that would flag where you are at and what your targets should be' (Participant 21; 26 weeks pregnant)

Some women suggested setting "goals" as an enabler to physical activity, providing them with targets to accomplish.

'I am very goal driven, I would love that, if someone said ' you need to walk three miles this week and you need to do four laps of the pool and something else, you know you would hit your targets and you know then that even if they say that was helping you, that you are going a good job. You're doing something good anyway' (Participant 18; 14 weeks pregnant)

Although women felt a pedometer or step count would help with motivation, other forms of technology did not have the same perceived benefit. Women disliked the idea of tracking physical activity (number of days, length of activity time) in a phone app if it was linked with the antenatal clinic. They felt like *'big brother'* would be watching or that it was a chance for their health care professionals to *'check up on me'* calling it an *'invasion of privacy'*. Furthermore some women felt that tracking physical activity would be a *'burden'* or like *'homework'* and that with their busy lifestyles they would just forget.

'I'm not actually that good of keeping track of anything really like that [PA] (laughs) I would try to write things down but I would just be so busy or I would forget and I wouldn't do it, so I wouldn't be a good user of those [pregnancy apps]' (Participant 13; 32 weeks pregnant)

Opportunity
Environmental context and resources
Women's opportunity to engage in physical activity in pregnancy was often hindered by work and family commitments. Even though they were motivated to be physically active, often constraints in the way of time and bad weather conditions justified not participating in physical activity.

'I suppose prior to the first pregnancy I could go from work to exercise and then come home. Whereas, now if I do that I don't see my son before he goes to bed. So I just can't fit it into my day to be honest, it's more challenging' (Participant 21; 26 weeks pregnant)

Some women identified a lack of financial means as well as a lack of targeted services specifically tailored for pregnancy as barriers to physical activity. Women suggested subsidised services as a solution to financial difficulties. Making services *'financially viable'* might encourage the use of a gym or exercise class's thus enabling physical activity.

'I mean I'm not going just because I have two kids I have a massive big mortgage and I actually can't afford the full membership to go swimming........Free gym membership for pregnant woman for 9 months (laughs) that would be great, even I would go then (laughs)' (Participant 16; 38 weeks pregnant)

Social influences
A commonly reported enabler was that of "social influences" which included family and friends encouragement of physical activity. Women's partner or husbands were the most influencing factor (e.g. *'always pushing me to go for a walk', 'he would drag me out for a walk'*).

The women's husbands were not seen as a barrier to PA while other family members were.

'Put your feet up' that's what I get especially over the last four weeks, from my mother in law' (Participant 16; 38 weeks pregnant)

Women also expressed an interest in pregnancy physical activity classes giving mothers a chance to *'talk'* comparing it to a *'support group'*.

'...it would be that extra motivation [PA classes]. Get out and make friends and talk more, and enjoy the activity more' (Participant 04; 28 weeks pregnant)

Motivation

Social role and identity
A clear justification for not engaging in physical activity was the 'individual'. It was commonly reported that *'every woman is different'* and *'every pregnancy is different'* and it was up to that 'individual' whether or not they would make healthy choices or be physically active.

'I think it definitely depends on the individual, I think it depends on the pregnant mother whether they want to be healthy or not...' (Participant 01; gestation unknown)

Belief about capability
When considering "belief about capability" pregnancy was viewed as a time for change particularly for the benefit of the baby *'I just have to... be as healthy as I can be now, I mean it's all for the baby' (Participant 13; 32 weeks pregnant)*. The foremost feelings that prevailed throughout the interviews were the sense of *'responsibility'* in providing the best for the baby in terms of healthy lifestyle behaviours.

'...every woman is different and every woman will take on board information differently [diet & PA]. I think it is very important when you're pregnant, you need to just take responsibility like, and you do. (Participant 19; 27 weeks pregnant)

Some women also described how they were changing behaviour to be healthy not only for the baby but for themselves.

'..when I came out of my doctor I knew I was going to do something that was going to help me and the baby and that my actions would make us healthier together ya know. (Participant 18; 14 weeks pregnant)

At the same time, pregnancy provided a reason to not make healthy changes (e.g. *'...like sure I'm pregnant. I'm going to be big anyway' (Participant 09; 39 weeks pregnant))*. Woman felt that pregnancy could be used as an *'excuse'* and that *'mind-set'* played a big part in whether or not you would make any changes. Some women stated they would have to have been physically active at the start of pregnancy in order to keep it up and that breaking bad habits in pregnancy is difficult.

> *'No I would have to have been doing it from the start [PA]. I wouldn't have picked it up half way through. I definitely would have had to have started at the beginning. I mean I told myself at the start, I actually wouldn't mind doing that [PA] and keeping it up but I just didn't and then I just stopped and sat and eat....it's hard to break that habit especially when you are pregnant as you do use it as an excuse' (Participant 02; gestation unknown)*

Intentions

Others reported being motivated when talking about after pregnancy and their implicit intentions to change (e.g *'I have it planned out in my head'*).

> *'I know I am not having any more and I tell myself afterwards I'll get back into it' (Participant 02; gestation unknown)*

> *'So I said right when this baby now is done...after I have recovered I'm going back to my [PA] classes' (Participant 05; 28 weeks pregnant)*

Emotion

In terms of "emotion", enablers to physical activity included feelings of *'guilt'* and *'concern'*.

> *'if I could get away with it [no PA], if I could I would definitely but I know I would feel pure guilty. I know I would have them [health care professionals] looking at me and I would feel fierce guilty' (Participant 18; 14 weeks pregnant)*

> *'...the first time round I could go for walks, I was taking care of my health and ya know, you kind of that bit worried the first time round, you make sure you are doing the best for the baby and yourself' (Participant 01; gestation unknown)*

A fear based on previous pregnancy outcomes was highlighted with women afraid to do anything in pregnancy due to previous miscarriage experiences.

> *'...from the moment I knew I was pregnant it has been terrifying for me. Because like I'm after having 3 miscarriages in 2 years it's not a nice thing to experience, I mean you're constantly waiting to see that heartbeat..' (Participant 05; 28 weeks pregnant)*

Discussion

The aim of this study was to systematically identify the barriers and enablers to physical activity for women who are overweight and obese in pregnancy using the TDF and COM-B model. A wide range of barriers and enablers were identified which influenced women's capability, motivation and opportunity to engage in physical activity with women providing more information about barriers than enablers.

In the current study, the most commonly reported barrier to physical activity during pregnancy was "knowledge". It was clear from the findings that women were unclear on what types of physical activity they could engage in while pregnant and whether physical activity was safe. This finding is similar to that of a qualitative study conducted in the US, in which pregnant women mentioned a lack of advice regarding physical activity [58]; the most information they received from their midwives was to 'carry on as usual' [59]. Perhaps this lack of information can explain why adherence to physical activity guidelines is so low particularly for pregnant women with a BMI > 25 kg/m^2 (6.4%) [24]. Health care professionals are key to enhancing pregnant women's knowledge of being physical active and the benefits of being active in pregnancy [60]. Furthermore, many women received little or no advice on appropriate weight management in pregnancy. Service providers [61], similar to the women here, considered verbal advice offered to women on topics such as lifestyle and weight management to be inconsistent and unsupported by written information [62]. This is perhaps not surprising given the lack of Irish guidance regarding weight management in pregnancy [22]. However, despite this the women actually expressed little concern about weight gain.

"Physical skills" such as pregnancy-related symptoms (e. g. morning sickness/nausea/pelvic pain) were common barriers to physical activity. However, research has shown that being physical active in early pregnancy can reduce these symptoms [11, 12]. Thus this information may be a useful motivational strategy to encourage overweight and obese women to be active early on. Furthermore, high risk pregnancies were identified as a barrier, yet, research has indicated that in the case of risk factors for preeclampsia, exercise has been seen to promote maternal circulation, improve maternal fetal vascularity and boost the immune system of women [63]. For women with high risk pregnancies, physical activity is recommended with some restrictions; but there are currently no clear recommendations available [64], therefore, evidence based guidelines are required for health care professionals in order for them to guide women about safe activity in pregnancy given their health status. Another barrier reported by the women was tiredness and a lack of energy due to being pregnant, work and family commitments. This is consistent with previous literature, feeling tired or having no energy are the most commonly reported reasons for not being active [58, 65–67].

The women identified "social influences" indicating the relative importance of advice received from family and friends in initiating physical activity behaviour. Also, the women enjoyed meeting other pregnant women and expressed interest in physical activity classes tailored for pregnancy. Healthcare professionals need to take a holistic approach to care, taking into consideration the women's social support network and influences to include their partners in group pregnancy sessions. Action planning and goal setting were identified by the women as a means of motivation and that pedometers and step counts could help with self-monitoring. A review, examining the use of pedometers to increase physical activity and improve health, concluded that pedometers were associated with significant increases in physical activity in an adult population [68]. Furthermore, in a study with pregnant women the pedometer was acceptable to the women [25]. Thus, future interventions should include some component of self-monitoring in order to improve physical activity levels in overweight and obese pregnant women.

Analysis using the TDF provided a detailed understanding of the barriers and enablers to physical activity for pregnant women and the refinement of the findings into the COM-B model has set the stage for developing a theory and evidence based intervention to increase physical activity levels in overweight and obese pregnant women. Using these frameworks added substantial strength to this study because it is composed of theoretically derived domains based on a comprehensive list of behavioural theories. This will help to identify potentially relevant domains and to select a set of relevant theories to investigate the target behaviour in depth at a later stage. While the study has some clear strengths, there were some potential limitations. While the TDF provided a comprehensive framework for understanding types of enablers and barriers to physical activity among this population, at times it was difficult to categorise themes due to lack of clarity in the definitions of the theoretical domains. Where this happened, the best solution was determined through discussion with members of the research team (CF) and (SMH). An additional limitation was the sampling frame for the study; all women were recruited through a public clinic in one maternity hospital setting potentially limiting diversity in study findings. Furthermore, even though this ethnically diverse sample of pregnant women shared similar views regarding physical activity, research is warranted to assess racial or cultural differences in overweight and obese pregnant women.

Conclusion

This research provides an important overview of the behavioural factors enabling or inhibiting physical activity and has also identified a system of behaviours that may be relevant in order to increase physical activity levels amongst overweight and obese pregnant women. Using the TDF and COM-B model is a theoretical starting point for understanding behaviour within specific contexts and to make a 'behavioural diagnosis' of what needs to change to alter behaviour. The COM-B model forms the hub of the Behaviour Change Wheel (BCW) which provides a systematic and transparent way to conduct a behavioural assessment, identify the target behaviour, select intervention functions and to develop theory based intervention strategies [45]. The findings suggest a lack of knowledge around safe types of physical activity in pregnancy and awareness of the potential benefits for mother and baby. Interventions which provide continuing support from health care professionals and involve partners and family members are potential approaches to consider for interventions in pregnancy. In future research, we will use the behaviour change wheel to identify intervention functions to systematically develop a lifestyle intervention to increase physical activity levels for overweight and obese pregnant women. Developing an antenatal intervention that targets these salient barriers to physical activity will have greater potential to change behaviour.

Abbreviations

BCW: Behaviour Change Wheel; COM-B: Capability, opportunity and motivation-behaviour; PW: Pregnant woman; TDF: Theoretical Domains Framework

Acknowledgements

The authors would like to acknowledge the midwives and staff at Cork University Maternity Hospital (CUMH) for their support and assistance with recruitment. We would also like to thank the pregnant women who agreed to be interviewed for this study.

Funding

This research was funded by the Health Research Board SPHeRE/2013/1. The Health Research Board (HRB) supports excellent research that improves people's health, patient care and health service delivery. The HRB aims to ensure that new knowledge is created and then used in policy and practice. In doing so, the HRB supports health system innovation and create new enterprise opportunities.

Authors' contributions

CF, SMH, PMK and MB conceived and designed the study. CF and SMH developed the topic guide and study protocol. LCK and MOR facilitated access to pregnant women for recruitment to the study. CF and AEA facilitated and transcribed the interviews. CF and SMH coded the transcripts and developed and refined the themes. MB provided TDF and COM-B model expertise. CF wrote the first draft of the paper. All other authors (EC and FMA) contributed to successive drafts and the revising of the manuscript. All authors (CF, SMH, AEA, EC, MOR, LCK, FMA, PMK and MB) read and approved the final manuscript.

Competing interests
The authors declare that they have no competing interests.

Author details
[1]Health Behaviour Change Research Group, School of Psychology, National University of Ireland, Galway, Ireland. [2]School of Public Health, University College Cork, Cork, Ireland. [3]Department of Nutrition & Dietetics, South Infirmary Victoria University Hospital, Cork, Ireland. [4]Department Obstetrics and Gynaecology, University College Cork, Cork, Ireland. [5]Department of Women's and Children's Health, Faculty of Health and Life Sciences, University of Liverpool, Liverpool, UK. [6]UCD Perinatal Research Centre, School of Medicine, University College Dublin, National Maternity Hospital, Dublin, Ireland.

References
1. Ramachenderan J, Bradford J, Mclean M. Maternal obesity and pregnancy complications: a review. Aust N Z J Obstet Gynaecol. 2008;48:228–35.
2. Guelinckx I, Devlieger R, Beckers K, Vansant G. Maternal obesity: pregnancy complications, gestational weight gain and nutrition. Obes Rev. 2008;9:140–50.
3. McDonald SD, Han Z, Mulla S, Beyene J. Overweight and obesity in mothers and risk of preterm birth and low birth weight infants: systematic review and meta-analyses. BMJ. 2010;341:c3428.
4. Catalano PM, Ehrenberg HM. Review article: the short- and long-term implications of maternal obesity on the mother and her offspring. BJOG. 2006;113:1126–33.
5. Galliano D, Bellver J. Female obesity: short- and long-term consequences on the offspring. Gynecol Endocrinol. 2013;29:626–31.
6. Weng SF, Redsell SA, Swift JA, Yang M, Glazebrook CP. Systematic review and meta-analyses of risk factors for childhood overweight identifiable during infancy. Arch Dis Child. 2012;97:1019–26.
7. Hawkins SS, Cole TJ, Law C. An ecological systems approach to examining risk factors for early childhood overweight: findings from the UK Millennium Cohort Study. J. Epidemiol. Community Health. 2008; jech. 2008.077917.
8. Luoto RM, Kinnunen TI, Aittasalo M, Ojala K, Mansikkamaki K, Toropainen E, Kolu P, Vasankari T. Prevention of gestational diabetes: design of a cluster-randomized controlled trial and one-year follow-up. BMC Pregnancy Childbirth. 2010;10:39.
9. Morisset AS, St-Yves A, Veillette J, Weisnagel SJ, Tchernof A, Robitaille J. Prevention of gestational diabetes mellitus: a review of studies on weight management. Diabetes Metab Res Rev. 2010;26:17–25.
10. Hill B, Skouteris H, Fuller-Tyszkiewicz M. Interventions designed to limit gestational weight gain: a systematic review of theory and meta-analysis of intervention components. Obes Rev. 2013;14:435–50.
11. Warburton DE, Nicol CW, Bredin SS. Health benefits of physical activity: the evidence. CMAJ. 2006;174:801–9.
12. Morris SN, Johnson NR. Exercise during pregnancy: a critical appraisal of the literature. J Reprod Med. 2005;50:181–8.
13. Tobias DK, Zhang C, van Dam RM, Bowers K, Hu FB. Physical Activity Before and During Pregnancy and Risk of Gestational Diabetes Mellitus. A meta-analysis. 2011;34:223–9.
14. Thangaratinam S, Rogozińska E, Jolly K, Glinkowski S, Roseboom T, Tomlinson J, Kunz R, Mol B, Coomarasamy A, Khan K. Effects of interventions in pregnancy on maternal weight and obstetric outcomes: meta-analysis of randomised evidence. BMJ. 2012;344:e2088.
15. Pivarnik JM, Chambliss H, Clapp J, Dugan S, Hatch M, Lovelady C, Mottola M, Williams M. Impact of physical activity during pregnancy and postpartum on chronic disease risk. Med Sci Sports Exerc. 2006;38:989–1006.
16. Clark M, Ogden J. The impact of pregnancy on eating behaviour and aspects of weight concern. Int J Obes Relat Metab Disord. 1999;23:18–24.
17. Hesketh KR, O'Malley C, Paes VM, Moore H, Summerbell C, Ong KK, Lakshman R, van Sluijs EMF. Determinants of change in physical activity in children 0–6 years of age: a systematic review of quantitative literature. Sports Med. 2017;47:1349–74.
18. Borodulin K, Evenson KR, Herring AH. Physical activity patterns during pregnancy through postpartum. BMC Womens Health. 2009;9:1–7.
19. RCOG: Recreational exercise and pregnancy: information for you. 2006. https://www.rcog.org.uk/globalassets/documents/patients/patient-information-leaflets/pregnancy/recreational-exercise-and-pregnancy.pdf. 21 Aug 2016.
20. SOGC/CSEP: Clinical Practice Guidelines: Exercise in pregnancy and the postpartum period. 2003. https://sogc.org/wp-content/uploads/2013/01/129E-JCPG-June2003.pdf. 19 Aug 2016.
21. HSE/ICGP. Healthy Weight Management Guidelines Before, During & After Pregnancy. http://www.icgp.ie/go/library/catalogue/item/73ACFC19-4195-4F57-91E5F973ED955D72. 2013;
22. HSE: Obesity and Pregnancy Clinical Practice Guideline. 2013. https://www.hse.ie/eng/services/publications/clinical-strategy-and-programmes/obesity-and-pregnancy-clinical-practice-guideline.pdf. 2 Sept 2016.
23. Walsh JM, McGowan C, Byrne J, McAuliffe FM. Prevalence of physical activity among healthy pregnant women in Ireland. Int J Gynaecol Obstet. 2011; 114:154–5.
24. O'Keeffe LM, Dahly DL, Murphy M, Greene RA, Harrington JM, Corcoran P, Kearney PM. Positive lifestyle changes around the time of pregnancy: a cross-sectional study. BMJ Open. 2016;6:e010233.
25. Renault K, Nørgaard K, Andreasen KR, Secher NJ, Nilas L. Physical activity during pregnancy in obese and normal-weight women as assessed by pedometer. Acta Obstet Gynecol Scand. 2010;89:956–61.
26. Sui Z, Moran LJ, Dodd JM. Physical activity levels during pregnancy and gestational weight gain among women who are overweight or obese. Health Promot J Austr. 2013;24:206–13.
27. Guelinckx I, Devlieger R, Mullie P, Vansant G. Effect of lifestyle intervention on dietary habits, physical activity, and gestational weight gain in obese pregnant women: a randomized controlled trial. Am J Clin Nutr. 2010;91:373–80.
28. Bogaerts A, Devlieger R, Nuyts E, Witters I, Gyselaers W, Van den Bergh B. Effects of lifestyle intervention in obese pregnant women on gestational weight gain and mental health: a randomized controlled trial. Int J Obes. 2013;37:814.
29. Harrison CL, Lombard CB, Strauss BJ, Teede HJ. Optimizing healthy gestational weight gain in women at high risk of gestational diabetes: a randomized controlled trial. Obesity. 2013;21:904–9.
30. Vinter CA, Jensen DM, Ovesen P, Beck-Nielsen H, Jorgensen JS. The LiP (lifestyle in pregnancy) study: a randomized controlled trial of lifestyle intervention in 360 obese pregnant women. Diabetes Care. 2011;34:2502–7.
31. Ong M, Guelfi K, Hunter T, Wallman K, Fournier P, Newnham J. Supervised home-based exercise may attenuate the decline of glucose tolerance in obese pregnant women. Diabetes Metab. 2009;35:418–21.
32. Rowlands I, Graves N, de Jersey S, McIntyre HD, Callaway L. Obesity in pregnancy: outcomes and economics. Semin Fetal Neonatal Med. 2010;15: 94–9.
33. Oteng-Ntim E, Varma R, Croker H, Poston L, Doyle P. Lifestyle interventions for overweight and obese pregnant women to improve pregnancy outcome: systematic review and meta-analysis. BMC Med. 2012;10:47.
34. Campbell F, Johnson M, Messina J, Guillaume L, Goyder E. Behavioural interventions for weight management in pregnancy: a systematic review of quantitative and qualitative data. BMC Public Health. 2011;11:491.
35. Claesson IM, Sydsjo G, Brynhildsen J, Cedergren M, Jeppsson A, Nystrom F, Sydsjo A, Josefsson A. Weight gain restriction for obese pregnant women: a case-control intervention study. BJOG. 2008;115:44–50.
36. Shirazian T, Monteith S, Friedman F, Rebarber A. Lifestyle modification program decreases pregnancy weight gain in obese women. Am J Perinatol. 2010;27:411–4.
37. Choi J, Fukuoka Y, Lee JH. The effects of physical activity and physical activity plus diet interventions on body weight in overweight or obese women who are pregnant or in postpartum: a systematic review and meta-analysis of randomized controlled trials. Prev Med. 2013;56:351–64.
38. Seneviratne S, Jiang Y, Derraik J, McCowan L, Parry G, Biggs J, Craigie S, Gusso S, Peres G, Rodrigues R. Effects of antenatal exercise in overweight and obese pregnant women on maternal and perinatal outcomes: a randomised controlled trial. BJOG. 2016;123:588–97.
39. Sanabria-Martínez G, García-Hermoso A, Poyatos-León R, Álvarez-Bueno C, Sánchez-López M, Martínez-Vizcaíno V. Effectiveness of physical activity interventions on preventing gestational diabetes mellitus and excessive maternal weight gain: a meta-analysis. BJOG. 2015;122:1167–74.
40. Craig P, Dieppe P, Macintyre S, Michie S, Nazareth I, Petticrew M. Developing and evaluating complex interventions: the new Medical Research Council guidance. BMJ. 2008;337:a1655.

41. Michie S, Johnston M, Francis J, Hardeman W, Eccles M. From theory to intervention: mapping theoretically derived behavioural determinants to behaviour change techniques. Appl Psychol. 2008;57:660–80.

42. Gaston A, Cramp A. Exercise during pregnancy: a review of patterns and determinants. J Sci Med Sport. 2011;14:299–305.

43. Currie S, Sinclair M, Murphy MH, Madden E, Dunwoody L, Liddle D. Reducing the decline in physical activity during pregnancy: a systematic review of behaviour change interventions. PLoS One. 2013;8:e66385.

44. French SD, Green SE, O'Connor DA, McKenzie JE, Francis JJ, Michie S, Buchbinder R, Schattner P, Spike N, Grimshaw JM. Developing theory-informed behaviour change interventions to implement evidence into practice: a systematic approach using the theoretical domains framework. Implement Sci. 2012;7:38.

45. Michie S, van Stralen MM, West R. The behaviour change wheel: a new method for characterising and designing behaviour change interventions. Implement Sci. 2011;6:42.

46. Michie S AL, West R . The Behaviour Change Wheel A guide to Designing Interventions Great Britain: Silverback Publishing 2014;

47. McSherry LA, Dombrowski SU, Francis JJ, Murphy J, Martin CM, O'Leary JJ, Sharp L. It'sa can of worms': understanding primary care practitioners' behaviours in relation to HPV using the theoretical domains framework. Implement Sci. 2012;7:1.

48. Rubinstein H, Marcu A, Yardley L, Michie S. Public preferences for vaccination and antiviral medicines under different pandemic flu outbreak scenarios. BMC Public Health. 2015;15:1–13.

49. Islam R, Tinmouth AT, Francis JJ, Brehaut JC, Born J, Stockton C, Stanworth SJ, Eccles MP, Cuthbertson BH, Hyde C. A cross-country comparison of intensive care physicians' beliefs about their transfusion behaviour: a qualitative study using the theoretical domains framework. Implement Sci. 2012;7(1)

50. Cadogan SL, McHugh SM, Bradley CP, Browne JP, Cahill MR. General practitioner views on the determinants of test ordering: a theory-based qualitative approach to the development of an intervention to improve immunoglobulin requests in primary care. Implement Sci. 2016;11:102.

51. Alexander KE, Brijnath B, Mazza D. Barriers and enablers to delivery of the healthy kids check: an analysis informed by the theoretical domains framework and COM-B model. Implement Sci. 2014;9:60.

52. Handley MA, Harleman E, Gonzalez-Mendez E, Stotland NE, Althavale P, Fisher L, Martinez D, Ko J, Sausjord I, Rios C. Applying the COM-B model to creation of an IT-enabled health coaching and resource linkage program for low-income Latina moms with recent gestational diabetes: the STAR MAMA program. Implement Sci. 2016;11:73.

53. Cork University Maternity Hospital. Cork University Maternity Hospital Annual Report 2015. Cork 2015.

54. Goodrich K, Cregger M, Wilcox S, Liu J. A qualitative study of factors affecting pregnancy weight gain in African American women. Maternal & Child Health Journal. 2013;17:432–40.

55. Lavender T, Smith DM. Seeing it through their eyes: a qualitative study of the pregnancy experiences of women with a body mass index of 30 or more. Health Expect. 2016;19:222–33.

56. Padmanabhan U, Summerbell CD, Heslehurst NA. Qualitative study exploring pregnant women's weight-related attitudes and beliefs in UK: the BLOOM study. BMC Pregnancy Childbirth. 2015;15:1–14.

57. Gale NK, Heath G, Cameron E, Rashid S, Redwood S. Using the framework method for the analysis of qualitative data in multi-disciplinary health research. BMC Med Res Methodol. 2013;13:1–8.

58. Evenson KR, Moos M-K, Carrier K, Siega-Riz AM. Perceived barriers to physical activity among pregnant women. Matern Child Health J. 2009;13:364–75.

59. Weir Z, Bush J, Robson SC, McParlin C, Rankin J, Bell R. Physical activity in pregnancy: a qualitative studyof the beliefs of overweight and obese pregnantwomen. BMC Pregnancy Childbirth. 2010;10:18–24.

60. van der Pligt P, Campbell K, Willcox J, Opie J, Denney-Wilson E. Opportunities for primary and secondary prevention of excess gestational weight gain: general Practitioners' perspectives. BMC Fam Pract. 2011;12:124.

61. Oteng-Ntim E, Pheasant H, Khazaezadeh N, Mohidden A, Bewley S, Wong J, Oke B. Developing a community-based maternal obesity intervention: a qualitative study of service providers' views. BJOG. 2010;117:1651–5.

62. Olander EK, Atkinson L, Edmunds JK, French DP. The views of pre- and post-natal women and health professionals regarding gestational weight gain: an exploratory study. Sex Reprod Healthc. 2011;2:43–8.

63. Mparmpakas D, Goumenou A, Zachariades E, Pados G, Gidron Y, Karteris E. Immune system function, stress, exercise and nutrition profile can affect pregnancy outcome: lessons from a Mediterranean cohort. Exp Ther Med. 2013;5:411–8.

64. Kasawara KT, Surita FG, Pinto e Silva JL, Pinto E Silva JL. Translational studies for exercise in high-risk pregnancy: pre-eclampsia model. Hypertens Pregnancy. 2016;35:265–79.

65. Downs DS, Hausenblas HA. Women's exercise beliefs and behaviors during their pregnancy and postpartum. J Midwifery Womens Health. 2004;49:138–44.

66. Leiferman J, Swibas T, Koiness K, Marshall JA, Dunn AL. My baby, my move: examination of perceived barriers and motivating factors related to antenatal physical activity. J Midwifery Womens Health. 2011;56:33–40.

67. Duncombe D, Wertheim EH, Skouteris H, Paxton SJ, Kelly L. Factors related to exercise over the course of pregnancy including women's beliefs about the safety of exercise during pregnancy. Midwifery. 2009;25:430–8.

68. Bravata DM, Smith-Spangler C, Sundaram V, Gienger AL, Lin N, Lewis R, Stave CD, Olkin I, Sirard JR. Using pedometers to increase physical activity and improve health: a systematic review. JAMA. 2007;298:2296–304.

A retrospective study of gestational weight gain in relation to the Institute of Medicine's recommendations by maternal body mass index in rural Pennsylvania from 2006 to 2015

Michael L. Power[1,2]* ⓘ, Melisa L. Lott[3], A. Dhanya Mackeen[3], Jessica DiBari[4] and Jay Schulkin[1,5]

Abstract

Background: In 2009, the Institute of Medicine (IOM) published guidance on gestational weight gain (GWG) modified by maternal pre-pregnancy body mass index (BMI). Estimates indicate that less than half of US pregnant women have GWG within recommendations. This study examined GWG from before (2006–2009) and after (2010–2015) the release of the IOM guidance in a rural, non-Hispanic white population to assess the proportion of women with GWG outside of IOM guidance, whether GWG became more likely to be within IOM guidance after 2010, and identify potential maternal factors associated with GWG outside of recommendations.

Methods: We examined GWG in 18,217 term singleton births between 2006 and 2015 in which maternal pre-pregnancy BMI could be calculated from electronic medical records at Geisinger, PA, and a subset of 12,912 births in which weekly GWG in the third trimester could be calculated. The primary outcome was whether GWG was below, within, or above recommendations based on maternal BMI. The relationships between GWG, maternal BMI, parity, age at conception, gestation length, and maternal blood pressure were examined.

Results: GWG declined with increasing maternal BMI, however, more than 50% of overweight and obese women gained above IOM recommendations. About one of five women gained below recommendations (21.3%) with underweight women the most likely to gain below recommendations (33.0%). The proportion of births with usable data increased after 2010, driven by a higher probability of recording maternal weight. However, the proportion of women who gained below, within or above recommendations did not change over the ten years. GWG above recommendations was associated with higher maternal BMI, lower parity, and longer gestation. GWG below recommendations was associated with lower maternal BMI, higher parity, shorter gestation, and younger age at conception. Maternal blood pressure was higher for GWG outside recommendations.

Conclusions: Despite the publication of IOM recommendations in 2009 and an apparent increase in tracking maternal weight after 2010, GWG in this population did not change between 2006 and 2015. A majority of overweight and obese women gained above recommendations. GWG below recommendations continues to occur, and is prevalent among underweight women.

Keywords: Pregnancy, Obstetrics, Guidelines, Body mass index, Gestational weight gain, Obesity

* Correspondence: mpower@acog.org
[1]Research Department, American College of Obstetricians and Gynecologists, PO Box 96920, Washington, DC 20090-6920, USA
[2]Smithsonian National Zoo and Conservation Biology Institute, Washington, DC, USA
Full list of author information is available at the end of the article

Background

Gaining an appropriate amount of weight during pregnancy has been shown to positively influence fetal and maternal health during pregnancy, immediately postpartum, and well into the future [1]. Gestational weight gain (GWG) in a woman's first pregnancy is a significant predictor of her weight gain in a subsequent pregnancy [2]. Excessive GWG is associated with an increased risk for maternal hypertensive disorders and macrosomia for all maternal body mass index (BMI) categories [3].

Two of the Maternal, Infant and Child Health (MICH) objectives listed in Healthy People 2020 are to increase the proportion of women who gain the recommended amount of weight during pregnancy (MICH 13) and to increase the proportion of women delivering a live birth who had a healthy weight prior to pregnancy (MICH 16.5) [4]. In 2009, the Institute of Medicine published revised guidance on GWG that took account of the mother's pre-pregnancy BMI for the suggested total GWG and weekly weight gain during the second and third trimester [5]. In 2013 the American College of Obstetricians and Gynecologists endorsed the 2009 IOM GWG by maternal BMI recommendations [6].

This retrospective study examines data on GWG in a population of women who received their prenatal health care at Geisinger between 2006 and 2015. The goals of the study are to characterize GWG for singleton term births in this largely non-Hispanic white, rural population, to assess whether there has been any change in the patterns of GWG in this population over the ten-year period in response to the 2009 IOM recommendations, and to identify maternal factors associated with GWG outside of the IOM recommendations.

Methods

Geisinger is an open integrated health care delivery system that employs roughly 700 physicians across more than 50 clinical practice sites dispersed over 41 largely rural counties in central and northeastern Pennsylvania. Geisinger serves a patient population of approximately 2.5 million people, both through its own health plan and by accepting payment from other payers both public (e.g. Medicaid) and private (e.g. Blue Cross). Geisinger adopted an electronic health record system in 1995, with access provided to patients as well as to health care providers and managers. Geisinger becomes an integrated "medical home" for its patients [7]. The protocols for this project were determined to meet the criteria for exemption by the Geisinger Institutional Review Board. Electronic medical records (EMR) from 35,758 term (gestation length 259–294 days) singleton births at Geisinger between calendar years 2006 and 2015 (01/01.2006–12/31/2015) were examined. Of those 35,758 births, there were 23,555 that had a valid recorded

maternal height and weight either from before the pregnancy or within 30 days of conception which could be used to calculate maternal pre-pregnancy BMI. Maternal BMI was categorized as: underweight (BMI < 18.5 kg/m^2), normal weight (18.5 kg/m^2 ≤ BMI < 25 kg/m^2), overweight (25 kg/m^2 ≤ BMI < 30 kg/m^2), and obese (BMI ≥ 30 kg/m^2). Obesity was further categorized as: class I (30 kg/m^2 ≤ BMI < 35 kg/m^2), class II (35 kg/m^2 ≤ BMI < 40 kg/m^2), and class III (BMI ≥ 40 kg/m^2). Of those births, 18,217 had a weight recorded both within the first 30 days of pregnancy and within 7 days of parturition (Table 1). These 18,217 singleton term births that occurred between 2006 and 2015 at Geisinger were examined for total GWG. Total GWG was calculated by the difference between the last weight recorded within seven days before birth and the earliest pregnancy weight recorded (within the first thirty days of pregnancy).

The beginning of the third trimester was defined to be within 10 days of day 184 of gestation. There were 12,912 births with at least one recorded weight between days 174 and 194 of gestation and within 7 days of parturition. The difference between the last weight recorded within seven days before birth and the weight recorded closest to day 184 of gestation was divided by the number of days between those weights and then multiplied by 7 to calculate the mean weekly weight gain in the third trimester. For each birth the total GWG and the weekly GWG in the third trimester was classified as below IOM recommendations, within IOM recommendations or above IOM recommendations [21] based on the calculated maternal pre-pregnancy BMI.

Statistical analysis

The data were analyzed using a personal computer-based software package (IBM SPSS 20.0; IBM Corp, Armonk NY). The main dependent variable for analysis was GWG, and the main independent parameters/covariates were maternal pre-pregnancy BMI, maternal pre-pregnancy blood pressure, the year the infant was born, parity, age at conception, presence/absence of certain pregnancy complications (e.g. depression, hypertension, gestational diabetes), and estimated gestation length.

Values for continuous parameters are given as mean ± SEM. Pearson correlation was used to examine relationships between continuous parameters. Linear regression was used to assess changes over the ten-year period in birth complications and cesarean deliveries. Analysis of covariance (ANCOVA) was used to examine factors affecting GWG. Multinomial logistic regression was used to examine factors that would influence GWG to be either under or above recommendations relative to within recommendations (reference category).

Table 1 Basic maternal demographic information for the birth data extracted from electronic medical records by year. There were no significant changes in these parameters between 2006 and 2015

Birth year (N)	Non-Hispanic white (%)	Age at conception (years)	Pre-pregnancy BMI[a]	Postpartum BMI (N = 12,581)[b]	Systolic blood pressure[c] (mmHg)	Gestation length (days)
2006 (418)	96.9	26.2 ± 0.3	27.3 ± 0.3	29.2 ± 0.4	113.2/69.6	275.0 ± 0.4
2007 (1224)	96.1	26.6 ± 0.2	27.7 ± 0.2	28.9 ± 0.2	112.9/69.3	275.7 ± 0.2
2008 (1063)	96.6	26.7 ± 0.2	27.9 ± 0.2	29.6 ± 0.3	112.0/68.8	275.1 ± 0.2
2009 (1242)	94.1	26.8 ± 0.2	27.4 ± 0.2	29.1 ± 0.2	112.1/69.0	276.2 ± 0.2
2010 (1103)	95.1	27.1 ± 0.2	27.5 ± 0.2	29.2 ± 0.2	112.6/69.1	276.2 ± 0.2
2011 (2328)	95.1	26.9 ± 0.1	27.8 ± 0.1	29.5 ± 0.2	112.5/68.6	277.1 ± 0.2
2012 (2486)	93.6	26.8 ± 0.1	27.7 ± 0.1	29.2 ± 0.2	113.3/69.4	276.5 ± 0.1
2013 (2640)	94.7	26.8 ± 0.1	28.2 ± 0.1	29.4 ± 0.2	113.5/69.5	276.7 ± 0.1
2014 (2915)	93.4	27.0 ± 0.1	27.8 ± 0.1	29.5 ± 0.2	113.5/68.9	276.7 ± 0.1
2015 (2798)	93.9	27.1 ± 0.1	28.2 ± 0.1	29.7 ± 0.2	113.5/69.6	276.9 ± 0.1
Total (18,217)	94.5	26.9 ± 0.1	27.8 ± 0.1	29.4 ± 0.1	113.1/69.2	276.5 ± 0.1

[a]Calculated from either a pre-pregnancy weight or the earliest prenatal visit weight within 30 days of estimated conception
[b]From the postpartum visit
[c]Calculated from either a pre-pregnancy measurement or a measurement taken at the earliest prenatal visit within 30 days of estimated conception

Results

The 18,217 births were divided among 15,326 women, with 12,717 contributing a single birth, 2355 two births, 226 three births, and 28 women contributing four births. Most births were to multiparous women (2010 births to primiparous women, and 1201 births in which maternal parity was not known). The limited demographic information available for the mothers is presented in Table 1. Mean maternal age at conception, pre-pregnancy BMI, postpartum BMI, pre-pregnancy blood pressure, and gestation length did not differ across these years (Table 1). Almost all (94.5%) of the women were non-Hispanic white. The mean age at conception was 26.9 ± 0.1 years (18–49 years old). The mean gestational length was 276.5 ± 0.1 days (259–294 days). Based on BMI, more than half of the women were overweight (25.4%) or obese (31.6%). Few (3.0%) were underweight. The mean number of weights recorded during the prenatal period for these births was 16, with a median of 15 and a mode of 14.

Patterns over the ten years

Between 2006 and 2010, the percentage of term singleton births that met our criteria for inclusion (i.e. data to calculate the pre-pregnancy maternal BMI and within 7 days of birth) averaged 33.4%. In 2011, the percentage increased to 52.4% and steadily continued to increase, reaching 77.2% in 2015 (Table 2). The increase was driven by a higher proportion of both recorded pre-pregnancy weights or weights within 30 days of estimated conception and weights within seven days of delivery.

Among the 18,217 births analyzed, 8730 had at least one complication reported (excluding cesarean delivery as a potential complication), leaving 9487 births with no reported complications. There was a small (just under

0.5 percentage points per year) but consistent increase in the proportion of births with at least one recorded complications over the ten years, from about 46% of births before 2009 to 49.7% in years 2014 and 2015 (Fig. 1). Recorded complications included pre-existing hypertension, gestational hypertension, preeclampsia, pre-existing diabetes, gestational diabetes, depression, and polycystic ovarian syndrome. Cesarean delivery accounted for 29% of deliveries. The cesarean rate declined by about 1.1 percentage points per year from above 30% from 2006 through 2009 to 26 and 25% in 2014 and 2015, respectively (Fig. 1).

Gestational weight gain

Mean total GWG for all 10 years averaged 30.2 ± 0.1 lb. (range = 29.4–31.4 lb). Significant factors affecting GWG were gestation length, pre-pregnancy BMI, pre-pregnancy systolic blood pressure, and parity. The year of birth, maternal age at conception, pre-pregnancy diastolic blood pressure, and complications during pregnancy were not significant factors with respect to GWG. Although significant, the associations between GWG and gestation length ($r = 0.095$, $P < 0.001$) and maternal systolic blood pressure ($r = -0.097$, $P < 0.001$) were low. The association with maternal pre-pregnancy BMI was greater ($r = 0.320$, $P < 0.001$). Parity also appeared to have a larger effect. The estimated marginal means for GWG evaluated at 276 days of gestation, maternal BMI of 28 kg/m^2, and systolic blood pressure of 113 mmHg were 33.6 ± 0.4 lb., 31.4 ± 0.2 lb., and 27.2 ± 0.2 lb. for the first birth, second birth, and for more than one previous birth, respectively.

Consistent with the positive correlation between gestation length and GWG, the proportion of women who gained above recommendations increased with weeks'

Table 2 Singleton term births between 2006 and 2015 from electronic medical records at Geisinger. Note: the lower number of births in 2006 derives from the fact that these births were conceived and delivered in 2006, while for later years the number represents all deliveries in that year regardless of year of conception

Year of birth	Births	Births with pre-pregnancy weight	Percent of births with pre-pregnancy weight	Births also with weight within 7 days of parturition	Percent of births also with weight within 7 days of parturition
2006	1470	706	48.0%	418	28.4%
2007	3626	1940	53.5%	1224	33.8%
2008	3249	1639	50.4%	1063	32.7%
2009	3351	1814	54.1%	1242	37.1%
2010	3133	1667	53.2%	1103	35.2%
2011	4440	3023	68.1%	2328	52.4%
2012	4440	3146	70.9%	2486	56.0%
2013	4256	3217	75.6%	2640	62.0%
2014	4170	3355	80.5%	2915	69.9%
2015	3623	3048	84.1%	2798	77.2%
Total	35,758	23,555	65.9%	18,217	50.9%

gestation for all BMI categories (Table 3). A majority of overweight women gained above recommendations regardless of gestation length, increasing from 60.6% in the 38th week to 75.2% in the 42nd week (Table 3).

Although GWG declined with increasing maternal BMI for all births and for births without complications, the proportion of women that gained above the IOM recommendations based on maternal BMI was highest in overweight and obese women (Table 4). These patterns of GWG did not vary over the ten years between 2006 and 2015, with no consistent change in the proportions of women gaining under, within or above IOM recommendations with respect to maternal BMI. Only 25.8% of women in this population gained within

recommendations (range = 24.3–27.7%) with an average of 21.3% gaining below recommendations (range = 17.3–24.0%) and 52.9% gaining above (range = 51.4–55.0%). A third of underweight women had a total GWG under IOM recommendations, with no change over these years (Fig. 2).

The results were similar for weekly weight gain in the third trimester. Despite a numerical decrease in mean weekly weight gain in obese women, the proportion that gained above recommendations exceeded 60% (Table 5). Underweight women (BMI < 18.5 kg/m²) was the only BMI category in which a majority of women did not gain above IOM recommendations. Almost half of underweight women (49.1%) gained below IOM recommendations in

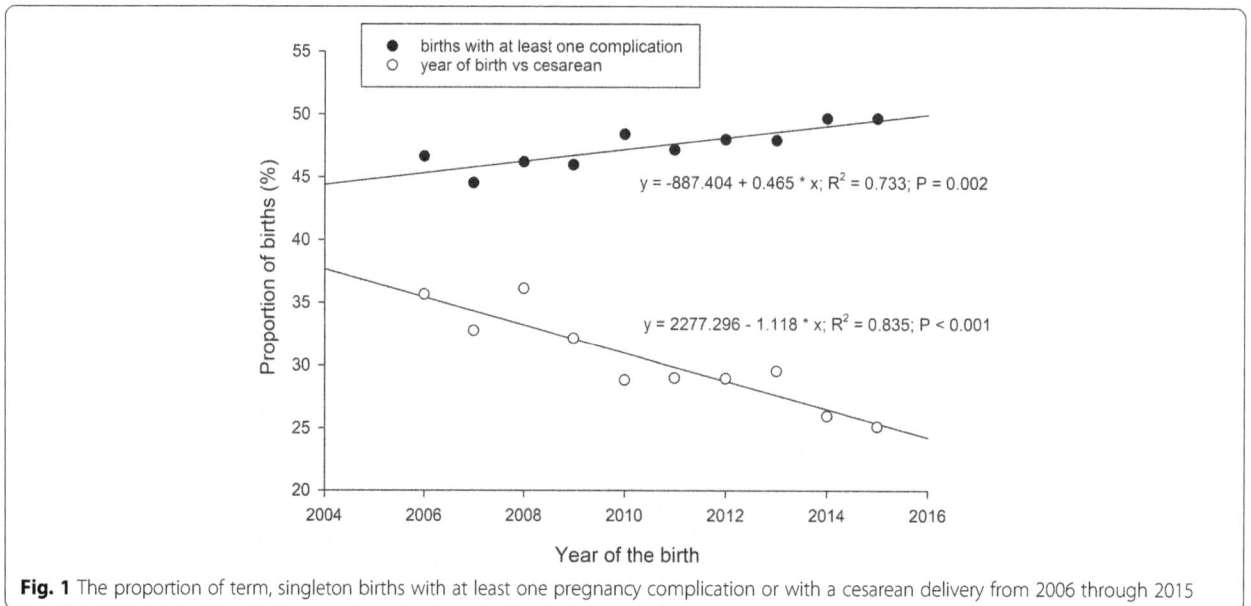

Fig. 1 The proportion of term, singleton births with at least one pregnancy complication or with a cesarean delivery from 2006 through 2015

Table 3 The proportion of women with GWG above recommendations by maternal BMI class and weeks of completed gestation. Both week of gestation and BMI class were significant factors for GWG above recommendations

Gestational age	All women	Underweight	Normal weight	Overweight	Obese
37^0–37^6	667	12	213	212	230
weeks	(47.1%)	(26.7%)	(37.0%)	(60.6%)	(47.1%)
38^0–38^6	1247	20	421	394	412
weeks	(47.5%)	(22.5%)	(38.6%)	(61.6%)	(51.2%)
39^0–39^6	3577	61	1116	1101	1299
weeks	(51.0%)	(28.6%)	(42.2%)	(63.6%)	(53.5%)
40^0–40^6	2876	49	1037	972	818
weeks	(56.0%)	(32.7%)	(48.4%)	(70.1%)	(56.2%)
41^0–41^6	1263	20	480	389	374
weeks	(62.4%)	(37.0%)	(56.4%)	(75.2%)	(62.1%)

the third trimester. Similar to total GWG, there was no change in the pattern of weekly weight gain in the third trimester for under, within or above recommendations across the 10 years, with only 12.9% gaining within recommendations over the ten-year period.

The multinomial logistic regression results indicated that gestation length, pre-pregnancy BMI, and parity were significant factors for both GWG below and above recommendations, although the effects were not large, except for parity (Table 6). Age at conception was a significant factor for those who were under recommendations, with younger women being more likely to gain under recommendations. Pre-pregnancy systolic blood pressure was significant for those who gained above recommendations, with higher blood pressure associated with a greater likelihood of exceeding GWG recommendations. Both of these effects were small (Table 6).

Women who gained within recommendations had both lower pre-pregnancy BMI (26.6 ± 0.1 kg/m^2; $P < 0.001$) and systolic blood pressure (112.0 ± 0.1 mmHg; P < 0.001) than either those who gained under (28.8 ± 0.1 kg/m^2 and 113.5 ± 0.2 mmHg) or above recommendations (28.0 ± 0.1 kg/m^2 and 113.4 ± 0.2 mmHg). Mean gestation length increased by 1.8 days from GWG under recommendations (275.3 ± 0.1 days) to GWG above recommendations (277.1 ± 0.1 days; P < 0.001), a statistically significant, but perhaps not clinically relevant finding. Parity had the largest effect on both gaining above and below recommendations (Table 6). Consistent with the declining estimated marginal means for GWG with increasing parity given above (controlling for gestation length, maternal BMI, and systolic blood pressure), the proportion of women who gained above recommendations consistently declined with parity (62.6, 56.4, and

Table 4 Gestational weight gain by BMI class for all term singleton births and for births without complications. Prepregnancy BMI had a significant effect on weight gain, with mean weight gain declining with BMI ($r = -0.329$, P < 0.001 for all births)

	IOM Recommendations (lb)	N	Mean GWG ± SEM (lb)	Proportion above IOM recommendations
All births		18,217	30.2 ± 0.1	52.9%
Underweight	28–40	551	35.0 ± 0.5	29.4%
Normal weight	25–35	7305	34.5 ± 0.2	44.7%
Overweight	15–25	4623	32.0 ± 0.2	66.4%
Obese class I	11–20	2815	26.0 ± 0.3	63.0%
Obese class II	11–20	1631	21.1 ± 0.4	50.6%
Obese class III	11–20	1292	17.7 ± 0.5	41.3%
Births with no complications		9487	31.6 ± 0.2	52.8%
Underweight	28–40	340	34.1 ± 0.6	26.5%
Normal weight	25–35	4541	34.7 ± 0.2	44.8%
Overweight	15–25	2461	32.6 ± 0.3	68.0%
Obese class I	11–20	1215	26.8 ± 0.5	65.3%
Obese class II	11–20	596	20.0 ± 0.7	48.2%
Obese class III	11–20	334	17.1 ± 1.1	38.9%

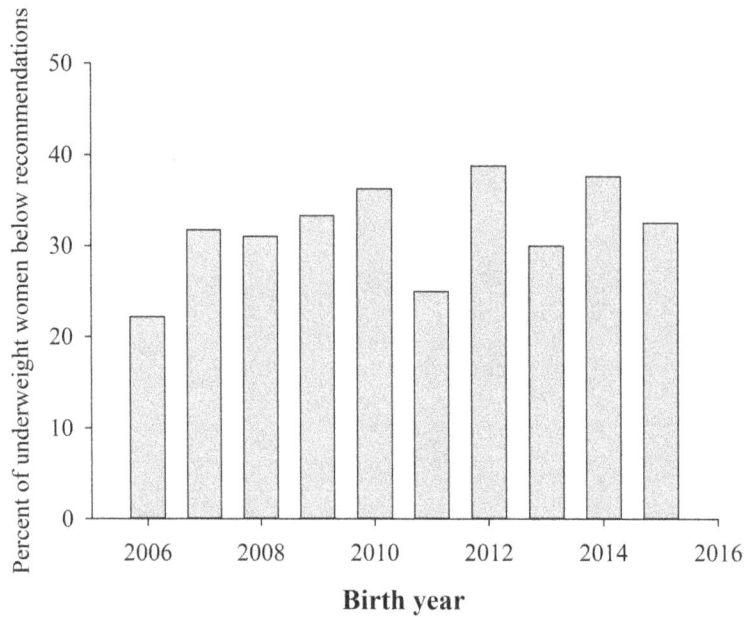

Fig. 2 The proportion of underweight women who gained below recommendations did not change over the ten-year period

46.3% for first birth, second birth, and more than one previous birth, respectively; P < 0.001). Conversely, the proportion of GWG below recommendations was lowest for a first birth (14%), almost doubling to 26% for women with two or more previous births.

Discussion

The pattern of GWG with respect to pre-pregnancy maternal BMI in this population is concerning. Only 25.8% of women in this population had total GWG within recommendations over the ten years of data, with only 12.9% gaining within recommendations in the third trimester. The majority of women in this population gained above IOM recommendations, especially in the third trimester, in which even a majority of women with a normal pre-pregnancy BMI gained above recommendations. Although overweight and obese women in this population had numerically lower GWG than did women with normal BMI, this reduced GWG still generally exceeded the GWG recommended by IOM, resulting in a

Table 5 Weekly weight gain in the third trimester by BMI class for all term singleton births and for births without complications

	IOM Recommendations (lb)	N	Mean weekly GWG ± SEM in the third trimester (lb/week)	Proportion above IOM recommendations
All births		12,912	1.06 ± 0.01	64.5%
Underweight	1–1.3	371	1.05 ± 0.03	28.6%
Normal weight	0.8–1.0	5085	1.12 ± 0.01	56.8%
Overweight	0.5–0.7	3230	1.12 ± 0.01	75.9%
Obese class I	0.4–0.6	2028	0.98 ± 0.02	71.8%
Obese class II	0.4–0.6	1230	0.89 ± 0.02	65.0%
Obese class III	0.4–0.6	968	0.90 ± 0.03	64.4%
Births with no complications		6473	1.11 ± 0.01	65.3%
Underweight	1–1.3	220	1.03 ± 0.03	25.9%
Normal weight	0.8–1.0	3098	1.14 ± 0.01	58.0%
Overweight	0.5–0.7	1666	1.17 ± 0.02	79.6%
Obese class I	0.4–0.6	837	1.04 ± 0.03	74.3%
Obese class II	0.4–0.6	420	0.87 ± 0.03	65.5%
Obese class III	0.4–0.6	232	0.96 ± 0.09	63.8%

Table 6 Significant factors in the multinomial logistic regression for GWG under, within (reference category) and above IOM recommendations

Parameter	Odds ratio	Standard error	95% confidence interval
Under recommendations versus within recommendations			
Maternal BMI	1.041	0.004	1.034–1.048
Age at conception	0.987	0.005	0.978–0.996
First birth	0.617	0.053	0.521–0.731
Second birth	0.794	0.042	0.716–0.879
Gestation length	0.989	0.003	0.982–0.995
Systolic blood pressure	1.001	0.002	0.998–1.005
Over recommendations versus within recommendations			
Maternal BMI	1.030	0.003	1.024–1.036
Age at conception	0.998	0.004	0.991–1.006
First birth	1.558	0.100	1.374–1.766
Second birth	1.372	0.059	1.261–1.493
Gestation length	1.016	0.003	1.010–1.021
Systolic blood pressure	1.005	0.002	1.001–1.008

large proportion of these women gaining above the IOM recommendations, especially in the third trimester (66.4 and 54.6%, respectively). The only group without a majority gaining above recommendations was underweight women, who disturbingly had a high percentage of GWG below recommendations.

Perhaps most disappointing is that there was no change in these outcomes over the 10 years. Surveys of obstetrician-gynecologists in 2012 and 2014 found widespread knowledge of the IOM recommendations (81.8%) and use of pre-pregnancy BMI to modify GWG recommendations (78.5%) [8]. There were several indications that providers in this study had appropriately counseled their patients regarding recommendations on GWG based on pre-pregnancy BMI. Overweight and obese women did have lower GWG, both total and in the third trimester compared to women with a normal BMI. The fact that women diagnosed with GDM were less likely to have GWG above recommendations potentially represents appropriate practice for these women, with more extensive counseling on diet and GWG. The increase in recorded maternal weights after 2010 indicates a focus on tracking weight in pregnant women and an increased ability to calculate pre-pregnancy and early pregnancy BMI. The fact that the median number of prenatal weights recorded was 15 implies that these women had significant contact with health care providers, and that their pattern of weight gain should have been known to both the women and their care providers. However, despite what appears to be widespread knowledge of the dangers of inappropriate GWG [8] and good tracking of weight during pregnancy, the pattern of inappropriate GWG by most of the women in this population was essentially unchanged over the ten-year period.

Data on mothers with inadequate GWG have unequivocally supported the benefits of increasing total weight gain recommendations for underweight women in reducing the risk of low birth weight babies [9, 10]. It is disconcerting that one third of underweight women gained below IOM recommendations during pregnancy, with almost half gaining below recommendations in the third trimester. Surveys of obstetrician-gynecologists in 2012 and 2014 found they likely underestimated the proportion of their pregnant patients with GWG below recommendations by more than half (7.8%) [8] compared with national data (20%) [11] or the data from this study (21.3%). A concern is that the large proportion of women with GWG above recommendations is resulting in providers failing to recognize women with GWG below recommendations.

Although several maternal factors were significantly associated with GWG outside of recommendations, most (age at conception, gestation length, and systolic blood pressure) had small effects. Even the effect of maternal pre-pregnancy BMI was moderate (Table 6). Parity had a strong effect on the likelihood of gaining an appropriate amount of weight during pregnancy, with the proportion of women gaining above recommendations declining with the number of previous births. This result is consistent with a recent prospective study in Brazil that found that GWG was highest in primiparous women [12]. Unfortunately, the decline of GWG above recommendations with parity did not result in a large increase of women gaining within recommendations. Rather, the proportion of GWG below recommendations increased with parity such that more than one-of-four women with two or more previous births gained below recommendations. Relatively little research appears to have focused on the effect of parity on GWG and how the two factors together might affect differences in health outcomes for mother and child. Higher parity is associated with higher infant birth weight and a greater risk of macrosomia [13]. Children of primiparous mothers have higher body fat at age thirty, and the effect of parity was independent of the effects of maternal BMI and GWG [14]. We suggest that an examination of whether GWG recommendations should be adjusted for maternal parity may be warranted.

The limitations of this study include its retrospective nature, which means the findings are associations and causality cannot be assumed, and the racial homogeneity of the population (94.4% non-Hispanic white), which may limit the extent to which the findings can be generalized to the entire US population. Also, the majority of women were overweight or obese, although, unfortunately, that may be representative of US women of childbearing age. The amount of usable data from the EMR system varied systematically across the years, primarily due to progressively higher incidence of recorded pre-pregnancy and early pregnancy weights after 2010, such that the characterization of GWG is based on less than 40% of term births between 2006 and 2010, and more than 50% of term births after 2010, reaching a maximum of more than 77% of term births in 2015. Thus, GWG is likely more reliably characterized for this population after 2010. However, based on the number of weights taken during pregnancy, the women included in this study were women that had consistent contact with health care providers. They represent women who would be expected to be appropriately counseled and monitored during their pregnancy, regardless of the year the birth occurred, and thus we argue they are comparable across years.

Our expectation was that any effects of the IOM GWG recommendations on patient behavior would be most evident in an integrated system with an extensive medical records system such as Geisinger. The lack of change in GWG across the ten years, despite the general acceptance of the IOM recommendations by obstetrician-gynecologists [8], and the apparent increase in weight tracking after 2010 at Geisinger, reinforces other studies that suggest that obstetrician-gynecologists require additional tools and strategies to encourage behavior change and modify their patients' GWG effectively [8, 15, 16]. Our data suggest that GWG is resistant to simple interventions, such as increased tracking and recording of weight during pregnancy. A prospective cohort study found little association between receiving provider advice on GWG and gaining within IOM recommendations, suggesting that current provider practice on GWG counseling is not effective [16]. A simple-in-concept health care practice that would improve

maternal and neonatal outcomes, helping patients regulate their weight gain during pregnancy within healthy limits, appears to be difficult to accomplish with the current tool set available to obstetrician-gynecologists.

Physicians' confidence in their ability to affect GWG in their patients was found to be associated with practice effort [8]. If provider counseling on GWG remains ineffective, this could lead to reduced efforts as confidence is lessened by observed lack of change in outcomes. A focus group study found that providers were aware of and concerned about the risks associated with excess GWG, but were concerned that their training was inadequate. A common motivation for participating in the focus groups was "...to find out what other people are doing", indicating an interest in learning new counseling methods [15]. This suggests the need for new tools to assist providers in communicating the importance of appropriate GWG to their patients and monitoring weight gain throughout pregnancy. Recent randomized trials of life-style modifications have produced encouraging results, resulting in lower GWG in overweight and obese women [17, 18]. Among women who were not low income, consistent GWG tracking was associated with lower GWG [19]. Developing provider tools to guide the management of GWG in patients may improve the quality of care, enhance provider efforts to monitor and manage GWG, and have a positive influence on both maternal and child health outcomes.

Conclusions

Despite the publication of IOM recommendations in 2009 and an apparent increase in tracking maternal weight after 2010, GWG in this population did not change between 2006 and 2015. The majority of women in this population gained above IOM recommendations, especially in the third trimester, in which even a majority of women with a normal pre-pregnancy BMI gained above recommendations. Overweight and obese women were especially likely to gain above recommendations. Although GWG above recommendations is the most common occurrence, GWG below recommendations continues to occur and is prevalent among underweight women.

Abbreviations
ANCOVA: Analysis of covariance; BMI: Body mass index; EMR: Electronic medical records; GDM: Gestational diabetes mellitus; GWG: Gestational weight gain; IOM: Institute of Medicine

Acknowledgements
This project is supported by the Health Resources and Services Administration (HRSA) of the U.S. Department of Health and Human Services (HHS) under UA6MC19010 and UA6MC31609. This information or content and conclusions are those of the author and should not be construed as the official position or policy of, nor should any endorsements be inferred by HRSA, HHS or the U.S. Government. The authors report no conflicts of interest.

Financial support

This project is supported by the Health Resources and Services Administration (HRSA) of the U.S. Department of Health and Human Services (HHS) under UA6MC19010 and UA6MC31609.

Funding

This research was supported by the Health Resources and Services Administration (HRSA) of the U.S. Department of Health and Human Services (HHS) under UA6MC19010 and UA6MC31609. HRSA did not play a role in the design, data collection, or analysis of the study. HRSA provided some technical assistance in the writing of the paper, however, the conclusions and opinions expressed in this paper represent the authors and not those of HRSA.

Authors' contributions

MLP performed the data analysis. MLP, MLL, and ADM designed the study. JD and JS provided interpretation and context for the results. All authors contributed to writing the manuscript and all read and approved the final version.

Competing interests

The authors declare that they have no competing interests.

Author details

[1]Research Department, American College of Obstetricians and Gynecologists, PO Box 96920, Washington, DC 20090-6920, USA. [2]Smithsonian National Zoo and Conservation Biology Institute, Washington, DC, USA. [3]Geisinger, Department of Obstetrics and Gynecology, Division of Maternal-Fetal Medicine, Danville, PA, USA. [4]Health Resources and Services Administration, Maternal and Child Health Bureau, Office of Epidemiology and Research, Division of Research, Rockville, MD, USA. [5]Department of Obstetrics and Gynecology, University of Washington School of Medicine, Seattle, WA, USA.

References

1. Phelan S. Pregnancy: a "teachable moment" for weight control and obesity prevention. Am J Obstet Gynecol. 2010;202(135):e1–8.
2. Chin JR, Krause KM, Østbye T, Chodhury N, Lovelady CA, Swamy GK. Gestational weight gain in consecutive pregnancies. Am J Obset Gynecol. 2010;203(279):e1–6.
3. Johnson J, Clifton RG, Roberts JM, et al. Pregnancy outcomes with weight gain above or below the 2009 Institute of Medicine guidelines. Obstet Gynecol. 2013;121:969–75.
4. Healthy People 2020. https://www.healthypeople.gov/2020/topics-objectives/topic/maternal-infant-and-child-health/objectives.
5. Institute of Medicine. Weight gain during pregnancy: reexamining the guidelines. Washington DC: National Academies Press; 2009.
6. American College of Obstetricians and Gynecologists. Committee opinion 548 weight gain during pregnancy. Obstet Gynecol. 2013;121:210–2.
7. Paulos RA, Davis K, Steele GD. Continuous innovation in health care: Implicatoins of the geisinger experience. Health Aff. 2008;27:1235–45.
8. Power ML, Schulkin J. Obstetrician/gynecologists' knowledge, attitudes and practices regarding weight gain during pregnancy. J Women's Health. 2017; 26:1169–75.
9. Abrams BF, Laros RK. Prepregnancy weight, weight gain. and birth weight Am J Obstet Gynecol. 1996;154(3):503–8.
10. Han Z, Lutsiv O, Mulla S, Rosen A, Beyene J, McDonald SD. Low gestational weight gain and the risk of preterm birth and low birthweight: a systematic review and meta-analyses. Acta Obstet Gynecol Scand. 2011;90(9):935–54. https://doi.org/10.1111/j.1600-0412.2011.01185.x.
11. Deputy NP, Sharma AJ, Kim SY. Gestational weight gain–United States, 2012 and 2013. Morb Mortal Wkly Rep. 2015;64:1215–20.
12. Paulino DSM, Surita FG, Peres GB, Nascimento SL, Morais SS. Association between parity, pre-pregnancy body mass index and gestational weight gain. J Matern Fetal Neonatal Med. 2016;29:880–4.
13. Ørskou J, Henriksen TB, Kesmodel U, Secher NJ. Maternal characteristics and lifestyle factors and the risk of delivering high birth weight infants. Obstet Gynecol. 2003;102:115–20.
14. Reynolds RM, Osmond C, Phillips DIW, Godfrey KM. Maternal BMI, parity, and pregnancy weight gain: influences on offspring adiposity in young adulthood. J Clin Endocrinol Metab. 2010;95:5365–9.
15. Stotland NE, Gilbert P, Bogetz A, Harper CC, Abrams B, Gerbert B. Preventing excessive weight gain in pregnancy: how do prenatal care providers approach counseling? J Women's Health. 2010;19:807–14.
16. Ferrari RM, Siega-Riz AM. Provider advice about pregnancy weight gain and adequacy of weight gain. Matern Child Health J. 2013;17:256–64.
17. Cahill AG, Haire-Joshu D, Cade WT, Stein RI, Woolfolk CL, Moley K, Mathur A, Schechtman K, Klein S. Weight control program and gestational weight gain in disadvantaged women with overweight and obesity: a randomized clinical trial. Obesity. 2018;26:485–91.
18. Gallaghar D, Rosenn B, Toro-Ramos T, Paley C, Gidwani S, Horowitz M, Crane J, Lin S, Thornton JC, Pi-Sunyer X. Greater neonatal fat-free mass and similar fat mass following a randomized trial to control excess gestational weight gain. Obesity. 2018;26:578–87.
19. Olson CM, Strawderman MSGraham ML. Association between consisten weight gain tracking and gestational weight Gan: secondary analysis of a randomized trial. Obesity. 2017;25:1217–27.

12

Impact of obesity and other risk factors on labor dystocia in term primiparous women

Tuija Hautakangas[1]* (iD), Outi Palomäki[2], Karoliina Eidstø[3], Heini Huhtala[4] and Jukka Uotila[2]

Abstract

Background: Purpose of this study was to investigate differences between primiparous term pregnancies, one leading to vaginal delivery (VD) and the other to acute cesarean section (CS) due to labor dystocia in the first stage of labor. We particularly wanted to assess the influence of body mass index (BMI) on CS risk.

Methods: A retrospective case-control study in a tertiary delivery unit with 5200 deliveries annually. Cases were 296 term primiparous women whose intended vaginal labor ended in acute CS because of dystocia. Controls were primiparas with successful vaginal delivery VD ($n = 302$). The data were retrieved from medical records. Multiple logistic regression analyses were used to assess the associations between BMI and covariates on labor dystocia.

Results: In the cases ending with acute CS, women were older (OR 1.06 [1.03–1.10]), shorter (OR 0.94 [0.91–0.96]) and more often had a chronic disease (OR 1.60 [1.1–2.29]). In this group fetal malposition (OR 42.0 [19.2–91.9]) and chorioamnionitis (OR 10.9 [5.01–23.6]) were more common, labor was less often in an active phase (OR 3.37 [2.38–4.76]) and the cervix was not as well ripened (1.5 vs. 2.5 cm, OR 0.57 [0.48–0.67] on arrival at the birth unit. BMI was higher in the dystocia group (24.1 vs. 22.6 kg/m^2, $p < 0.001$), and rising maternal pre-pregnancy BMI had a strong association with dystocia risk. If BMI increased by 1 kg/m^2, the risk of CS was 10% elevated. Among obese primiparas, premature rupture of membranes, chorioamnionitis and induction of labor were more common. Their labors were less often in an active phase at hospital admission. Severely obese primiparas (BMI ≥ 35 kg/m^2) had 4 hours longer labor than normal-weight parturients.

Conclusions: Labor dystocia is a multifactorial phenomenon in which the possibility to ameliorate the condition via medical treatment is limited. Hospital admission at an advanced stage of labor is recommended. Pre-pregnancy weight control in the population at reproductive age is essential, as a high BMI is strongly associated with labor dystocia.

Keywords: Dystocia, Primipara, Obesity, Cesarean section, Case control

Background

The rate of cesarean section (CS) has increased worldwide during the last few decades [1, 2] and even during the on-going decade: the global CS rate in 2000–2008 was 13.9%, and it rose in 2007–2014 to 17%. In Europe as a whole the CS rate in 2007–2014 was 25% and in Finland it was 16% [1]. The CS rate has risen among both primiparous and multiparous women [2, 3]. The rate of intrapartum CS has increased significantly as well [2], the main indications being fetal distress and labor dystocia [4, 5].

Some risk factors of labor dystocia have been recognized or suggested. One of the contributors may be the increasing number of cases of labor induction [2, 3, 6]. A high body mass index (BMI) is associated with dystocia and intrapartal CS [7–9], as is advanced maternal age [3, 5].

Although CS can be a lifesaving operation, it can cause severe maternal morbidity, and sometimes lead to complications in the next pregnancy [10]. Thus, measures should be taken to reduce the number of unnecessary CSs, especially in primiparous women, as CS after the

* Correspondence: tuija.hautakangas@ksshp.fi
[1]Department of Obstetrics and Gynecology, Central Hospital of Central Finland, Keskussairaalantie 19, 40620 Jyväskylä, Finland
Full list of author information is available at the end of the article

first pregnancy is prone to lead to repeat CSs in following pregnancies [2, 11].

The aim of this study was to assess the differences between two types of primiparous labor, one leading to vaginal delivery and the other to acute CS due to labor dystocia in the first stage of labor. We particularly wanted to investigate the influence of an overweight condition on the risk factors of labor dystocia.

Methods

This was a retrospective parity-matched case-control study in a tertiary delivery unit (Tampere University Hospital) with an annual delivery rate of 5200. The study period was from February 2009 to December 2012. Data were obtained from medical files of the mother and newborn. Ethical approval for the study was given by the Ethics Committee of Pirkanmaa Hospital District (R12522S), 3rd April 2012.

The study group consisted of 296 term primiparous women whose intended vaginal labor ended in acute cesarean section as a result of dystocia, i.e. Robson groups 1 and 2A [12]. To obtain data for the study group, the birth register was searched for primiparas with WHO International Classification of Diseases (ICD)-10 diagnosis O82.10 (acute CS excluding emergency CS) with at least one of the dystocia-diagnoses O62, O63 or O64. One of the doctors form the study group checked the medical files of these primiparas to exclude the cases with twins and premature (< H37 + 0) labors. Pathological findings in cardiotocography (CTG) as the main indication for CS represented an exclusion criterion as was diagnosis of dystocia made after full dilatation of the cervix.

Primiparous women at term, with vertex presentation and singleton pregnancies attending the delivery unit and with successful vaginal delivery were selected as controls ($n = 302$). Deliveries were spontaneous or augmented. A flow chart of the collected study cohorts is shown in Fig. 1.

Variables related to maternal background, labor characteristics and neonatal outcome were recorded and compared between groups. To study the effects of obesity on labor outcome and on the risk factors of dystocia, the parturients were divided into subgroups according to WHO BMI classification [13]. The weights of the primiparas were self-reported in the first antenatal visit in primary health care in gestational weeks 6 to 8. If there was discrepancy between self-reported and measured weight in this antenatal visit, or women were not aware of their pre-pregnancy weight, the weight measured by health professional was used. The BMI was calculated by the formula: weight (kg) ÷ height^2 (cm). Almost every parturient was screened for gestational diabetes mellitus according to Finnish Current Guidelines during the pregnancy. The 2 h 75-g oral glucose tolerance test was made for all except the lowest risk primiparas (age under 25 years, BMI ≤ 25 kg/m^2 or no family history of diabetes mellitus). If fasting blood glucose level was ≥5,3 mmol/l or 1 hour's level ≥ 10 mml/l or 2 hours level ≥ 8,6 mmol/l, the diagnosis of gestational diabetes (GDM) was made. The fear of childbirth (FOC) was defined by a separate diagnose code used in Finland for that disorder in the medical records. All the parturients with this diagnosis had been visited maternity clinic of birth hospital to get treatment for FOC.

As our study was retrospective, it had not influence on the treatment of labor. Labors were treated by the hospital's guidelines. During this period, a modified active management of labor- protocol was used and the maximum oxytocin dose limit was 15 mIU/min. Partograms were used in delivery rooms. Intrauterine pressure catheters were used, if external tocodynamometry did

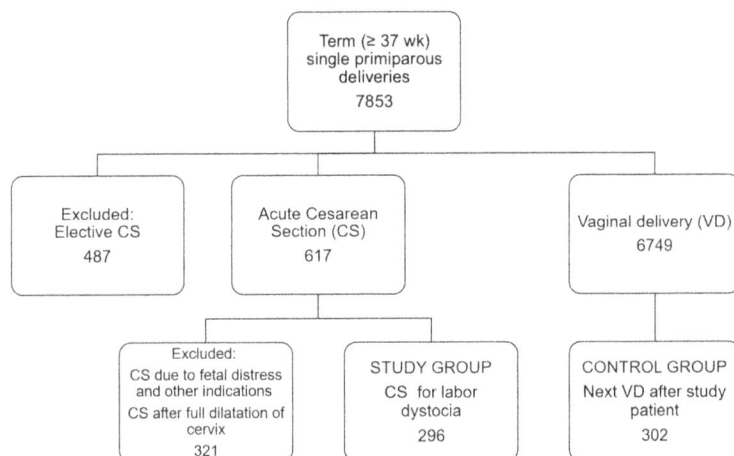

Fig. 1 Number of singleton primiparous deliveries during the study period and the application of exclusion and inclusion criteria

not provide enough information, and liberally among oxytocin augmented labors. Chorionamnionitis was defined by intrapartum temperature more than 38.0 or a combination of fetal tachycardia and maternal C-reactive protein more than 20 g/l.

All statistical analyses were performed using SPSS for Windows 23 (IBM SPSS Statistics for Windows, Version 23.0. Armonk, NY: IBM Corp.). Continuous variables were expressed as means with standard deviations, or medians with quartiles. Categorical variables were expressed as frequencies and percentages. Comparisons were made between the intrapartum CS and successful VD groups. The Mann–Whitney U-test, Fisher's exact test and the chi-squared test were used, as appropriate. Associations between risk factors and the mode of delivery were analyzed separately. Multivariable analyses were performed separately as regards maternal background variables and intrapartum variables that were significant in univariate analyses. The results of logistic regression analyses were expressed as adjusted odds ratios (aORs) and 95% confidence intervals (95% CIs). A p-value of < 0.05 was considered statistically significant. All p-values were two-sided.

Results

Table 1 shows maternal characteristics in the study groups. In multivariable analysis of the background variables, maternal age, height, BMI and chronic disease (e.g. asthma, thyroid, neurological or psychiatric disorders)

remained as independent risk factors. Women in the dystocia group had a higher BMI, and if BMI increased by 1 kg/m^2, the risk of CS was elevated by 10%. A 1 year increase in maternal age or a 1 cm decrease in maternal height increased CS risk by 6%.

Intrapartum factors possibly associated with acute CS due to labor dystocia are presented in Table 2. In multivariable analysis, longer gestational age, less advanced cervical status at admission, chorioamnionitis and malposition remained as independent risk factors of CS. The great majority of malpositions were occipitoposterior positions (89%). The most common indications for induction of labor (IOL) were post term pregnancy (26.8% of inductions) and rupture of membranes with no contractions within 24 h of PROM (27.6%).

Neonatal outcome was good in both groups. Newborns in the CS group were slightly heavier than those in the control group (3655 g vs. 3503 g; OR 1.11 [1.07–1.15]). 94% of newborns whose birthweight was over 4500 g, were born by CS. There were five newborns, whose birthweight was under 2500 g, two of them in CS group and three were born vaginally. In CS group newborns had a higher umbilical artery pH (7.33 vs. 7.24; OR 1.11 [1.08–1.15]) but slightly poorer 5-min Apgar scores (8.81 vs. 8.88; OR 0.56 [0.41–0.77]). Admission to the pediatric care unit was low in both groups (5.7% vs. 5.0%, NS). Fetal scalp blood sample was taken during 19.6% of labors.

Table 1 Maternal characteristics in the study groups

	CS (n = 296)	VD (n = 302)	univariate			multivariable		
			p-value	OR	95% CI	p-value	OR	95% CI
Maternal age (years, mean)	28.9	27.3	< 0.001	1.06	1.03–1.10	< 0.001	1.07	1.03–1.11
Maternal height (cm, mean)	163.3	165.8	< 0.001	0.94	0.91–0.96	< 0.001	0.93	0.90–0.95
Maternal pre-pregnancy weight (kg, median)	64.0	61.5	0.012	1.02	1.01–1.03			
Maternal pre-pregnancy BMI (kg/m^2) (median)	24.1	22.6	< 0.001	1.10	1.06–1.14	< 0.001	1.10	1.06–1.14
Diabetes (GDM or DM) (%)	17.6	7.9	0.001	2.47	1.48–4.13			
GDM, diet treatment	10.8	5.3						
GDM, medical treatment	5.8	2.3						
Chronic DM	1	0.3						
Infertility treatment (%)	12.2	6.8	0.033	1.89	1.05–3.39			
IVF/ICSI	7.0	3.6						
Ovarian stimulation	3.8	1.8						
Insemination	1.4	1.4						
Chronic disease (%), excl. DM, HT	33.8	24.2	0.010	1.60	1.12–2.29	< 0.001	1.52	1.02–2.25
Hypertension (HT) (%)[a]	14.5	11.9	0.347	1.26	0.78–2.02			
Gestational HT	8.8	7.0						
Pre-eclampsia	6.8	5.6						
Chronic HT	0.7	1.0						
Fear of childbirth (%)	5.7	5.0	0.67	1.17	0.57–2.38			

[a]8 primiparas, who had chronic or gestational HT had also pre-eclampsia

Table 2 Intrapartum factors according to delivery route

	CS (n = 296)	VD (n = 302)	univariate			multivariable		
			p-value	OR	95% CI	p-value	OR	95% CI
Gestational age (days, median)	285	281	< 0.001	1.06	1.04–1.08	< 0.001	1.08	1.03–1.12
Spontaneous contractions at admission (n)	106	195	< 0.001	0.30	0.21–0.42			
PROM (n)	101	66	0.001	1.85	1.29–2.67			
IOL (PG or balloon) (n)	90	42	< 0.001	2.71	1.80–4.07			
Indication for IOL								
Postterm pregnancy	28	7						
PROM	22	15						
Pre-eclampsia or HT	16	7						
Diabetes	6	6						
LGA	7	0						
SGA	0	2						
Other	11	5						
Cervix dilatation at admission (mean, cm)	1.5	2.6	< 0.001	0.57	0.48–0.67	0.002	0.65	0.50–0.85
Head position in birth canal at admission (mean, cm)	−2.7	−2.1	< 0.001	0.47	0.36–0.60	0.003	0.56	0.39–0.82
Chorioamnionitis (n)	95	10	< 0.001	10.9	5.01–23.6	< 0.001	21.3	6.86–65.9
Fetal malposition (n)	148	7	< 0.001	42.0	19.2–91.9	< 0.001	70.9	24.2–207
Oxytocin during labor (n)	281	220	< 0.001	6.98	3.92–12.5			
Amniotomy in labor (n)	129	148	0.183					
CTG abnormality (n)	123	12	< 0.001	17.3	9.28–32.2			
Fetal blood sample (n)	103	15	< 0.001	10.2	5.78–18.0			
Meconium-stained fluid (n)	101	40	< 0.001	3.31	2.20–5.00			
Use of IUPC (n)	202	10	< 0.001	63.4	32.2–125			
Epidural analgesia (n)	280	214	< 0.001	7.20	4.10–12.6			
PCB (n)	65	102	0.001	0.55	0.38–0.79			
Duration of delivery (mins, median)	960	620	< 0.001	1.19	1.14–1.23			

PROM = premature rupture of membranes
IOL = induction of labor
LGA = suspected Large for Gestational Age
SGA = suspected Small for Gestational Age
IUPC = intrauterine pressure catheter
PCB = paracervical block
The multivariable p-values and ORs are from logistic regression analyses carried out among the factors related to dystocia, i.e. the first eight main factors in the table

Although the parturients with abnormal CTG findings as a primary reason for CS were excluded from the study, CTG pathology was a secondary finding in many CS cases. To avoid an adverse effect on the results, we performed a subgroup analysis, where we removed parturients with any abnormal CTG findings. The results in univariate and multivariable analysis were otherwise similar with the original study group except for maternal age which did not differ significantly between the subgroups.

Significant differences were found between the study groups as regards pre-pregnancy BMI (Tables 3 and 4). Most parturients (64.2%) were of normal weight before pregnancy and in this BMI class the women experienced more VDs than CSs. When BMI was above normal, the risk of dystocia and intrapartum CS increased almost

linearly (Fig. 2). Severely obese parturients (BMI ≥ 35 kg/m^2) needed 4 hours longer to achieve successful VD when compared with normal-weight primiparas and almost 6 hours longer when compared with underweight primiparas (BMI < 18.5 kg/m^2). Among moderate obese (BMI ≥30–35) primiparas, the most common indication for induction was post term pregnancy (n = 6; 42.9%), and among severe obese primiparas it was hypertension (including pre-eklampsia, n = 5; 33.3%).

Premature rupture of membranes (PROM) was associated with obesity. In severely obese parturients (BMI > 35 kg/m^2) PROM preceded labor in 41.9% of cases, while PROM occurred in 13.6 and 27.6% of cases in BMI classes of < 18.5 and 18.5–25 kg/m^2, respectively – this trend was significant (p = 0.046). Obesity did not affect newborn outcome.

Table 3 Route of delivery according to WHO BMI classes

BMI	Total		CS (291)		VD (299)		univariate			multivariable		
	n	%	n	%	n	%	p	OR	95% CI	p	OR	95% CI
< 18.5	22	3.7	5	1.71	17	5.69	0.073	0.39	0.14–1.09	0.791	0.82	0.20–3.44
≥18.5–25	379	64.2	162	55.7	217	72.6		1		0.011	1	
≥25–30	113	19.2	67	23.0	46	15.4	0.002	1.95	1.27–2.99	0.262	1.41	0.78–2.55
≥30–35	45	7.6	33	11.3	12	4.01	< 0.001	3.68	1.85–7.35	0.005	3.36	1.44–7.84
≥35	31	5.3	24	8.25	7	2.34	0.001	4.59	1.93–10.9	0.016	3.82	1.29–11.3

8 BMIs were missing

The multivariable p-values and ORs are from logistic regression analyses carried out among the most marked factors affecting delivery route, i.e. BMI class, maternal age, diabetes, chronic disease, induction of labor, chorioamnionitis, fetal malposition, gestational age, birth weight

In multivariable analysis, obesity remained as an independent risk factor of labor dystocia when BMI was 30 kg/m^2 or more.

Discussion

In line with the results of previous studies, advancing maternal age [3, 5, 6, 14, 15], high BMI [6, 7, 14–16] and maternal chronic disease [6, 17] were independently associated with labor dystocia and intrapartal CS in our study. Our finding of short stature being associated with dystocia has been shown in previous studies [15, 18], but there are also converse results [14].

The age of primiparas has risen during the last few decades, which may be one reason for the increased CS rate worldwide. In Finland the mean age of all primiparas was 28.6 years in 2014 [19], which is slightly lower

Table 4 Maternal characteristics and intrapartum factors according to BMI WHO classification in the whole study population

BMI	< 18.5 (22)	≥18.5–25 (379)	≥25–30 (113)	≥30–35 (45)	≥35 (31)	p-value
Maternal age (y, mean)	24.5	27.9	28.6	28.8	28.9	0.007
Diabetes (GDM or DM) (%)	0	7.1	18.6	24.4	51.6	< 0.001
Chronic disease (%)	27.3	27.4	27.4	35.6	41.9	0.396
Thyroid disorder (%)	0	4	7.1	2.2	16.1	0.039
Gestational age (d, median)	281	283	285	289	286	[a]
Infertility treatment %	5	8.1	12.8	9.3	14.3	0.264
Admission dilatation (mean, cm)	2.8	2.2	1.9	1.8	1.4	0.007
Head position in birth canal at admission (mean, cm)	−1.9	−2.2	−2.6	−2.6	−2.8	< 0.001
Spontaneous contractions (%)	77.3	56.4	38.1	33.3	32.3	< 0.001
Induction of labor (%)	9.1	17.4	29.2	31.1	45.2	< 0.001
Duration of labor in VD excl. CS (h:min, median)	8:50	10:20	10:31	10:39	14:35	0.51
Oxytocin during labor (%)	68.2	81.5	89.4	93.3	87.1	0.024
Chorionamnionitis (%)	4.5	15.3	19.5	20.0	35.5	0.002
Fetal malposition (%)	13.6	23.8	31.9	28.9	38.7	0.113[b]
Use of IUPC (%)	18.2	29.1	42.5	57.8	61.3	< 0.001
PROM (%)	13.6	27.2	30.0	29.5	41.9	0.23[c]
Time between ROM and delivery (h:min)	4:05	8:02	8:50	8:47	11:40	[d]
CTG pathology	9.1	23.0	24.8	22.2	22.6	0.878
Birth weight (g, mean)	3245	3518	3667	3816	3718	< 0.001
LGA > 4500 g (%)	0	2.1	2.7	11.1	3.2	
SGA < 2500 g (%)	4.5	1.1	0	0	0	
5 min Apgar	8.86	8.85	8.90	8.93	8.39	0.307
Umb. artery pH	7.28	7.28	7.30	7.31	7.28	NS

[a]p-value was significant (< 0.05) when normal BMI (18.5–25) was compared to BMI group ≥ 25–30 or ≥ 30–35
[b]Significant trend (p = 0.014)
[c]Significant trend (p = 0.046)
[d]p-values between BMI groups < 18.5– ≥35 p = 0.001 and ≥ 18.5–25 p = 0.023

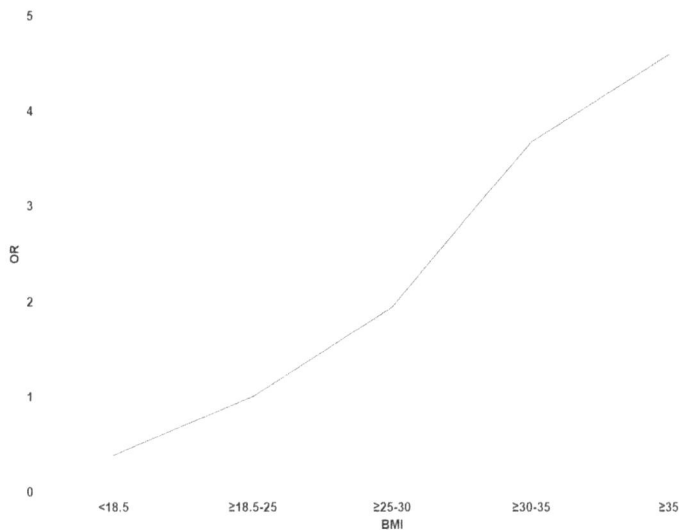

Fig. 2 Influence of BMI on the risk of cesarean section due to labor dystocia

than the mean age of the dystocia group in our study. Surprisingly, fear of childbirth did not increase the incidence of intrapartum CS for labor dystocia in our study population. In a Swedish study, FOC was associated with an increased emergency CS rate even after psychiatric counseling [20]. On the other hand, in a Finnish randomized trial, when fear of childbirth was treated in a psychoeducational group, treatment decreased the emergency CS rate [21]. In our study population, the incidence of FOC was in line with the national prevalence of FOC. This prevalence may reflect Finland's health care system's aim to recognize and treat parturients with FOC early in pregnancy. Besides these background factors, several intrapartum factors were also found to differ between groups, some of which may be regarded rather as a consequence of dystocia than a cause of it.

The results of the present study confirmed previous findings that admission to hospital at an early stage of labor, and induction of labor, are related to intrapartal CS [6, 15]. However, the indication for induction, such as prolonged pregnancy, rather than induction itself, may carry a risk of dystocia. Likewise, admission to hospital at an early stage of cervical dilatation [14, 15] may be a result of a diminished capacity of labor to proceed in some cases.

Oxytocin, intrauterine pressure catheters and epidural analgesia are used in the treatment of prolonged labor, which probably explains their greater use in the CS group. In the dystocia group, there was a greater need of analgesia, such as epidural analgesia, opiates and nitrous oxide, and many parturients needed several modes of analgesia. On the other hand, in successful VD, there was significantly more use of paracervical blocks. Our intrapartal findings support the clinical experience that

prolonged labor is a sum of many factors, and it is hard to say which is first: lack of progress, fetal malposition, or chorioamnionitis.

The increased risk of labor dystocia brought about by obesity may be direct or the consequence of associated risk factors. In our multivariable test, mild obesity [BMI 25–30 kg/m^2] did not appear to be an independent risk factor, but beyond that, BMI independently increased the risk of CS almost fourfold. As a new finding in our study, we noticed that among obese women PROM preceded labor more often than in normal-weight parturients. In addition, in line with the results of previous studies, overweight women came to hospital at an earlier stage of cervical dilatation, they less frequently had spontaneous contractions before admission to hospital, their labors were more often induced and they more often needed oxytocin during labor [6–8, 15, 16]. The reason for these findings is obscure, but they may reflect relative myometrial inactivity related to the unfavorable metabolic circumstances in obese parturients [22], possibly associated with endothelial dysfunction [22, 23]. It has also been speculated that oxytocin receptors might be influenced by maternal obesity [8].

Successful vaginal deliveries of obese parturients lasted 4 hours longer than among normal-weight parturients. This is in line with the results of previous studies, which have suggested that obese parturients need 2 hours more to progress in the first stage of labor, especially before 7 cm dilatation [8, 24]. It can be speculated that in our study population some severely obese women could have achieved vaginal delivery if they had been given more time in the first stage of labor.

A strength of our study is that the fairly large study material from a single center is homogeneous. The data on maternal background and deliveries is reliable and of good quality, being collected from the patients' medical records. In the literature we found only one case-control study of labor abnormalities [25], and none regarding the risk of dystocia among term primiparas [14].

A limitation of the study is that diagnoses such as chorioamnionitis, fetal malposition and CTG pathology may not always have been registered in connection with successful VD. As this study was retrospective, we could not control the indication for CS and the diagnosis of dystocia in the delivery room. Dystocia is often a complex, multifactorial phenomenon. Hence, there is an unavoidable challenge as regards causality.

Conclusions

Because CS can be problematic for the parturient and newborn, and also in regard to subsequent pregnancy and delivery, it is worth trying VD. Clinical possibilities to avoid dystocia are limited. Maternal pre-pregnancy BMI is one of the contributors that could be influenced before pregnancy. This way, clinicians could try to avoid dystocia and prevent CS. To prevent CS further, primiparas should be encouraged to delay admission to hospital until the cervix is properly dilated and IOL of primiparas with an unfavorable cervix should be avoided. When there is an obese parturient in the delivery room, clinicians should recognize this risk factor and allow considerably more time in the first stage of labor before diagnosing dystocia.

List of abbreviations: CS, cesarean section; VD, vaginal delivery; BMI, body mass index; CTG, cardiotocography; GDM, gestational diabetes mellitus; FOC, fear of childbirth; IOL, induction of labor; PROM, premature rupture of membranes.

Funding

Financial support from the Orion Research Foundation and Special Grant funding of the Government of Finland. Funding sources have not involved in the collection, analysis or interpretation of data or writing of the manuscript.

Authors' contributions

All authors have taken part in manuscript writing. TH: Project development, Data analyses. OP: Protocol/project development, Data analyses. KE: Data collection, Data analyses. JU: Protocol/project development, Data analyses. HH: Protocol development, Statistical analyses. All authors read and approved the final manuscript.

Consent for publication

Not applicable.

Competing interests

The authors declare that they have no competing interests.

Author details

[1]Department of Obstetrics and Gynecology, Central Hospital of Central Finland, Keskussairaalantie 19, 40620 Jyväskylä, Finland. [2]Department of Obstetrics and Gynecology, Tampere University Hospital, Tampere, Finland. [3]Kangasala Health Center, Kangasala, Finland. [4]School of Health Sciences, Tampere University, Tampere, Finland.

References

1. World Health Organization. World Health Statistics 2010 and 2015. Available at: http://www.who.int/gho/publications/world_health_statistics/EN_WHS10_Part2.pdf/EN_WHS2015_Part2.pdf, 2010, 2015.
2. Brennan DJ, Murphy MR, Robson MS, O'Herlihy C. The singleton, cephalic, nulliparous woman after 36 weeks of gestation: contribution to overall cesarean delivery rates. Obstet Gynecol. 2011;117(2, Part 1):273–9.
3. Klemetti R, Gissler M, Sainio S, Hemminki E. Associations of maternal age with maternity care use and birth outcomes in primiparous women: a comparison of results in 1991 and 2008 in Finland. BJOG. 2014;121(3):356–62.
4. Stjernholm YV, Petersson K, Eneroth E. Changed indications for cesarean sections. Acta Obstet Gynecol Scand. 2010;89(1):49–53.
5. Herstad L, Klungsyr K, Skjaerven R, et al. Maternal age and emergency operative deliveries at term: a population-based registry study among low-risk primiparous women. BJOG. 2015;122(12):1642–51.
6. Ehrenthal DB, Jiang X, Strobino DM. Labor induction and the risk of a cesarean delivery among nulliparous women at term. Obstet Anesth Digest. 2011;31(3):162.
7. Arrowsmith S, Wray S, Quenby S. Maternal obesity and labour complications following induction of labour in prolonged pregnancy. BJOG. 2011;118(5):578–88.
8. Vahratian A, Zhang J, Troendle JF, Savitz DA, SiegaRiz AM. Maternal Prepregnancy overweight and obesity and the pattern of labor progression in term nulliparous women. Obstet Gynecol. 2004;104(5, Part 1):943–51.
9. Zhang J, Bricker L, Wray S, Quenby S. Poor uterine contractility in obese women. BJOG. 2007;114(3):343–8.
10. Pallasmaa N, Ekblad U, Gissler M. Severe maternal morbidity and the mode of delivery. Acta Obstet Gynecol Scand. 2008;87(6):662–8.
11. Mozurkewich E, Hutton E. Elective repeat cesarean delivery versus trial of labor: a meta-analysis of the literature from 1989 to 1999. Am J Obstet Gynecol. 2000;183(5):1187–97.
12. Robson MS. Can we reduce the caesarean section rate? Best Pract Res Clin Obstet Gynaecol. 2001;15(1):179–94.
13. WHO. World Health Organization BMI classification. 2016; Available at: http://www.euro.who.int/en/health-topics/disease-prevention/nutrition/a-healthy-lifestyle/body-mass-indexbmi.
14. Wu C, Chen C, Chien C. Prediction of dystocia-related cesarean section risk in uncomplicated Taiwanese nulliparas at term. Arch Gynecol Obstet. 2013; 288:1027.
15. Kominiarek MA, VanVeldhuisen P, Gregory K, Fridman M, Kim H, Hibbard JU. Intrapartum cesarean delivery in nulliparas: risk factors compared by two analytical approaches. J Perinatol. 2015;35(3):167–72.
16. Denison FC, Price J, Graham C, Wild S, Liston WA. Maternal obesity, length of gestation, risk of postdates pregnancy, and spontaneous onset of labor at term. Obstet Anesth Digest. 2009;29(1):20.
17. Linton A, Peterson MR. Effect of preexisting chronic disease on primary cesarean delivery rates by race for births in U.S. military hospitals, 1999-2002. Birth. 2004;31(3):165–75.
18. Sheiner E, Levy A, Katz M, Mazor M. Short stature - an independent risk factor for cesarean delivery. Eur J Obstet Gynecol Reprod Biol. 2005;120(2):175–8.
19. National Institute for Health and Welfare of Finland. Perinatal statistics 2014: Parturients, deliveries and newborns. 2015; Available at: http://urn.fi/URN:NBN:fi-fe2015093014270.
20. Sydsjo G, Sydsjo A, Gunnervik C, Bladh M, Josefsson A. Obstetric outcome for women who received individualized treatment for fear of childbirth during pregnancy. Acta Obstet Gynecol Scand. 2012;91(1):44–9.
21. Rouhe H, SalmelaAro K, Toivanen R, Tokola M, Halmesmaki E, Saisto T. Obstetric outcome after intervention for severe fear of childbirth in nulliparous women - randomised trial. BJOG Int J Obstet Gynaecol. 2013; 120(1):75–84.

22. Ramsay JE, Ferrell WR, Crawford L, Wallace AM, Greer IA, Sattar N. Maternal obesity is associated with dysregulation of metabolic, vascular, and inflammatory pathways. J Clin Endocrinol Metab. 2002;87(9):4231–7.

23. Chaemsaithong P, Madan I, Romero R, Than NG, Tarca AL, Draghici S, et al. Characterization of the myometrial transcriptome in women with an arrest of dilatation during labor. J Perinat Med. 2013;41(6):665–81.

24. Kaplan-Sturk R, Akerud H, Volgsten H, Hellstrom-Westas L, Wiberg-Itzel E. Outcome of deliveries in healthy but obese women: obesity and delivery outcome. BMC Res Notes. 2013;6:50.

25. Abraham W, Berhan Y. Predictors of labor abnormalities in university hospital: unmatched case control study. BMC Pregnancy Childbirth. 2014;14:256.

13

Evaluation of an activity monitor for use in pregnancy to help reduce excessive gestational weight gain

Paul M. C. Lemmens[1][*] [iD], Francesco Sartor[1], Lieke G. E. Cox[1], Sebastiaan V. den Boer[1] and Joyce H. D. M. Westerink[1,2]

Abstract

Background: Excessive weight gain during pregnancy increases the risk for negative effects on mother and child during pregnancy, delivery, and also postnatally. Excessive weight gain can be partially compensated by being sufficiently physically active, which can be measured using activity trackers. Modern activity trackers often use accelerometer data as well as heart rate data to estimate energy expenditure. Because pregnancy affects the metabolism and cardiac output, it is not evident that activity trackers that are calibrated to the general population can be reliably used during pregnancy. We evaluated whether an activity monitor designed for the general population is sufficiently accurate for estimating energy expenditure in pregnant women.

Methods: Forty pregnant women (age: 30.8 ± 4.7 years, BMI: 25.0 ± 4.0) from all three trimesters performed a 1-h protocol including paced and self-paced exercise activities as well as household activities. We tracked reference energy expenditure using indirect calorimetry and used equivalence testing to determine whether the estimated energy expenditure from the activity monitor was within the limits of equivalence.

Results: Overall we found an averaged underestimation of 10 kcal (estimated energy expenditure was 97% of the reference measurement). The 90% CI for the cumulative total energy expenditure was 94–100%. The activities of self-paced cycling, household activities, stair-walking, and yoga had one of their equivalence boundaries outside a 80–125% range of equivalence; for exercise on a cross-trainer, for self-paced and fixed-pace walking, fixed-paced cycling, and resting, the estimations were within the limits of equivalence.

Conclusions: We conclude that the activity monitor is sufficiently accurate for every-day use during pregnancy. The observed deviations can be accounted for and are acceptable from a statistical and an applied perspective because the positive and negative deviations that we observed cancel out to an accurate average energy expenditure over a day, and estimations during exercise are sufficiently accurate to enable coaching on physical activity. The positive and negative deviations themselves were relatively small. Therefore, the activity monitor can be used to help in preventing excessive weight gain during pregnancy by accurately tracking physical activity.

Keywords: Activity monitor, Heart rate, Accelerometer, Validation, Energy expenditure, MET

* Correspondence: paul.lemmens@philips.com
[1]Philips Research, High Tech Campus 34, 5656 AE Eindhoven, the Netherlands
Full list of author information is available at the end of the article

Background

Excessive Gestational Weight Gain (eGWG) is defined as a weight gain of more than 10 kg for women of normal pre-pregnancy weight, more than 9 kg in pregestationally overweight women, or a more than 6 kg weight increase in pregestationally obese women [1, 2]. eGWG is an increasingly prevalent health risk for pregnant women that affects more than 50% of all pregnancies in the United States (US) [3, 4]. It has been shown to be an independent risk factor for multiple medical conditions including gestational diabetes mellitus (GDM), gestational hypertension and pre-eclampsia [5, 6]. Physical *inactivity* is the main contributors to eGWG, and is relatively common in our increasingly obesogenic environment [7, 8]. In contrast, physical *activity* has been shown to have protective effects against GDM and pre-eclampsia [9–11], while not affecting fetal growth [11] or triggering premature delivery [11].

Concerning physical activity during pregnancy, guidelines recommend a minimum of three 15-min sessions per week up to a maximum of four 30-min sessions per week at a moderate to hard exertion level [2, 12, 13]. These exertion levels are considered safe, provided that there is no medical contraindication [2]. The targets that the various guidelines propose vary from 16 to 28 Metabolic Equivalent of Task (MET) hours per week (1 MET is equivalent to energy expenditure during rest). For a 71 kg person on a schedule of 4 days of exercise per week, this corresponds to an energy expenditure between 300 to 525 kcal during exercise [12]. However, these recommendations are often not met [14, 15] partly because these abstract guidelines in terms of METS or kcals are often difficult to translate into real-life exercise targets that, cumulatively over the duration of the pregnancy, will result in achieving sufficient physical activity to prevent eGWG.

A possible solution would be to accurately and objectively measure expended energy during physical activities, and to provide feedback about it in terms of activity minutes of activity or energy expended [16–18] in free-living settings [19, 20]. Accelerometer and heart-rate based activity monitors have become available that provide such an accurate yet unobtrusive estimation of energy expenditure [21–25]. The combination of accelerometer and heart-rate provides improved accuracy compared to questionnaires [20] as well as compared to accelerometer-only or HR-only estimations of energy expenditure [25, 26]. Such products could help pregnant women to determine whether their expended energy matches the proposed physical activity guidelines and become more compliant to them. It is paramount that the estimated energy expenditure is sufficiently accurate to enable appropriate guidance to minimize eGWG when physical activity is observed to be insufficient.

To our knowledge, however, none of the consumer-grade devices exploiting a combination of accelerometer and heart rate based estimation of energy expenditure has been validated for use during pregnancy. This is remarkable because it is known that a pregnancy has distinct effects on physiological and metabolic processes [27, 28]. For instance, resting metabolic rate (RMR) has been shown to be significantly different in pregnant women compared to matched controls [29], and even within pregnancy significant differences between the first, second and third trimesters have been observed on, for instance, cardiac output [30, 31]. Thus, a validation on the general population might not suffice.

Here, we aim to validate whether an existing activity monitor combining accelerometry and heart rate information to estimate energy expenditure, is sufficiently accurate to be used in guiding and monitoring pregnant women in achieving the activity levels set out in the guidelines to prevent or minimize the effects of eGWG and its comorbidities. Because of the noted differences on physiological parameters over trimesters, the validation was performed on women of all gestational ages.

Methods

Participants

We included 51 pregnant women from all gestational ages (12–35 weeks pregnant). Participants were required to be in primary care which excluded high-risk pregnancies. Of this set of 51 participants, the data of 40 participants were used in the statistical analyses (see Fig. 1). The data of eleven participants could not be used due to equipment failure or inability to properly synchronize the data from the sensors. The mean age of the 40 participants was 30.8 $\pm$ 4.7 years, average height was 169.5 $\pm$ 7.8 cm, and the average weight was 71.7 $\pm$ 12.6 kg. For each participant we estimated VO_{2max} using the equation in Fig. 1 of Sady et al. [32] using HR_{60W} and $VO_{2,60W}$ from the last minute of the 6-min cycling activity in the protocol (see below). The average value for VO_{2max} was 33.0 $\pm$ 6.8 ml/kg/min. The

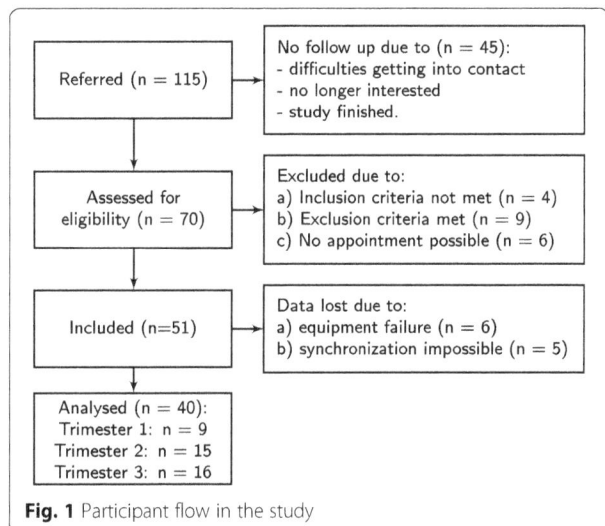

Fig. 1 Participant flow in the study

study was approved by our institutional review board (Philips Research IRB dossier ICBE-2-3895; formal medical-ethical review was waived) and written informed consent was obtained from all participants prior to collecting any data. Participants were recruited and referred by a local recruiting agency.

Materials

We used two devices to measure and estimate energy expenditure. The reference measurements were taken by a Cosmed K4b^2 calorimeter (Cosmed, Italy) that uses a breath-by-breath pulmonary gas exchange (VO$_2$, VCO$_2$) analyzer to calculate (total) energy expenditure [33]. The K4b^2 was calibrated according to the manufacturer's instructions by first performing a room-air calibration, then a reference-gas calibration using a gas tank with a 16% O$_2$ and 5% CO$_2$ mix, and finally a flow-turbine calibration using a 3.0 L syringe.

The second device was a watch (referred to as Optical Heart Rate Monitor, OHRM) that was worn on the participants' left wrist. The OHRM is based on the Philips Cardio and Motion Monitoring Module (CM3-Generation-1) that is an accelerometer and optical heart rate sensor module developed by Philips [21, 34]. It estimates energy expenditure using contributions of measured heart rate and accelerometry. Additional devices were employed to make sure that protocol timing and synchronization of the various data streams was possible. One of these devices was a Garmin Forerunner 620 that we used as master clock and to set markers at the beginning and end of each activity.

Protocol

Participants were asked to fill out the International Physical Activity Questionnaire (IPAQ) to evaluate their baseline physical activity level of the last seven days. Age, height, weight and gestational age were recorded. Then a series of physical activities was performed that each lasted for 1–3 min and one activity lasting for 6 min (see Table 1). Each activity was followed by 1–3 min of (seated) rest to prevent fatigue. The durations of activities and rest were based on striking a balance between the need for a minimum duration to achieve steady state (based on pilots and earlier studies) and keeping the overall duration and exertion level acceptable for pregnant women. During the indoor laboratory protocol, exercises with high and low intensity were alternated to balance overall physical exertion. Based on pilots and earlier studies, we defined high intensity activities as those where participants were expected to achieve a heart rate of at least 60% of maximal heart rate which Zavorsky and Long set as definition of vigorous activity during pregnancy [2]. Half of the participants performed the indoors activities in the reversed order. During the outdoor part, cycling and various forms of walking were

Table 1 Overview of the protocol that was used in the study with durations of the activity and rest immediately after the activity indicated in square brackets

Heart rate at rest [5]
Indoor activities
1. Stacking groceries [3, 1]
2. Desk work [2, 1]
3. Vacuuming [3, 2]
4. Sitting resting [3, 1]
5. [a]Cycling fitness test (60 W) [6, 5]
6. [a]Walking treadmill - 3 km/h – 0% incline [3, 2]
7. Standing resting [1, 1]
8. [a]Walking treadmill - 5 km/h – 0% incline [3, 2]
9. Folding towels [3, 1]
10.[a]Walking treadmill - 5 km/h - 0% incline - carrying 4 kg [3, 3]
11. Cooking or Washing dishes [3, 1]
12. [a]Walking treadmill - 3 km/h - 5% [3, 3]
13. Cleaning table [3, 1]
14. [a]Cross trainer - 60 W [3, 5]
15. Yoga [3, 1]
Switch to self-paced/outdoor activities
16. Walking upstairs (indoors) [1, 2]
17. Walking downstairs (indoors) [1, 2]
18. Walking, hands free [2, 1]
19. Walking, hands in pockets [2, 1]
20. Walking, carrying a bag [2, 1]
21. Cycling [3, 2]

After step 15, a pause of 5–10 min was required to replace the battery of the K4b^2 and to prepare participants for doing the self-paced activities that were executed indoors and outdoors. Before the activities, all participants started with a 5-min measurement of heart rate at rest so all participants started at a similar steady state in rest. Note that, due to weather conditions, for some participants, the self-paced activities were performed indoors. Also note that cooking and dishwashing (11) were "role-playing" activities mimicking the actual activities. Activities marked with an 'a' were fixed paced activities enforced by either setting a specific speed of the respective exercise machine or by monitoring by the study assistant

required. The total duration of the activities was 61 min, excluding rest and a break between the indoor and outdoor part. Heart rate was monitored continuously to ensure participants did not exceed 85% of their maximal HR.

Data synchronization, preprocessing, and statistical analysis

We used a series of steps to synchronize all separate data sets. Because most devices did not have the option to place a marker in their data to synchronize the devices, we used a 1-min shaking protocol during which all sensors containing accelerometers were shaken vigorously to introduce a signal in their accelerometer data that could be easily recognized. This shaking protocol was performed before the sensors were placed on the participants.

We started the preprocessing with converting the K4b^2 data by linear interpolation from a breath-by-breath frequency to a time-series with a sampling frequency of 1 Hz. Then we synchronized the data sets first based on heart rate and subsequently based on accelerometer data using cross-correlation techniques with possible fine-tuning based on visual assessment. We used the Garmin as master clock and synchronized the data of the ORHM and the K4b^2 to the Garmin's heart rate.

Next, we extracted the cumulative total energy expenditure (TEE in kcal) for both devices from the recorded and estimated energy expenditure at the end of the laboratory protocol. We calculated the average (total) energy expenditure (kcal/h). The average bias (kcal/h) was determined by subtracting the reference from the estimated energy expenditure. Mean absolute percentage error (MAPE) for each individual activity was calculated by extracting the data for the individual activities from the synchronized data using the markers and their associated time stamps that we set using the Garmin. Finally, we calculated for each activity, 10-s non-overlapping windows of averaged TEE to compute root-mean-squared errors (RMSE) on the differences between reference and estimated expenditure. We chose non-overlapping windows because this was consistent with how one would use the averaged TEE samples to calculate the cumulative TEE over each activity or even the full protocol.

We based the statistical analysis on equivalence testing [35] and tested whether the ratio of the OHRM-based estimated energy expenditure and the K4b^2-based reference measurements thereof was within an acceptable interval around 100% [36, 37]. As acceptable interval, we used the 20% margin that has international consensus [38–40] but also used a tighter 10% margin. We determined equivalence based on the differences in log-transformed energy expenditure because this is mathematically equivalent to a ratio of untransformed values. This transformation is required because the equivalence testing procedure only works on differences. Therefore, a symmetric 20% margin translates as a range of values from 80 to 125% (= 1/0.8) for the assessment of equivalence in log-transformed units [41]. That is, when the 90% confidence interval for the ratio of the OHRM's estimations and the measured TEE of the K4b^2 was within the interval ranging from 80 to 125%, we declared the monitor's estimation as equivalent.

We implemented the equivalence testing using the two one-sided tests (TOST) procedure. It requires calculating $(100 - 2\alpha) = 90\%$ confidence intervals (90% CI) [42, 43] for the observed difference between reference and estimated scores to determine whether that 90% CI falls within the pre-established equivalence margin. Tryon and colleagues [44, 45] have analytically shown that the TOST procedure and the visualizations that we use are equivalent. Therefore, we refrained from using p-values throughout the

equivalence analysis, but instead we focused on visualizations of the observed confidence intervals against the regions of equivalence of 80–125% as well as a more restrictive 90–111% interval, concluding equivalence only if the observed confidence interval was fully included in the 80–125% region of equivalence. Note that we carried out the analysis on differences of log-transformed energy expenditure but that the visualizations are presented on back-transformed ratios expressed as percentage of the reference.

In addition to equivalence tests, we also calculated bias (difference in kcal/h) between the OHRM and indirect calorimetry from the K4b^2, and errors (in terms of mean percentage errors, and mean absolute percentage errors) for total energy expenditure. We used the visual technique of Bland-Altman plots [46, 47] to determine the degree of agreement, and to evaluate the bias for aspects like proportional error (heteroscedasticity). In addition, Bland-Altman plots provide an overall view of the data, including outliers, and enables, via the limits of agreement (LOAs), the assessment of the relevance of potential outliers by showing whether the LOAs are influenced mostly by the general quality of the agreement or also by outliers. Thus a Bland-Altman plot provides more information than, for instance, a concordance correlation coefficient.

Based on similarity of activities and whether activities were self-paced or not, we created nine clusters of activities: cycling (paced, indoors), cycling (self-paced, outdoors), walking (paced, indoors), walking (self-paced, outdoors), resting, stair walking, household activities, yoga, and cross training; The latter two clusters actually comprised a single activity. We based our statistical analyses on these activity clusters.

Results

We found that the estimations of TEE by the OHRM averaged over all activities were at 96.8% (SD: ± 12.0) of the reference measurements (90% CI: 93.8–99.8%). It was clear that the 90% confidence interval around the OHRM-estimated cumulative TEE for the duration of the lab protocol fell well within the boundaries for equivalence of the conventional 80–125% case as well as of the more restrictive 90–111% (see the left-hand panel in Fig. 2).

Next, we determined whether the average TEE estimation from the OHRM was equivalent to the averaged reference measurements from the K4b^2 for each cluster of activities (see Fig. 2, right-hand panel). This shows that the 90% CI's for the walking activities (fixed pace as well as self-paced), resting, fixed pace cycling, and the cross training were well within the conventional 80–125% boundaries of equivalence, although the OHRM's estimations were too high or too low for some participants. Only the cross-training activity achieved an accuracy with a 90% CI that was within the more restrictive 90–111% boundary.

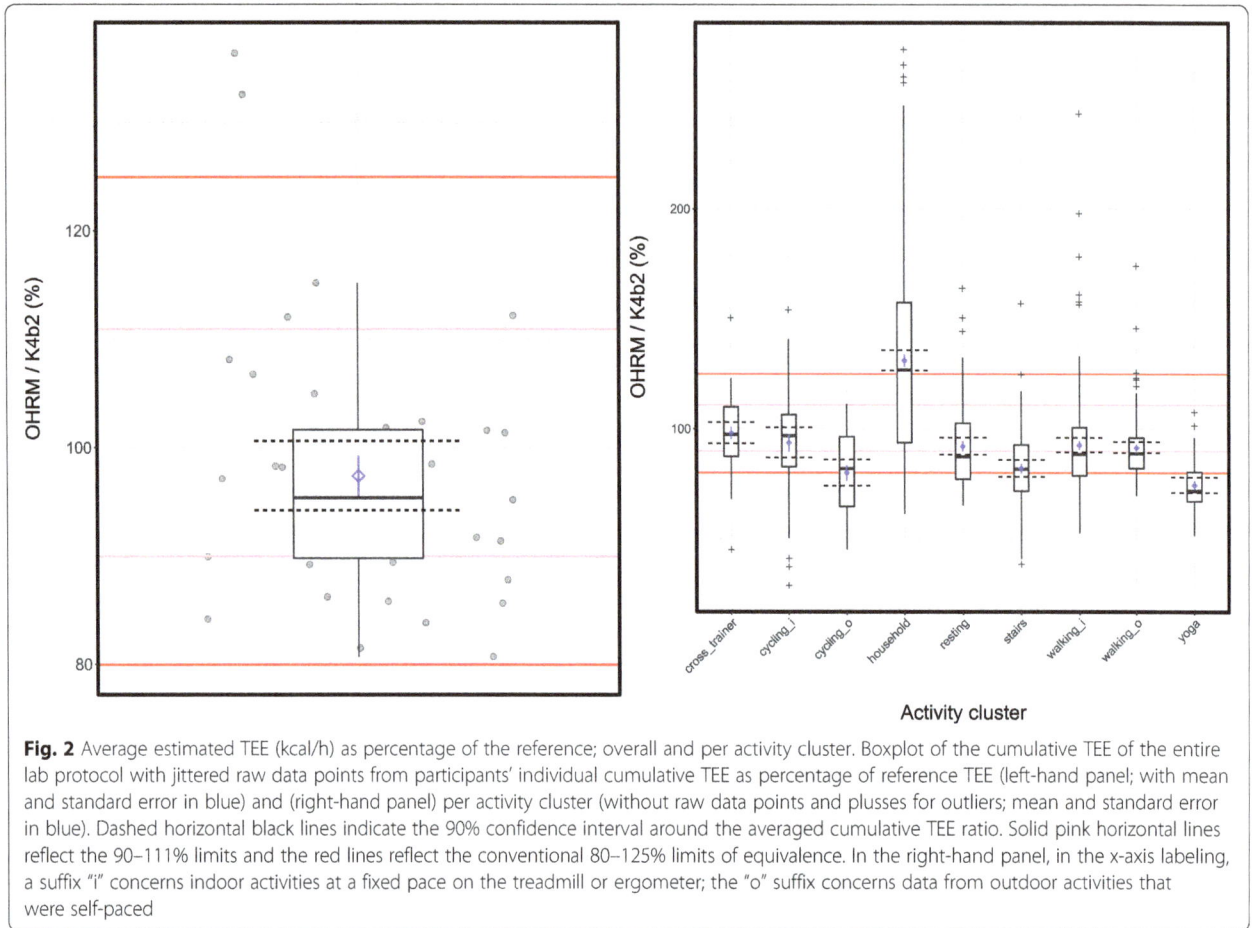

Fig. 2 Average estimated TEE (kcal/h) as percentage of the reference; overall and per activity cluster. Boxplot of the cumulative TEE of the entire lab protocol with jittered raw data points from participants' individual cumulative TEE as percentage of reference TEE (left-hand panel; with mean and standard error in blue) and (right-hand panel) per activity cluster (without raw data points and plusses for outliers; mean and standard error in blue). Dashed horizontal black lines indicate the 90% confidence interval around the averaged cumulative TEE ratio. Solid pink horizontal lines reflect the 90–111% limits and the red lines reflect the conventional 80–125% limits of equivalence. In the right-hand panel, in the x-axis labeling, a suffix "i" concerns indoor activities at a fixed pace on the treadmill or ergometer; the "o" suffix concerns data from outdoor activities that were self-paced

We found that for four activity clusters, the upper or lower limit of the 90% CI of the OHRM's estimations were higher or lower than the 80–125% range of equivalence. For the household activities we observed that the upper CI limit was larger than 125% and that, with the median approximately equal to the 125% limit, a little over half of the data fell above the 125% equivalence limit. This indicated that the OHRM overestimated energy expenditure for this activity cluster. On the other hand, we observed that for outdoor (self-paced) cycling as well as stair walking the lower limit of the 90% CI was below the 80% equivalence limit, reflecting estimations that were too low compared to the K4b^2's reference measurement. The yoga activity was the only activity cluster that was completely outside of the 80–125% equivalence boundaries. There, the estimations were too low compared to the reference measurements.

To study whether the observed deviations in estimated energy expenditure could be detrimental to, for instance, physical activity programs to reduce (e)GWG, we considered the deviations in terms of kcal/h because those programs aim for a specific exercise intensity to expend a certain amount of kilocalories. A series of Bland-Altman plots for the activity clusters showed that the bias (the

difference) between TEE estimation and the TEE reference measurement ranged, on average, from − 68.0 kcal/h (SD: 68.7; self-paced cycling) to + 46.2 kcal/h (SD: 60.1; household activities; see Fig. 3). The best estimations of TEE of the OHRM were obtained during the cross-trainer activity and during rest with average deviations as small as − 7.1 (62.7) kcal/h and − 10.3 (19.8) kcal/h, respectively.

The Bland-Altman plots showed several interesting patterns: for instance, the marked difference in estimation accuracy for upstairs versus downstairs walking. Whereas the estimations for the latter were quite accurate with an error close to zero on average, the estimations for the former were too low compared to the reference measurements and this underestimation resulted in the overall underestimation for the activity cluster of stair walking that we observed in Fig. 3 (right-hand panel).

Another striking pattern in the Bland-Altman plots was the concentrated cluster of data points in the lower left part of the (middle-left) panel of Fig. 3 that concerned the household activities comprising (computer) desk work, stacking groceries, vacuuming, folding clothes, cleaning a table, and cooking and dish washing. This cluster of data points was from the desk-work activity that, relative to activities like grocery stacking, cooking, and dish washing,

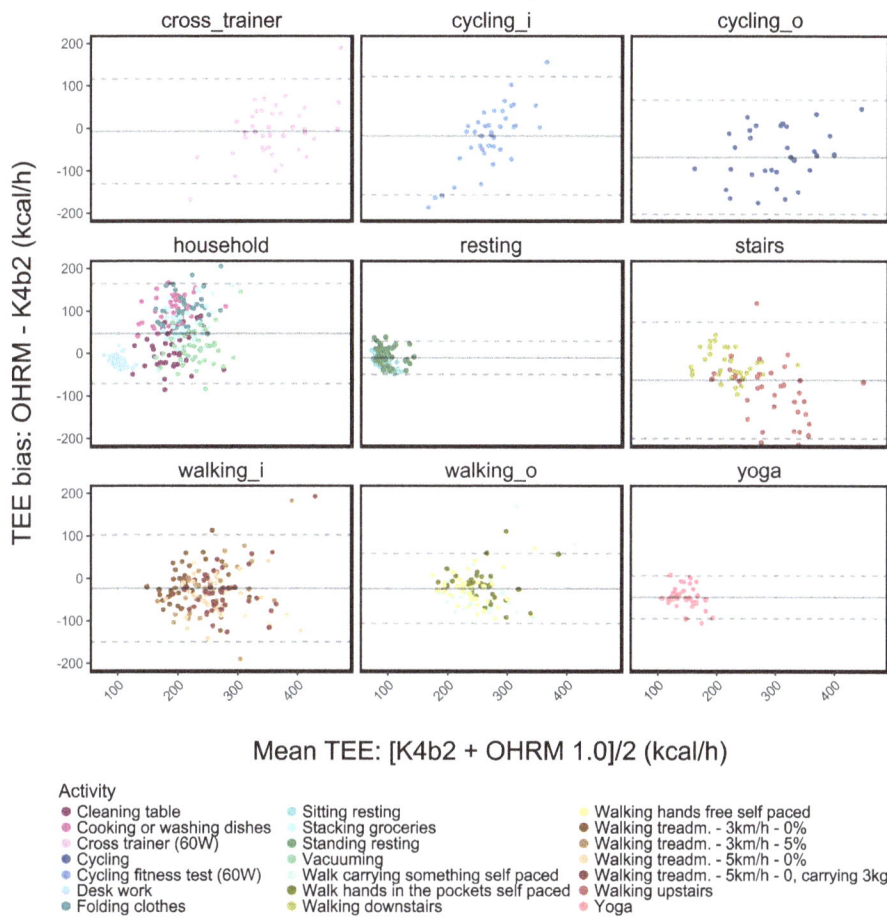

Fig. 3 Bland-Altman plots of TEE (kcal/h) for each activity cluster. Solid grey lines indicate the cluster's average TEE bias and dashed lines reflect the 95% limits of agreement (LoA). Colored dots are participants' averaged TEE biases for each activity. Average biases and LoA's were calculated for the collective data of each cluster. In the panel labels, a suffix "i" concerns indoor activities at a fixed pace on the treadmill or ergometer; the "o" suffix concerns data from outdoor activities that were self-paced

was a static activity with minimal hand and body movements resulting in very low energy expenditure. The other household activities were characterized by many repetitive hand movements and little body movement resulting in an overestimation by the OHRM.

The third interesting pattern is the one related to the indoor cycling (top-middle panel) that seems to show a correlation between the bias and TEE, indicative of a proportional error [46, 47]. However, this seems to be caused largely by the four data points around the LoA that overemphasize the proportional error. When we removed these data points, the apparent proportional error was no longer evident. Overall, we did not find further consistent or considerable flaws in the TEE-estimations by the OHRM indicated by the absence of patterns in the Bland-Altman plots.

From the biases calculated for the Bland-Altman plots, we determined that the average overall bias was – 10.6 kcal (Fig. 4, left-hand panel; without the outlier – 14.4 kcal) for the 61 min protocol which amounted to a mean percentage

error of – 2.6% and a mean absolute percentage error of 9.4%. This indicated that on average the OHRM's estimations were 10.6 kcal too low which was a – 3% error. RMSE's for each activity cluster ranged from 26.0 kcal/h (0.35 MET; resting activities) to 98.1 kcal/h (1.3 MET) for the self-paced cycling activity.

Discussion

Commercial solutions for estimating energy expenditure exist but to the extent of our knowledge have not been validated for use by pregnant women. We performed a study to determine whether the OHRM activity monitor [21], that estimates energy expenditure based on accelerometer and heart rate data at the wrist, is sufficiently accurate for use during pregnancy. This monitor has been developed based on data from the general population and it is known that a pregnancy changes some of the key biophysiological parameters upon which the OHRM builds its estimations [27–30]. In a protocol that combined a series of paced and

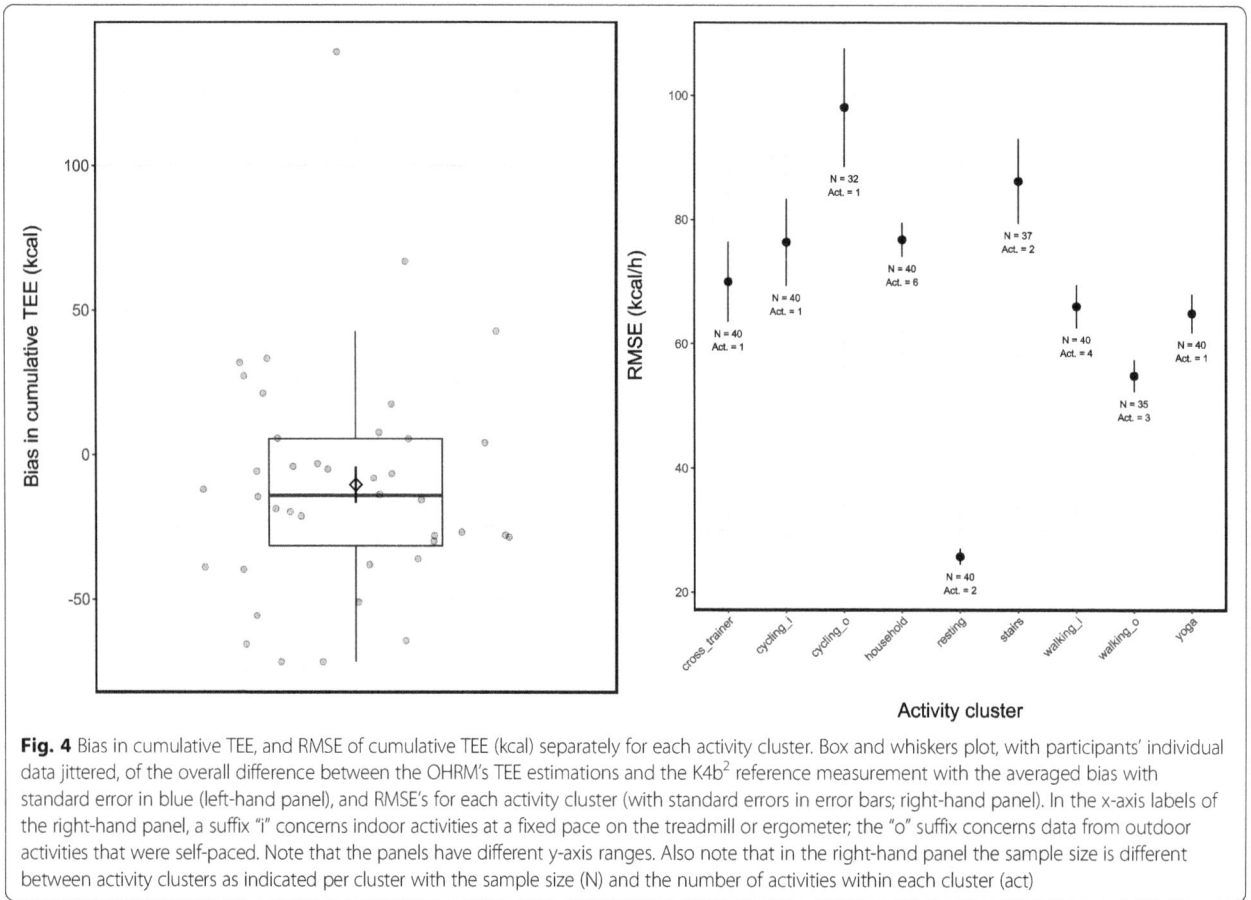

Fig. 4 Bias in cumulative TEE, and RMSE of cumulative TEE (kcal) separately for each activity cluster. Box and whiskers plot, with participants' individual data jittered, of the overall difference between the OHRM's TEE estimations and the K4b^2 reference measurement with the averaged bias with standard error in blue (left-hand panel), and RMSE's for each activity cluster (with standard errors in error bars; right-hand panel). In the x-axis labels of the right-hand panel, a suffix "i" concerns indoor activities at a fixed pace on the treadmill or ergometer; the "o" suffix concerns data from outdoor activities that were self-paced. Note that the panels have different y-axis ranges. Also note that in the right-hand panel the sample size is different between activity clusters as indicated per cluster with the sample size (N) and the number of activities within each cluster (act)

self-paced activities mimicking exercise activities as well as everyday life activities, participants used the OHRM and the activity monitor's estimated energy expenditure was compared against reference measurements from indirect calorimetry.

The data that we have gathered show that for cumulative total energy expenditure (TEE) the OHRM's estimations are on par with the reference K4b^2's measurements for a range of equivalence of 90–111%, which is stricter than the conventional 80–125% range [38–40]. On average, the estimated cumulative TEE is at 97% of the reference value from the K4b^2. When considering clusters of highly similar activities, on average, the estimations are within the conventional limits of equivalence of 80–125% for cross-trainer activities, indoor cycling, resting, and indoor and outdoor walking.

When converting the observed errors into METS, we find values that are below or a little over 1 MET which is equivalent to the energy expenditure at rest. For a 73 kg person, the largest errors in TEE estimation equated to –0.91 MET (self-paced cycling) and 0.62 MET (household activities) and around 0.1 MET for the smallest errors of cross training and resting. These small errors should enable appropriate guidance on physical activity in a program to minimize or prevent excessive weight gain during pregnancy.

However, four activities had 90% CI's for their averaged TEE that are partially or fully outside the region of equivalence. For outdoor cycling, stair walking, and yoga we observed underestimations whereas energy expenditure during household activities was overestimated. A possible reason for the overestimation above the 125% border of equivalence (see Fig. 2) of TEE for the household activities is that the activities that participants performed involved relatively stationary yet manually intensive activities. Because the OHRM was positioned at the wrist, our hypothesis is that the overestimation by the OHRM occurs because the contribution of the accelerometer data in the energy expenditure estimation is too high due to the mostly manual activities with intensive hand and wrist movements whereas the reference measurement hardly changes due to the low overall intensity of the activities. This pattern of overestimation due to manually-intensive activities is visible in the Bland-Altman plot (see Fig. 3) for the household activities, with a large cluster of data points with a positive bias of about 50 kcal/h and a spread that ranges from –72 to 163 kcal/h.

The estimations for self-paced cycling were lower than the 80% border of equivalence. The speed data from the GPS sensor that the participants wore during the outdoor activities showed an average speed of about 12.6 km/h during cycling. This is a low speed for cycling that may have further reduced the already limited movement of the wrist and that may have resulted in an accelerometer contribution that is too low, thus resulting in underestimation of energy expenditure. An additional explanation is proposed by Hendrikx and colleagues [34] that also applies to our study due to (also) having been performed during winter time. Their explanation revolves around cold outside temperatures that result in (additional) vasoconstriction that, in turn, excessively reduces the amount of time in which the estimated heart rate is within a reasonable distance from the reference heart rate thus increasing the difference between reference and estimated energy expenditure.

The last activity for which the 90% confidence interval was partially outside of the 80–125% range of equivalence was stair walking. The Bland-Altman plot for the stair walking activities in Fig. 3 shows a clear difference in estimation accuracy between walking upstairs (when the OHRM underestimated energy expenditure) versus walking downstairs (when the OHRM was on par with the reference energy expenditure). We speculate that this difference is related to not having properly controlled whether participants used the hand rail of the stairs. That is, when the wrist is hardly moving due to using the hand rail the accelerometer based contribution to energy expenditure estimation is too low.

The one activity having a 90% confidence interval fully outside of the equivalence region was the yoga activity for which the OHRM estimates TEE, on average, at 74.4% of the reference measurement. Our hypothesis for the underestimation is that the yoga activity comprised six 30-s stationary yoga positions. Due to the stationary nature of the yoga positions, the contribution of accelerometry to the estimation of energy expenditure is too low. This situation is exacerbated by the fact that holding the yoga positions is an activity of moderate to high intensity for pregnant women resulting in an increased difference between reference measurements and estimations of energy expenditure.

Overall, we find that the OHRM activity monitor, when used in pregnant women, provides energy expenditure estimations that, on average, are about 10 kcal too low for a 61 min protocol of activities, which amounts to an averaged error of −2.6% (MAPE, 9.4%). This low overall error also highlights that although some types of activities are overestimated and others underestimated, these average out over the day to achieve an estimated energy expenditure very close to the reference value(s). Because effective prevention of eGWG is based on being sufficiently active throughout the entire day, the overall estimation error is the most relevant error to consider;

additionally, the OHRM does accurately monitor energy expenditure during exercise activities. The overall underestimation is similar to the − 3% (and 10% MAPE) error reported by Hendrikx and colleagues [34] when they validated a medical class-2a activity monitor in the general population in a 48 min protocol. The high similarity of these observed errors highlights that the OHRM can be readily used in pregnant women as well as in the general population.

Our main finding therefore is that the OHRM can be reliably used in pregnant women to provide accurate lifestyle and activity coaching to prevent or minimize the detrimental effects of excessive gestational weight gain. This finding is limited by the following aspects of our study. The most important limitation is that our analyses and conclusions are based on extrapolations of data obtained during a laboratory protocol of limited duration whereas the intended use case would be a 24 × 7 scenario. Although the technology around indirect calorimetry is improving and is enabling longer recording times with smaller devices, the limitations of indirect calorimetry still preclude recording true 24 × 7 reference data. Another limitation is the fact that we did not deploy a longitudinal design involving repeated measurements of the participants in all three trimesters of their pregnancy. This would have enabled us to assess the within-person reliability of the energy expenditure estimations within and over trimesters of pregnancy. Nevertheless, our sample is representative for the Dutch population on aspects like age and BMI, and its coverage of the complete pregnancy duration.

Conclusion

We have shown that the OHRM activity monitor accurately estimates energy expenditure for use in activity coaching for pregnant women. Overall, the data from our study show an average error of about − 3% percent. Overestimation for specific (sets of) activities cancel out with underestimations for other activities and the observed errors translate to negligible values of around 1 MET. The average error is comparable in accuracy to the average error of a similar (medical class-2a) activity monitor that is validated on the general population. We therefore conclude that the OHRM can be readily used in pregnant women to help minimize or prevent excessive gestational weight gain.

Abbreviations
eGWG: Excessive gestational weight gain; GDM: Gestational diabetes mellitus; HR: Heart rate; IPAQ: International Physical Activity Questionnaire; MET(S): Metabolic equivalent of task; OHRM: Optical heart rate monitor; RMSE: Root-mean-squared error; TEE: Total energy expenditure

Acknowledgements
We would like to acknowledge Helma de Morree, Rob van der Straaten, Charlotte Lunsingh Scheurleer, and Bram Geerets for their help in the data acquisition. Stef Janssen worked on the tooling for synchronizing the data. Tim Tijs arranged the funding for the study.

Funding

Funding was provided by Philips Group Innovation; they were not involved in the design of the study, data collection, analysis, interpretation of the data, or writing of the manuscript.

Authors' contributions

PL: analysis and reporting; FS: study design, analysis, and reporting; LC: analysis and reporting; SdB: study design, data acquisition, and reporting; JW: study design and reporting. All authors read and approved the final manuscript.

Competing interests

All authors are employees of Philips Research, an entity of Philips Group Innovation which is part of Philips. Funding for the study was provided by Philips Group Innovation but they were not involved in the design, analysis, and reporting of the study.

Author details

[1]Philips Research, High Tech Campus 34, 5656 AE Eindhoven, the Netherlands. [2]Eindhoven University of Technology, Het Eeuwsel, 5612 AZ Eindhoven, the Netherlands.

References

1. Cedergren MI. Optimal Gestational Weight Gain for Body Mass Index Categories. Obstet Gynecol. 2007;110:759–64. https://doi.org/10.1097/01. AOG.0000279450.85198.b2.
2. Zavorsky GS, Longo LD. Exercise guidelines in pregnancy: new perspectives. Sports Med. 2011;41:345–60. https://doi.org/10.2165/11583930-000000000-00000.
3. Rasmussen KM, Yaktine AL, Institute of Medicine (U.S.), editors. Weight gain during pregnancy: reexamining the guidelines. Washington, DC: National Academies Press; 2009.
4. Truong YN, Yee LM, Caughey AB, Cheng YW. Weight gain in pregnancy: does the Institute of Medicine have it right? Am J Obstet Gynecol. 2015;212: 362.e1–8. https://doi.org/10.1016/j.ajog.2015.01.027.
5. Carreno CA, Clifton RG, Hauth JC, Myatt L, Roberts JM, Spong CY, et al. Excessive Early Gestational Weight Gain and Risk of Gestational Diabetes Mellitus in Nulliparous Women. Obstet Gynecol. 2012;119:1227–33. https:// doi.org/10.1097/AOG.0b013e318256cf1a.
6. Macdonald-Wallis C, Tilling K, Fraser A, Nelson SM, Lawlor DA. Gestational weight gain as a risk factor for hypertensive disorders of pregnancy. Am J Obstet Gynecol. 2013;209:327.e1–327.e17. https://doi.org/10.1016/j.ajog.2013.05.042.
7. Booth FW, Roberts CK, Laye MJ. Lack of exercise is a major cause of chronic diseases. Compr Physiol. 2012;2:1143–211.
8. Stuebe AM, Oken E, Gillman MW. Associations of diet and physical activity during pregnancy with risk for excessive gestational weight gain. Am J Obstet Gynecol. 2009;201:58.e1–8.
9. Dempsey FC, Butler FL, Williams FA. No Need for a Pregnant Pause: Physical Activity May Reduce the Occurrence of Gestational Diabetes Mellitus and Preeclampsia. Exerc Sport Sci Rev. 2005;33:141–9. https://doi.org/10.1097/ 00003677-200507000-00007.
10. Dye TD, Knox KL, Artal R, Aubry RH, Wojtowycz MA. Physical activity, obesity, and diabetes in pregnancy. Am J Epidemiol. 1997;146:961–5.
11. Hegaard HK, Pedersen BK, Nielsen BB, Damm P. Leisure time physical activity during pregnancy and impact on gestational diabetes mellitus, pre-eclampsia, preterm delivery and birth weight: a review. Acta Obstet Gynecol Scand. 2007;86:1290–6. https://doi.org/10.1080/00016340701647341.
12. Bredin SSD, Gledhill N, Jamnik VK, Warburton DER. PAR-Q+ and ePARmed-X +. Can Fam Physician. 2013;59:273–7.
13. Committee CPO. Exercise in pregnancy and the postpartum period. Jt SOGCCSEP Clin Pract Guidel. 2003;129:1–7. https://sogc.org/wp-content/ uploads/2013/01/129E-JCPG-June2003.pdf
14. Borodulin K, Evenson KR, Herring AH. Physical activity patterns during pregnancy through postpartum. BMC Womens Health. 2009;9 https://doi. org/10.1186/1472-6874-9-32.
15. Evenson KR, Wen F. National trends in self-reported physical activity and sedentary behaviors among pregnant women: NHANES 1999–2006. Prev Med. 2010;50:123–8. https://doi.org/10.1016/j.ypmed.2009.12.015.
16. Davidsson L. International Atomic Energy Agency. Assessment of body composition and total energy expenditure in humans using stable isotope techniques. Vienna: International Atomic Energy Agency; 2009. http://www-pub.iaea.org/books/IAEABooks/7982/Assessment-of-Body-Composition-and-Total-Energy-Expenditure-in-Humans-Using-Stable-Isotope-Techniques
17. Leonard WR. Laboratory and field methods for measuring human energy expenditure. Am J Hum Biol. 2012;24:372–84. https://doi.org/10.1002/ajhb.22260.
18. Schoeller DA, van Santen E. Measurement of energy expenditure in humans by doubly labeled water method. J Appl Physiol. 1982;53:955–9.
19. Hills AP, Mokhtar N, Byrne NM. Assessment of physical activity and energy expenditure: an overview of objective measures. Nutr Methodol. 2014;1:5. https://doi.org/10.3389/fnut.2014.00005.
20. Westerterp KR. Assessment of physical activity: a critical appraisal. Eur J Appl Physiol. 2009;105:823–8. https://doi.org/10.1007/s00421-009-1000-2.
21. Stankevičius D, Marozas V. A brief review of Accelerometry and heart rate measurements based physical activity monitoring. Biomed Eng. 2016;2013: 17.
22. Valenti G, Westerterp KR. Optical heart rate monitoring module validation study. IEEE. 2013;195–6. https://doi.org/10.1109/ICCE.2013.6486856.
23. Bernmark E, Forsman M, Pernold G, Wiktorin C. Validity of heart-rate based measurements of oxygen consumption during work with light and moderate physical activity. Work. 2012;41(Supplement 1):5475–6. https://doi. org/10.3233/WOR-2012-0857-5475.
24. Bonomi AG, Goldenberg S, Papini G, Kraal J, Stut W, Sartor F, et al. Predicting energy expenditure from photo-plethysmographic measurements of heart rate under beta blocker therapy: Data driven personalization strategies based on mixed models. In: 2015 37th Annual International Conference of the IEEE Engineering in Medicine and Biology Society (EMBC); 2015. p. 7642–6.
25. Kraal JJ, Sartor F, Papini G, Stut W, Peek N, Kemps HM, et al. Energy expenditure estimation in beta-blocker-medicated cardiac patients by combining heart rate and body movement data. Eur J Prev Cardiol. 2016; 2047487316667786 https://doi.org/10.1177/2047487316667786.
26. Kim D, Cho J, Oh H, Chee Y, Kim I. The estimation method of physical activity energy expenditure considering heart rate variability. In: 2009 36th Annual Computers in Cardiology Conference (CinC); 2009. p. 413–6.
27. Artal R, O'Toole M. Guidelines of the American College of Obstetricians and Gynecologists for exercise during pregnancy and the postpartum period. Br J Sports Med. 2003;37:6–12. https://doi.org/10.1136/bjsm.37.1.6.
28. King JC. Physiology of pregnancy and nutrient metabolism. Am J Clin Nutr. 2000;71:1218s–25s.
29. Melzer K, Schutz Y, Boulvain M, Kayser B. Pregnancy-related changes in activity energy expenditure and resting metabolic rate in Switzerland. Eur J Clin Nutr. 2009;63:1185–91. https://doi.org/10.1038/ejcn.2009.49.
30. Robson SC, Hunter S, Boys RJ, Dunlop W. Serial study of factors influencing changes in cardiac output during human pregnancy. Am J Physiol - Heart Circ Physiol. 1989;256:H1060–5.
31. Van Oppen ACC, Stigter RH, Bruinse HW. Cardiac output in normal pregnancy: a critical review. Obstet Gynecol. 1996;87:310–8.
32. Sady SP, Carpenter MW, Sady MA, Haydon B, Hoegsberg B, Cullinane EM, et al. Prediction of VO2max during cycle exercise in pregnant women. J Appl Physiol. 1988;65:657–61.
33. Elia M, Livesey G. Energy Expenditure and Fuel Selection in Biological Systems: The Theory and Practice of Calculations Based on Indirect Calorimetry and Tracer Methods. In: Simopoulos AP, Karger AG S, editors. World Review of Nutrition and Dietetics; 1992. p. 68–131. http://www.karger. com/?doi=10.1159/000421672. Accessed 27 Oct 2016.
34. Hendrikx J, Ruijs LS, Cox LG, Lemmens PM, Schuijers EG, Goris AH. Clinical evaluation of the measurement performance of the Philips health watch: a within-person comparative study. JMIR MHealth UHealth. 2017;5:e10. https:// doi.org/10.2196/mhealth.6893.
35. Wellek S. Testing statistical hypotheses of equivalence and noninferiority, Second Edition. New York: CRC Press; 2010.
36. Hauschke D, Kieser M, Diletti E, Burke M. Sample size determination for proving equivalence based on the ratio of two means for normally distributed data. Stat Med. 1999;18:93–105. https://doi.org/10.1002/ (SICI)1097-0258(19990115)18:1<93::AID-SIM992>3.0.CO;2-8.
37. Kieser M, Hauschke D. Statistical methods for demonstrating equivalence in crossover trials based on the ratio of two location parameters. Drug Inf J. 2000;34:563–8. https://doi.org/10.1177/009286150003400224.
38. Committee for Proprietary Medicinal Products (CPMP). Note for guidance on the investigation of bioavailability and bioequivalence. 2001.

39. Food and Drug Administration (FDA). Guidance on statistical procedures for bioequivalence studies using a standard two-treatment crossover design. Informal Commun Div Bioequivalence Off Generic Drugs Rockv MD. 1992.

40. Qia I. Stability testing guidelines: stability testing of new drug substances and products: ICH Steer Comm; 2003. http://www.ich.org/products/guidelines/quality/quality-single/article/stability-testing-of-new-drug-substances-and-products.html

41. Stegner BL, Bostrom AG, Greenfield TK. Equivalence testing for use in psychosocial and services research: an introduction with examples. Eval Program Plann. 1996;19:193–8. https://doi.org/10.1016/0149-7189(96)00011-0.

42. Barker L, Rolka H, Rolka D, Brown C. Equivalence testing for binomial random variables. Am Stat. 2001;55:279–87. https://doi.org/10.1198/000313001753272213.

43. Walker E, Nowacki AS. Understanding equivalence and noninferiority testing. J Gen Intern Med. 2011;26:192–6. https://doi.org/10.1007/s11606-010-1513-8.

44. Tryon WW. Evaluating statistical difference, equivalence, and indeterminancy using inferential confidence intervals: an integrated alternative method of conducting null hypothesis statistical tests. Psychol Methods. 2001;6:371–86. https://doi.org/10.1037//1082-989X.6.4.371.

45. Tryon WW, Lewis C. An inferential confidence interval method of establishing statistical equivalence that corrects Tryon's (2001) reduction factor. Psychol Methods. 2008;13:272–7. https://doi.org/10.1037/a0013158.

46. Bland JM, Altman DG. Measuring agreement in method comparison studies. Stat Methods Med Res. 1999;8:135–60.

47. Giavarina D. Understanding Bland Altman analysis. Biochem Medica. 2015;25:141–51. https://doi.org/10.11613/BM.2015.015.

14

Factors associated with gestational weight gain

Edyta Suliga[1]* ⓘ, Wojciech Rokita[2], Olga Adamczyk-Gruszka[2], Grażyna Pazera[3], Elżbieta Cieśla[4] and Stanisław Głuszek[5]

Abstract

Background: The aim of this study was to describe the dietary patterns in pregnant women and determine the association between diet factors, pre-pregnancy body mass index, socio-demographic characteristics and gestational weight gain.

Methods: The analysis was conducted on a group of 458 women. Cut-off values of gestational weight gain adequacy were based on recommendations published by the US Institute of Medicine and were body mass index-specific. Logistic regression analysis was used to assess the risk of the occurrence of inadequate or excessive gestational weight gain. Dietary patterns were identified by factor analysis.

Results: Three dietary patterns characteristic of pregnant women in Poland were identified: 'unhealthy', 'varied' and 'prudent'. The factor associated with increased risk of inadequate gestational weight gain was being underweight pre-pregnancy (OR = 2.61; $p = 0.018$). The factor associated with increased risk of excessive weight gain were being overweight or obese pre-pregnancy (OR = 7.00; $p = 0.031$) and quitting smoking (OR = 7.32; $p = 0.019$). The risk of excessive weight gain was decreased by being underweight pre-pregnancy (OR = 0.20; $p = 0.041$), being in the third or subsequent pregnancy compared to being in the first (OR = 0.37; $p = 0.018$), and having a high adherence to a prudent dietary pattern (OR = 0.47; $p = 0.033$).

Conclusions: Women who were overweight or obese pre-pregnancy and those who quit smoking at the beginning of pregnancy should be provided with dietary guidance to prevent excessive gestational weight gain.

Keywords: Dietary patterns, Body mass index, Excessive weight gain

Background

Abnormal gestational weight gain (GWG) is currently a serious obstetric problem. The prevalence of inadequate GWG varies among populations. In the US, GWG was *within the recommended range for 32% of women giving birth to full-term babies*. In 48% of cases, the increase in weight was higher, and in 21% of the cases, weight gain was lower than that recommended by the US Institute of Medicine (IOM) [1, 2]. A survey conducted between 2006 and 2015 on over 18,000 women in rural Pennsylvania showed that only 25.3% of women in this population gained weight within the recommended range – 21.3% gained an amount below and 52.9% gained an amount above the range in the IOM guidelines [3]. In a group of over 14,000 Italian women, the recommended GWG was found in 40.8%, in 30.1% of the women, GWG was lower, and in 29.1%, it was higher than the guidelines [4]. In German studies, 37.0% of women had excessive and 27.4% had inadequate GWG, according to the US IOM criteria [5]. Studies conducted in Poland showed that 40 to 48% of patients attain a GWG above the IOM guidelines and 14 to 23% attain a lower GWG [6, 7].

Abnormal GWG can have significant importance for both short-term pregnancy outcomes [1, 8, 9] and for the long-term health of the offspring [10–13] and the mother [8, 14, 15]. Health risks related to inadequate weight gain during pregnancy involve, first and foremost, a greater risk of premature birth and a low birth weight baby and/or intrauterine hypotrophy and, consequently, an increased risk of mortality and morbidity [1, 9, 16].

* Correspondence: edyta.suliga@ujk.edu.pl
[1]Department of Nutrition and Dietetics, Faculty of Medicine and Health Sciences, Jan Kochanowski University, Kielce, Poland
Full list of author information is available at the end of the article

Excessive weight gain is indicated as a risk factor for giving birth to a high birth weight baby compared with its gestational age [9, 17], giving birth to a baby with macrosomia [4, 9, 18], gestational diabetes [19, 20], pregnancy-induced hypertension [21, 22], caesarean delivery [23, 24], longer infant hospital stays [22] and the persistence of a higher postpartum weight for the mother after childbirth, which predisposes one to obesity later in life [8, 14, 15, 25, 26].

Maternal pre-pregnancy body mass index (BMI) [1, 27], diet [28–30], physical activity [27, 29], smoking status [31] and socio-demographic factors [1, 32–34] are listed as the main determinants of GWG. Women who were overweight or obese prior to pregnancy were significantly more likely to exceed weight guidelines [1, 27, 34]. Tielemans et al. [35] confirmed that specific dietary patterns (DP) may play a role in early pregnancy but are not consistently associated with GWG. In the meta-analysis carried out by Streuling et al. [28], five studies suggested significant positive associations between energy intake and GWG, whereas three found no significant associations. Women who remain physically active during their pregnancies have a lower risk for excessive weight gain [27, 29]. However, some of the studies did not confirm any significant associations between physical activity and GWG [36, 37]. Current smokers are at an increased risk for insufficient weight gain, and former smokers are at an increased risk for excess GWG, compared to women who have never smoked [31]. It is worth noting that some studies did not confirm the relationship between smoking and GWG [38]. Therefore, the relationship between lifestyle and GWG is inconclusive.

Studies of the impact of socio-economic factors on GWG show that in the US, women with lower incomes gained more than the recommended weight compared to women with higher incomes [31, 39]. Women with less than a high school education had higher odds of inadequate GWG [40]. Huynh et al. showed that having a college or higher education was associated with a decreased GWG for non-Hispanic white women, but an increased GWG for Hispanic women [41]. Abbasalizad Farhangi states that in Iran women with high educational attainment have a significantly higher GWG compared with low-educated women [32]. As we can see, the presented research results are ambiguous and indicate that the risk of incorrect GWG in different populations may be determined by various cultural and socio-economic factors. Thus, they should always be taken into account when examining weight gain in pregnant women.

Very few papers have been published on GWG within the Polish female population [6, 7, 42], and the relationship between dietary patterns and GWG has not been studied thus far. Dietary patterns are specific to particular populations, since they may vary with age, sex, ethnicity, cultural traditions, socioeconomic status, and food availability. Research confirms that there are important differences in dietary habits between and within Eastern and Western European countries [43, 44]. Thus, it is important to analyse them in different populations. Therefore, we have formulated a hypothesis that specific dietary patterns can be identified The aim of this study was to describe the dietary patterns in pregnant Polish women and determine the association between dietary factors, pre-pregnancy body mass index, smoking, socio-demographic characteristics and gestational weight gain.

Materials and methods
Study setting and population
This cross-sectional study was conducted within 12 months between 2014 and 2015. The data were collected through a self-administered questionnaire and completed with information from the women's medical documentation collected by a trained midwife.

The material consisted of the data of 505 women who, after childbirth, were patients of the Clinic of Obstetrics and Gynaecology of the Provincial Polyclinic Hospital in Kielce, Poland. The women who participated in the study aged 18–42 had given birth to a healthy child (without birth defects) and had labour that occurred after a full-term pregnancy, i.e., after the 37th week of pregnancy. The following patients were excluded from further analysis: four women with twin pregnancies, 18 patients whose labour occurred before the completion of the 37th week, and 25 patients lacking data. Finally, the analysis was conducted on a group of 458 women. This group comprised 12.1% of all women delivering during the year at the hospital where the study was conducted.

Study measures
The diet of the study participants during their most recent pregnancy was evaluated with the use of the authors' original semi-quantitative questionnaire of food frequency (FFQ) (Additional file 1). It was based on the principles of adequate nutrition of pregnant women, developed at the Institute of Food and Nutrition in Warsaw [45]. It has been used in previous studies, the results of which have been published in several papers [7, 46, 47]. The questionnaire was completed by all the women at the same time, i.e., 1 day before their scheduled discharge from the hospital. The FFQ assessed the consumption of vegetables (in total), fruit (in total), legumes, meat and meat-based products, sea fish, milk and dairy products, total grain food, whole grains, total fat, sweets and cakes, fast food, total drinks, fruit juice, sugary fizzy drinks, coffee, beer and/or wine, and strong liquors. The questions regarding the intake of particular

groups of products and drinks during pregnancy concerned the number of standard portions consumed in a day and a week. The size of a portion was determined according to the guidelines defined in the literature [45]. The questionnaire also contained questions related to some eating habits, i.e., the number of meals consumed in a day, snacking between meals, and sweetening with sugar.

The nutritional status of the subjects before pregnancy was assessed on the basis of self-reported data on height and weight before pregnancy, which were used to calculate the BMI. The following groups were distinguished: the underweight group (BMI $< 18.5 \, \text{kg/m}^2$; $N = 37$), those with a normal body mass ($18.5–24.9 \, \text{kg/m}^2$; $N = 377$), and those who were overweight or obese (BMI $\geq 25.0 \, \text{kg/m}^2$; $N = 44$). Due to the small number of obese participants ($N = 6$), the analyses were carried out in the combined groups of overweight and obese. The data concerning prenatal body mass and duration of the pregnancy were obtained based on the analysis of medical documentation. The total GWG of each woman was calculated as the difference between their last weight prior to delivery minus their weight before pregnancy. A self-administered questionnaire was used to collect information about age, parity (first, second, third, or subsequent labour), the occurrence of persistent vomiting during the pregnancy (no; yes, in the 1st trimester of pregnancy; or yes, during the whole pregnancy), smoking (never, passive, current smoker or quit smoking after conception), the place of residence (large city: ≥ 50 thousand residents; small city: < 50 thousand residents; or countryside), education (lower than secondary school, secondary school, or university), and always having adequate money to buy necessary food (yes or no).

Data analysis

Factor analysis by principal component analysis was used to determine dietary patterns (DP). Information about the frequency of consumption of certain portions of products included in the FFQ was the basis for the selection of variables for the analysis. The data obtained in this way were transformed into daily food intake and then normalized using the z-score procedure. The Bartlett Test of Sphericity and the Kaiser–Meyer–Olkin Measure of Sampling Adequacy were used to assess data adequacy for factor analysis. The applied procedure excluded sweetening with sugar from the analysis, which did not show any relationship with any other items. Factors were rotated using the Varimax procedure to improve the interpretation of the results. The number of the determined factors was established using Kaiser criterion (> 1). Additionally, it was verified by Cattell's criterion (scree plot test). Food items were retained in the pattern if the factor loading value was above 0.30. On

this basis, three factors were determined, and their own values were calculated for each of them. In the dietary pattern analysis, the majority of respondents are in the 'middle'- range of the indicator values and have little characteristic nutritional features, which causes difficulty in interpretation. Therefore we divided these dietary pattern data into quartiles. Study participants were assigned to the factor for which they obtained the highest score (i.e., 4th, the highest quartile).

The total GWG of each woman was calculated as the difference between their last weight prior to delivery minus their weight before pregnancy. GWG was classified as inadequate, adequate, or excessive. Cut-off values of gestational weight gain adequacy were based on the recommendations published by the US Institute of Medicine and were BMI-specific [1]. Adequate weight gain in women who were underweight before pregnancy should be 12.5–18.0 kg; in women with normal body weight it should be 11.5–16.0 kg; and in women who are overweight and obese it should be 7–11.5 kg and 5–9 kg, respectively. In the three GWG categories, for categorical data (place of residence, level of education, adequate money to buy food, persistent vomiting, smoking, and dietary patterns I–III), the structure indicators were calculated. The chi-square test was calculated for each factor to evaluate the relationships between structure indicators. Distributions of normality were checked for continuous variables (age and BMI of the subjects). The significance of differences between the means in three GWG categories was assessed by means of one factor analysis of variance (ANOVA) or Kruskal-Wallis one-way analysis of variance, depending on the distribution of the characteristics and the homogeneity of the variance. Inter-group differences between the means were evaluated by means of a post-hoc Bonferroni test. To assess the risk of the occurrence of inadequate or excessive GWG, logistic regression analysis was used (OR and 95% CI). Two models, crude and adjusted, were calculated for both categories of weight gain (inadequate and excessive). Adequate GWG was adopted as the reference level (1.0). The covariates included in the models were age, place of residence, education, having adequate money to buy necessary food, pre-pregnancy BMI, persistent vomiting, smoking, and dietary patterns. The following reference levels were adopted: for place of residence it was large city, for education it was university, for having adequate money to buy necessary food it was the answer "yes", for pre-pregnancy BMI it was normal ($18.5–24.9 \, \text{kg/m}^2$), for age it was < 30 years, for persistent vomiting it was the answer "no", for smoking it was never smokers, and for DP it was the lowest quartile (Q1).

Because all of the patients in the group with low GWG marked the same answer category for the variable "having adequate money to buy necessary food", the OR indicator and 95% CI were not calculated. The statistical analysis was carried out using SPSS software version 16.0. The p values $p < 0.05$ were considered statistically significant.

Results

Table 1 presents the characteristics of the socio-demographic variables and lifestyle of the study participants, depending on the GWG category. The women with excessive GWG were characterized by higher pre-pregnancy BMI compared with women with adequate and inadequate weight gain. Moreover, it was found that excessive GWG was significantly more often related to giving up smoking in the first weeks of pregnancy. Women who continued.

to smoke during pregnancy more often had an inadequate GWG, compared with those who quit smoking. In women with excessive GWG, a lower adherence to prudent patterns was noted in comparison to other participants in the study. Other lifestyle elements and socio-demographic characteristics did not differ in each GWG category.

Three DPs were identified, which, in total, accounted for 33.2% of the variance (Table 2). These patterns describe mutual associations between consumed food groups, and they were named according to the food groups loading highest on the respective DP. The first one, 'unhealthy', is characterized by high intakes of fast food, alcohol, sugary fizzy drinks, cake, sweets, and coffee. The second pattern, 'varied', is characterized by high intakes of fruit and vegetables, fruit juice, fats, grain products, milk and dairy products, meat and meat-based products, and snacking between meals. The third pattern, 'prudent', was characterized by high consumption of whole grains, vegetables, legumes, sea fish, milk and dairy products and by having meals more often, as well as drinking greater total amounts of liquids; it was negatively correlated with snacking between meals.

In the crude model, the risk of inadequate GWG was significantly higher in women underweight before pregnancy (OR = 2.14; $p = 0.037$) (Table 3). An increased risk of excessive GWG was positively associated with a pre-pregnancy BMI equal to $\geq 25 \, \text{kg/m}^2$ (OR = 6.44; $p < 0.001$), with giving up smoking (OR = 9.07; $p = 0.004$), and with a high score (Q4) of varied DP (OR = 1.89; $p = 0.036$). A lower risk of excessive GWG was associated with being underweight pre-pregnancy compared with having normal body mass (OR = 0.17; $p = 0.020$) and a high adherence (Q4) to prudent DP (OR = 0.047; $p = 0.016$).

In the adjusted model, the factor increasing the risk of inadequate GWG was being underweight pre-pregnancy (OR = 2.61; $p = 0.018$), whereas this risk was significantly lower in the third or subsequent pregnancy compared with the first one (OR = 0.39; $p = 0.042$) (Table 4). The

factors increasing the risk of excessive GWG were being overweight or obese pre-pregnancy (OR = 7.00; $p = 0.031$) and giving up smoking in the first weeks of pregnancy (OR = 7.32; $p = 0.019$) (Table 4); however, the risk of excessive GWG was decreased by being underweight pre-pregnancy (OR = 0.20; $p = 0.041$), being the third or subsequent pregnancy compared to the first (OR = 0.37; $p = 0.018$) and with having high adherence (Q4) to the prudent DP (OR = 0.47; $p = 0.033$).

Discussion

To the best of our knowledge, this is the first paper to identify the DP of pregnant women in Poland. In women in the highest quartile of the 'prudent' pattern, characterized by high intakes of whole grains, vegetables, legumes, sea fish, milk and dairy products, and avoiding snacking between meals, the risk of excessive GWG was significantly lower. Dietary patterns, as is well known, can differ between countries and populations, which accounts for the fact that the results obtained are not always comparable with the results of studies by other authors. Lai et al. found that the highest tertile of plant-based protein food intake was associated with a 60% lower likelihood of inadequate GWG and a 34% lower likelihood of excessive GWG [48]. Stuebe et al. [49] showed that a vegetarian diet in the first trimester is inversely associated with excessive GWG. Studies conducted in Norway showed that adherence to a regional diet rich in fruits and vegetables, potatoes, whole grains, fish, game, milk, and drinking water during pregnancy may facilitate the maintenance of optimal GWG in normal-weight women [50]. Tielemans et al. found that specific DP can play a significant role in early pregnancy but is not subsequently related to GWG [35]. However, these authors noted more moderate GWG in normal-weight women with higher scores on the 'nuts, high-fibre cereals, and soy' pattern than in women with a low score for this pattern. Wrottesley et al. noted that an increased intake of a traditional diet pattern high in whole grains, vegetables, legumes, traditional meats, and of a decreased intake of sugar and fat was related to a lower risk of excessive GWG [51]. Chuang et al. confirmed that appropriate GWG was related to intentional planning of meals and snacks [52]. Additionally, the results of intervention studies quite explicitly show that rationale eating habits among pregnant women contributes to the optimization of their GWG [29, 36, 53].

Several authors have shown that an unhealthy DP is significantly correlated with excessive GWG [49, 51, 54], although our study did not confirm such a relationship. Unambiguous scores related to the abovementioned associations may have occurred because dietary patterns vary according to age, ethnicity, culture, and other lifestyle factors. In a study conducted among Swedish

Table 1 The characteristics of the study participants in three categories of GWG (N%; X ± SD)

Variables	Gestational weight gain			p value
	Inadequate (N = 100) 9.49 ± 2.01 kg	Adequate (N = 207) 13.76 ± 1.66 kg	Excessive (N = 151) 19.60 ± 4.04 kg	
Age (X ± SD)	29.19 ± 4.87	29.62 ± 4.93	30.43 ± 3.80	0.090[A]
Pre-pregnancy BMI (X ± SD)	20.92 ± 2.46	21.32 ± 2.50	22.82 ± 3.57[a,b]	**< 0.001**[A]
Place of residence				
village	33 (33.0)	80 (38.6)	61 (40.4)	0.700[C]
town	19 (19.0)	42 (20.3)	31 (20.5)	
city	48 (48.0)	85 (41.1)	59 (39.1)	
Education				
lower than secondary school	6 (6.0)	10 (4.8)	12 (7.9)	0.729[C]
secondary school	30 (30.0)	55 (26.6)	39 (25.8)	
university	64 (64.0)	142 (68.6)	100 (66.2)	
Having adequate money to buy necessary food			1	
yes	100 (100.0)	202 (97.6)	47 (98.0)	0.306[C]
no	0 (0.0)	5 (2.4)	3 (2.0)	
Smoking				
non-smokers	55 (55.0)	120 (58.0)	86 (57.0)	**0.003**[C]
passive smokers	28 (28.0)	65 (31.4)	42 (27.8)	
current smokers	15 (15.0)	20 (9.7)	10 (6.6)	
women who quit smoking after conception	2 (2.0)	2 (1.0)	13 (8.6)	
Persistent vomiting				
no	60 (60.0)	119 (57.5)	98 (65.3)	0.411[C]
yes, in the 1st trimester of pregnancy	36 (36.0)	75 (36.2)	48 (32.0)	
yes, during the whole pregnancy	4 (4.0)	13 (6.3)	4 (2.7)	
Parity				
first	54 (54.0)	102 (49.3)	80 (51.5)	0.243[C]
second	36 (36.0)	69 (33.3)	56 (37.1)	
third or subsequent labour	10 (10.0)	36 (17.4)	15 (9.9)	
Unhealthy DP				
Q1	21 (21.0)	52 (25.1)	42 (27.8)	0.715[C]
Q2	27 (27.0)	57 (27.5)	32 (21.2)	
Q3	28 (28.0)	46 (22.2)	39 (25.8)	
Q4	24 (24.0)	52 (25.1)	38 (25.2)	
Varied DP				
Q1	26 (26.0)	59 (28.5)	30 (19.9)	0.246[C]
Q2	30 (30.0)	50 (24.2)	35 (23.2)	
Q3	25 (25.0)	49 (23.7)	39 (25.8)	
Q4	19 (19.0)	49 (23.7)	47 (31.1)	
Prudent DP				
Q1	20 (20.0)	47 (22.7)	48 (31.8)	**0.036**[C]
Q2	30 (30.0)	47 (22.7)	39 (25.8)	
Q3	18 (18.0)	57 (27.5)	37 (24.5)	
Q4	32 (32.0)	56 (27.1)	27 (17.9)	

Q represents quartile; DP represents dietary pattern; [A] represents one-way ANOVA; and [C] represents the chi-square test. The numbers in **bold** indicate statistically significant results; [a] represents the Bonferroni post hoc test $p < 0.001$ (adequate–excessive; and [b] represents the Bonferroni post hoc test $p < 0.001$ (inadequate–excessive)

Table 2 Factor-loading matrix for major dietary patterns*

Food groups	Factor I Unhealthy	Factor II Varied	Factor III Prudent
Fast food	0.682		
Beer or wine	0.682		
Strong liquors	0.600		
Sugary fizzy drinks	0.652		
Sweets, cakes	0.487		
Coffee	0.410		
Fruit		0.661	
Fat in total		0.612	
Cereals in total		0.556	
Snacking between meals		0.468	−0.412
Vegetables		0.443	0.421
Milk and dairy products		0.363	0.355
Fruit juice		0.330	
Meat and meat-based products		0.300	
Whole grains			0.710
Number of meals a day			0.502
Legumes			0.497
Sea fish			0.382
Drinks in total			0.305
Percentage of variance explained (%)	13.4	11.1	8.7

*Values <0.30 were excluded for simplicity

women, their intakes of caloric beverages, snacks, fish, and bread were positively related to excessive GWG [30]. Uusatilo et al. found that greater adherence to a 'fast food' DP, characterized by high intakes of fast food items such as hamburgers and pizza, as well as sweets, soft drinks and added sugar, was positively associated with GWG [54].

The results of our study showed that the factors related to inadequate GWG were pre-pregnancy BMI, smoking and parity. Being underweight pre-pregnancy was significantly correlated with gaining too little weight compared to gaining weight within the guidelines. It is commonly emphasized that being underweight results in a higher risk of insufficient GWG, whereas being overweight and/or obese at the time of conception is related to a higher risk of excessive gain [1, 6, 27, 30]. Fontaine et al. showed that 33 to 50% of healthy weight women and 50 to 75% of overweight and obese women had excessive GWG [55]. Heerman et al. found excessive GWG in 55.0% of mothers who were overweight before pregnancy, in 43.7% of those who were obese, and only in 37.5% of mothers who were underweight before pregnancy [56]. The results of our analyses agree with those of other authors.

The factor that strongly determined GWG in our study was quitting smoking. The results of several other papers also confirmed that women who quit smoking after conception gain much more weight than women who had never smoked [57–59]. Research carried out in the general population suggests, that heavy smokers (≥25 cigarettes per day) and those who were obese before quitting gain the most weight [60]. Although quitting smoking is a significant health-promoting change in lifestyle, it can also lead to negative metabolic consequences. Bush et al., on the basis of a literature review, found that weight gain related to quitting smoking results mainly from a decline in resting-state basal metabolism [61]. Furthermore, nicotine in cigarettes is an appetite suppressant. Depriving oneself of it results in an increase in appetite and in emotional eating, calorie misperception, and a greater craving for sweets, which may lead to excessive calorie intake.

The results of our study are consistent with reports of other authors that primiparous women gain more weight and that the probability of the occurrence of excessive GWG is higher compared to their multiparous counterparts [36, 62]. Only Hill et al. did not find any differences in GWG between primiparous and multiparous women [63]. In several papers, there were no significant associations reported between age and GWG [64–66], which is in agreement with the results of our study. In other studies, it is emphasized that a lower GWG is present in older women [1, 36, 67]. However, the results obtained by these authors usually concern women aged up to > 35 and not ≥30, as is the case in our analysis.

Despite the large number of publications regarding the association between socioeconomic status and GWG, the literature is inconsistent [32, 33, 39–41, 68, 69]. Women with low income have an increased risk for both excessive and inadequate GWG [69]. The reason for this is largely due to a lack of understanding of the importance of a healthy diet during pregnancy as well as limited access to healthy food. However, Guilloty et al. found that socio-demographic characteristics were not associated with GWG, which is consistent with the results of our studies [70]. Among the participants in our study, there were few women (only 1.75%) who reported a lack of adequate money to buy necessary food. Therefore, the results obtained should be considered with great caution. In most studies, a higher risk of gaining weight outside of the recommendations was found in women with a lower level of education [32, 40, 71, 72]. Cohen et al. suggested that higher education plays a role in healthier GWG for some, but not all, groups of pregnant women [33]. In most cases, higher education was associated with a lower chance of inadequate GWG. Educational attainment was also associated with excessive GWG; however, ethnicity and pre-pregnancy

Table 3 Factors determining the risk of inadequate and excessive GWG (unadjusted)

Variables	Gestational weight gain		
	Inadequate (N = 100)	Adequate (N = 207)	Excessive (N = 151)
Age			
< 30 years	1.0		1.0
≥30 years	1.02 (0.63–1.64)	1.0	1.36 (0.89–2.08)
p value	0.940		0.159
Pre-pregnancy BMI			
< 18.5 kg/m²	**2.14** (1.05–4.36)	1.0	**0.17** (0.04–0.76)
p value	**0.037**		**0.020**
18.5–24.9 kg/m²	1.0		1.0
≥25.0 kg/m²	0.85 (0.22–3.28)	1.0	**6.44** (2.87–14.42)
p value	0.812		**<0.001**
Place of residence			
city	1.0		1.0
town	0.80 (0.42–1.53)	1.0	1.06 (0.60–1.88)
p value	0.502		0.833
village	0.73 (0.43–1.25)	1.0	1.10 (0.69–1.76)
p value	0.253		0.695
Education			
university			
secondary school	1.21 (0.71–2.06)	1.0	1.01 (0.62–1.63)
p value	0.484		0.978
lower	1.33 (0.46–3.82)	1.0	1.70 (0.71–4.10)
p value	0.595		0.234
Having adequate money to buy necessary food			
yes	1.0		1.0
no	-*	1.0	0.82 (0.19–3.51)
p value	–		0.794
Smoking			
non-smokers	1.0		1.0
passive smokers	0.94 (0.54–1.62)	1.0	0.90 (0.56–1.45)
p value	0.824		0.670
current smokers	1.64 (0.78–3.44)	1.0	0.70 (0.31–1.57)
p value	0.193		0.383
women who quit smoking after conception	2.18 (0.30–15.89)	1.0	**9.07** (1.20–41.23)
p value	0.441		**0.004**
Persistent vomiting			
no	1.0		1.0
yes, in the 1st trimester of pregnancy	0.95 (0.58–1.58)	1.0	0.78 (0.50–1.22)
p value	0.848		0.272
yes, during the	0.61 (0.19–1.95)	1.0	0.37 (0.12–1.18)

Table 3 Factors determining the risk of inadequate and excessive GWG (unadjusted) *(Continued)*

Variables	Gestational weight gain		
	Inadequate (N = 100)	Adequate (N = 207)	Excessive (N = 151)
whole pregnancy			
p value	0.405		0.094
Parity			
first	1.0		1.0
second	0.99 (0.59–1.66)	1.0	1.03 (0.65–1.64)
p value	0.956		0.884
third or subsequent labour	0.49 (0.20–1.20)	1.0	0.61 (0.30–1.27)
p value	0.118		0.186
Unhealthy DP			
Q1	1.0		1.0
Q₂	1.17 (0.59–2.32)	1.0	0.69 (0.38–1.26)
p value	0.647		0.230
Q₃	1.51 (0.75–3.01)	1.0	1.05 (0.58–1.89)
p value	0.245		0.872
Q₄	1.14 (0.57–2.30)	1.0	0.91 (0.51–1.62)
p value	0.709		0.737
Varied DP			
Q1	1.0		1.0
Q₂	1.36 (0.71–2.60)	1.0	1.38 (0.74–2.55)
p value	0.349		0.309
Q₃	1.16 (0.59–2.26)	1.0	1.57 (0.85–2.88)
p value	0.667		0.149
Q₄	0.88 (0.44–1.78)	1.0	**1.89** (1.04–3.42)
p value	0.721		**0.036**
Prudent DP			
Q1	1.0		1.0
Q₂	1.50 (0.75–3.01)	1.0	0.81 (0.45–1.46)
p value	0.253		0.486
Q₃	0.74 (0.35–1.56)	1.0	0.64 (0.36–1.13)
p value	0.432		0.124
Q₄	1.34 (0.68–2.65)	1.0	**0.47** (0.26–0.87)
p value	0.396		**0.016**

The numbers in **bold** indicate statistically significant results; DP represents dietary pattern; Q represents quartile; * represents the number of individuals in the category 'having adequate money to buy necessary food, answer no', and the reference group is "adequate" GWG

overweight status both modified this association, sometimes in different directions. In addition, the correlation analysis among the participants in our study suggests that a high adherence to the unhealthy DP negatively correlated with a higher level of education (Spearman's rank correlation coefficient = − 0.28; $p < 0.05$; data not shown). Thus, although there is no direct relationship

Table 4 Factors determining the risk of inadequate and excessive GWG (adjusted)

Variables	Gestational weight gain		
	Inadequate (N = 100)	Adequate (N = 207)	Excessive (N = 151)
Age			
< 30 years	1.0		1.0
≥30 years	1.30 (0.70–2.44)	1.0	1.67 (0.97–2.88)
p value	0.410		0.065
Pre-pregnancy BMI			
< 18.5 kg/m^2	**2.61** (1.17–5.78)	1.0	**0.20** (0.04–0.94)
p value	**0.018**		**0.041**
18.5–24.9 kg/m^2	1.0		1.0
≥25.0 kg/m^2	0.88 (0.21–3.73)	1.0	**7.00** (2.87–17.08)
p value	0.872		**<0.001**
Place of residence			
city	1.0		1.0
town	0.70 (0.34–1.44)	1.0	1.27 (0.65–2.49)
p value	0.330		0.488
village	0.68 (0.36–1.29)	1.0	1.13 (0.62–2.08)
p value	0.240		0.689
Education			
university	1.0		1.0
secondary school	1.41 (0.75–2.65)	1.0	0.86 (0.46–1.59)
p value	0.289		0.627
lower	1.82 (0.52–6.42)	1.0	1.70 (0.54–5.39)
p value	0.350		0.365
Having adequate money to buy necessary food			
yes	1.0		1.0
no	-*	1.0	1.09 (0.20–6.04)
p value	–		0.924
Smoking			
non-smokers	1.0		1.0
passive smokers	0.88 (0.47–1.63)	1.0	0.96 (0.54–1.70)
p value	0.683		0.879
current smokers	1.64 (0.64–4.20)	1.0	1.08 (0.39–2.98)
p value	0.305		0.878
women who quit smoking after conception	2.08 (0.24–18.02)	1.0	**7.32** (1.39–38.56)
p value	0.506		**0.019**
Persistent vomiting			
no	1.0		1.0
yes, in the 1st trimester of pregnancy	0.90 (0.51–1.60)	1.0	0.63 (0.37–1.08)
p value	0.732		0.094
yes, during the whole pregnancy	0.48 (0.13–1.79)	1.0	0.44 (0.12–1.60)
p value	0.276		0.214
Parity			
first	1.0		1.0

Table 4 Factors determining the risk of inadequate and excessive GWG (adjusted) *(Continued)*

Variables	Gestational weight gain		
	Inadequate (N = 100)	Adequate (N = 207)	Excessive (N = 151)
second	0.91 (0.47–1.77)	1.0	0.74 (0.42–1.29)
p value	0.789		0.289
third or subsequent labour	**0.39** (0.16–0.96)	1.0	**0.37** (0.16–0.84)
p value	**0.042**		**0.018**
Unhealthy DP			
Q1	1.0		1.0
Q2	1.43 (0.68–3.00)	1.0	0.62 (0.26–1.04)
p value	0.342		0.066
Q3	1.45 (0.65–3.21)	1.0	0.97 (0.49–1.95)
p value	0.362		0.942
Q4	1.15 (0.49–2.71)	1.0	1.00 (0.48–2.08)
p value	0.754		0.996
Varied DP			
Q1	1.0		1.0
Q2	1.53 (0.76–3.09)	1.0	1.41 (0.70–2.85)
p value	0.234		0.332
Q3	1.04 (0.49–2.21)	1.0	1.38 (0.69–2.78)
p value	0.916		0.367
Q4	0.83 (0.36–1.80)	1.0	1.85 (0.92–2.78)
p value	0.640		0.085
Prudent DP			
Q1	1.0		1.0
Q2	1.27 (0.60–2.69)	1.0	0.70 (0.35–1.39)
p value	0.532		0.301
Q3	0.62 (0.28–1.39)	1.0	0.72 (0.38–1.39)
p value	0.247		0.329
Q4	1.38 (0.66–2.91)	1.0	**0.47** (0.23–0.97)
p value	0.394		**0.033**

The numbers in **bold** indicate statistically significant results, DP represents dietary pattern, Q represents quartile, * represents the number of individuals in the category 'having adequate money to buy necessary food, answer "no", and the reference group is "adequate" GWG

between education and GWG, this factor may affect the GWG indirectly by modifying the diet. This issue requires confirmation with a larger group of women.

The main limitation of the study is the lack of data concerning the physical activity of the women subjects, which can have an influence on GWG [27, 29]. However, some of the studies did not confirm any significant associations between physical activity and GWG [36, 37]. Moreover, for the evaluation of food intake, a non-validated, authors' original semi-quantitative questionnaire was applied. Standard questionnaires are very long and extensive, and in the opinion of the management of the hospital, they could be an excessive burden for women shortly after delivery. They could also contribute to lower response rates among women. The results obtained should also be treated with caution because of the small number of obese participants ($N = 6$; 1.31%), as well as the small number of those who were overweight ($N = 38$; 8.30%). However, it is known that in the Polish population, excessive body mass occurs least often among young women. In a representative group (i.e., 1129 female university students aged 20–24 years from the south of Poland), it was noted that 6.5% were overweight and only 0.5% were obese (BMI was calculated on the basis of the measurements of body height and mass) [73]. There was also a small number of women who quit smoking during pregnancy ($N = 17$; 3.7%). Therefore, the smoking results should also be approached with great caution.

Conclusions

Three dietary patterns, characteristic of pregnant women in Poland, were identified: 'unhealthy', 'varied' and 'prudent'. The risk of excessive GWG was lower in women with a high adherence to the prudent DP, which was characterized by a high intake of vegetables, legumes, whole grains, sea fish, milk, and dairy products, as well as a larger amount of total drinks, the consumption of a larger number of planned meals, and avoiding snacking between meals. The factors that was positively associated with a higher risk of excessive GWG in the study population were quitting smoking at the beginning of pregnancy and excessive body mass at the time of conception. The risk of inappropriate GWG (both too low and excessive) was smaller in the third and subsequent pregnancies compared to the first. Being underweight pre-pregnancy increased the risk of inadequate GWG and decreased the risk of excessive weight gain. Women who were overweight or obese pre-pregnancy and those who quit smoking at the beginning of pregnancy should be provided dietary guidance to prevent them from excessive GWG. Prevention programmes for pregnant women, developed to optimize their GWG, should include socio-economic factors, cultural traditions, and dietary patterns that are specific to a given population.

Abbreviations

BMI: Body mass index; DP: Dietary pattern; FFQ: Food frequency questionnaire; GWG: Gestational weight gain; IOM: Institute of medicine; OR: Odds Ratio; Q: Quartile; US: United States of America

Acknowledgements

The study was conducted with the support of the Regional Polyclinic Hospital in Kielce. The authors would like to thank AJE (http://www.aje.cn/) for the English language review.

Funding

The study was supported by The Ministry of Science and Higher Education from the funds received within the statutory financing activity for the Faculty of Medicine and Health Sciences, Jan Kochanowski University, research project No. 615507.00. The funding body was not involved in the study design; collection, analysis, or interpretation of data; or manuscript writing.

Author's contributions

ES conceptualized the project, participated in the statistical analysis, and wrote the manuscript. WR provided clinical expert oversight to the gynaecologic components of the survey development and analysis. OAG and GP carried out survey development and recruitment and are involved in analysis and interpretation of data and drafting the manuscript. EC participated in the statistical analysis and reviewed the manuscript. SG reviewed the manuscript and revised it critically for important intellectual content. All authors read and approved the final version of the manuscript.

Author details

[1]Department of Nutrition and Dietetics, Faculty of Medicine and Health Sciences, Jan Kochanowski University, Kielce, Poland. [2]Department of Gynecological and Obstetric Prophylaxis, Faculty of Medicine and Health Sciences, Jan Kochanowski University, Kielce, Poland. [3]Clinic of Neonatology at the Regional Polyclinic Hospital, Kielce, Poland. [4]Department of Developmental Age Research, Faculty of Medicine and Health Sciences, Jan Kochanowski University, Kielce, Poland. [5]Department of Surgery and Surgical Nursing with the Scientific Research Laboratory, Faculty of Medicine and Health Sciences, Jan Kochanowski University, Kielce, Poland.

References

1. Rasmussen KM, Pregnancy YALWGD. Reexamining the guidelines. Institute of Medicine. Washington D.C: National Research Council of the National Academies; 2009.
2. Branum AM, Sharma AJ, Deputy NP. Gestational weight gain among women with full-term, singleton births, compared with recommendations – 48 states and the District of Columbia, 2015. Morb Mortal Wkly Rep. 2016;65:1121.
3. Power ML, Lott ML, Mackeen A, AD DBJ, Schulkin J. A retrospective study of gestational weight gain in relation to the Institute of Medicine's recommendations by maternal body mass index in rural Pennsylvania from 2006 to 2015. BMC Pregnancy & Childbirth. 2018;18:239.
4. Alberico S, Montico M, Barresi V, Monasta L, Businelli C, Soini V, et al. The role of gestational diabetes, pre-pregnancy body mass index and gestational weight gain on the risk of newborn macrosomia: results from a prospective multicentre study. BMC Pregnancy Childbirth. 2014;14:23.
5. Beyerlein A, Nehring I, Rzehak P, Heinrich J, Müller MJ, et al. Gestational weight gain and body mass index in children: results from three German cohort studies. PLoS One. 2012;7:e33205.
6. Wierzejska R, Jarosz M, Stelmachów J, Sawicki W, Siuba M. Gestational weight gain by pre-pregnancy BMI. Postępy Nauk Med. 2011;9:718–23.
7. Suliga E, Adamczyk-Gruszka OK. Health behaviours of pregnant women and gestational weight gains – a pilot study. Med Stud./Studia Medyczne. 2015; 31:161–7.
8. Rong K, Yu K, Han X, Szeto IM, Qin X, Wang J, et al. Pre-pregnancy BMI, gestational weight gain and postpartum weight retention: a meta-analysis of observational studies. Public Health Nutr. 2015;18:2172–82.
9. Goldstein RF, Abell SK, Ranashina S, Misso M, Boyle JA, Black MH, et al. Association of gestational weight gain with maternal and infant outcomes: a systematic review and meta-analysis. JAMA. 2017;317: 2207–25.
10. de Boo HA, Harding JE. The developmental origins of adult disease (barker) hypothesis. Aust N Z J Obstet Gynaecol. 2006;46:4–14.
11. Contreras ZA, Ritz B, Virk J, Cockburn M, Heck JE. Maternal pre-pregnancy and gestational diabetes, obesity, gestational weight gain, and risk of cancer in young children: a population-based study in California. Cancer Causes Control. 2016;27:1273–85.

12. Mourtakos SP, Tambalis KD, Panagiotakos DB, Antonogeorgos G, Alexis CD, Georgoulis M, et al. Association between gestational weight gain and risk of obesity in preadolescence: a longitudinal study (1997-2007) of 5125 children in Greece. J Hum Nutr Diet. 2017;30:51–8.

13. Freitas-Vilela AA, Pearson RM, Emmett P, Heron J, Smith ADAC, Emond A, et al. Maternal dietary patterns during pregnancy and intelligence quotients in the offspring at 8 years of age: findings from the ALSPAC cohort. Matern Child Nutr. 2018;14. https://doi.org/10.1111/mcn.12431.

14. Nehring I, Schmoll S, Beyerlein A, Hauner H, von Kries R. Gestational weight gain and long-term postpartum weight retention: a meta-analysis. Am J Clin Nutr. 2011;94:1225–31.

15. Mannan MS, Doi A, Mamun AA. Association between weight gain during pregnancy and postpartum weight retention and obesity: a bias-adjusted meta-analysis. Nutr Rev. 2013;71:343–52.

16. Terada M, Matsuda Y, Ogawa M, Matsui H, Satoh S. Effects of maternal factors on birth weight in Japan. J Pregnancy. 2013;2013:172395.

17. Berggren EK, Stuebe AM, Boggess KA. Excess maternal weight gain and large for gestational age risk among women with gestational diabetes. Am J Perinatol. 2015;32:251–6.

18. Yang S, Zhou A, Xiong C, Yang R, Bassig BA, Hu R, et al. Parental body mass index, gestational weight gain, and risk of macrosomia: a population-based case-control study in China. Paediatr Perinat Epidemiol. 2015;29:462–71.

19. Hantouzadeh S, Sheikh M, Bosaghzadeh Z, Ghotbizadeh F, Tarafdari A, Panahi Z, et al. The impact of gestational weight gain in different trimesters of pregnancy on glucose challenge test and gestational diabetes. Postgrad Med J. 2016;92:520–4.

20. MacDonald SC, Bodnar LM, Himes KP, Hutcheon JA. Patterns of gestational weight gain in early pregnancy and risk of gestational diabetes mellitus. Epidemiology. 2017;28:419–27.

21. Cho E-H, Hur J, Lee K-J. Early gestational weight gain rate and adverse pregnancy outcomes in Korean women. PLoS One. 2015;10:e0140376.

22. Baugh N, Harris DE, Aboueissa AM, Sarton C, Lichter E. The impact of maternal obesity and excessive gestational weight gain on maternal and infant outcomes in Maine: analysis of pregnancy risk assessment monitoring system results from 2000 to 2010. J Pregnancy. 2016;2016:5871313.

23. Mamun AA, Kinarivala M, O'Callaghan MJ, Williams GM, Najman JM, Callaway LK. Associations of excess weight gain during pregnancy with long-term maternal overweight and obesity: evidence from 21 y postpartum follow-up. Am J Clin Nutr. 2010;91:1336–41.

24. Xiong C, Zhou A, Cao Z, Zhang Y, Qiu L, Yao C, et al. Association of pre-pregnancy body mass index, gestational weight gain with cesarean section in term deliveries of China. Sci Rep. 2016;22, 6.

25. Moll U, Olsson H, H M, Landin-Olsson M. Impact of pregestational weight and weight gain during pregnancy on long-term risk for diseases. PLoS One. 2017;2:e0168543.

26. Szczekala KM, Slusarska BJ, Gos AB. Motivational interviewing in obesity reduction. Med Stud/Studia Medyczne. 2017;33:73–80.

27. Samura T, Steer J, Michelis DL, Carroll L, Holland E, Perkins R. Factors associated with excessive gestational weight gain: review of current literature. Glob Adv Health Med. 2016;5:87–93.

28. Streuling I, Beyerlein A, Rosenfeld E, Schukat B, von Kries R. Weight gain and dietary intake during pregnancy in industrialized countries — a systematic review of observational studies. J Perinat Med. 2011;39:123–9.

29. Muktabhant B, Lawrie TA, Lumbiganon P, Laopaiboon M. Diet or exercise, or both, for preventing excessive weight gain in pregnancy (review). Cochrane Database Syst Rev. 2015;15:CD007145. https://doi.org/10.1002/14651858.CD007145.pub3.

30. Bärebring L, Brembeck P, Löf M, Brekke HK, Winkvist A, Augustin H. Food intake and gestational weight gain in Swedish women. Springerplus. 2016;5:377.

31. Lindberg S, Anderson C, Pillai P, Tandias A, Arndt B, Hanrahan L. Prevalence and predictors of unhealthy weight gain in pregnancy. WMJ. 2016;115:233–7.

32. Abbasalizad Farhangi M. Gestational weight gain and its related social and demographic factors in health care settings of rural and urban areas in Northwest Iran. Ecol Food Nutr. 2016;55:258–65.

33. Cohen AK, Kazi C, Headen I, Rehkopf DH, Hendrick CE, Patil D, et al. Educational attainment and gestational weight gain among U.S. mothers. Womens Health Issues. 2016;26:460–7.

34. Akgun N, Keskin HL, Ustuner I, Pekcan G, Avsar AF. Factors affecting pregnancy weight gain and relationships with maternal/fetal outcomes in Turkey. Saudi Med J. 2017;38:503–8.

35. Tielemans MJ, Erler NS, Leermakers ET, van den Broek M, Jaddoe VW, Steegers EA, et al. A priori and a posteriori dietary patterns during pregnancy and gestational weight gain: the generation R study. Nutrients. 2015;7:9383–99.

36. Rogozińska E, Marlin N, Jackson L, Rayanagoudar G, Ruifrok AE, Dodds J, et al. Effects of antenatal diet and physical activity on maternal and fetal outcomes: individual patient data meta-analysis and health economic evaluation. Health Technol Assess. 2017;21:1–158.

37. Schlaff RA, Holzman C, Mudd LM, Pfeiffer K, Pivarnik JM. Body mass index is associated with appropriateness of weight gain but not leisure-time physical activity during pregnancy. J Phys Act Health. 2014;11:1593–9.

38. Weisman CS, Hillemeier MM, Downs DS, Chuang CH, Dyer AM. Preconception predictors of weight gain during pregnancy: prospective findings from the Central Pennsylvania Women's Health Study. Womens Health Issues. 2010;(2):126–32.

39. Olson CM, Strawderman MS. Modifiable behavioral factors in a biopsychosocial model predict inadequate and excessive gestational weight gain. J Am Diet Assoc. 2003;103:48–54.

40. Deputy NP, Sharma AJ, Kim SY, Hinkle SN. Prevalence and characteristics associated with gestational weight gain adequacy. Obstet Gynecol. 2015;125(4):773–81.

41. Huynh M, Borrell LN, Chambers EC. Maternal education and excessive gestational weight gain in new York City, 1999–2001: the effect of race/ethnicity and neighborhood socioeconomic status. Matern Child Health J. 2014;18:138–45.

42. Borkowski W, Mielniczuk H. Wpływ wybranych czynników społecznych i zdrowotnych, w tym tempa przyrostu masy ciała w ciąży i masy przed ciążą, na małą masę urodzeniową noworodka. Ginekol Pol. 2008;79:415–21 (in polish).

43. Boylan S, Lallukka T, Lahelma E, Pikhart H, Malyutina S, Pajak A, et al. Socio-economic circumstances and food habits in eastern, central and Western European populations. Public Health Nutr. 2011;14:678–87.

44. Stefler D, Pajak A, Malyutina S, Kubinova R, Bobak M, Brunner EJ. Comparison of food and nutrient intakes between cohorts of the HAPIEE and Whitehall II studies. Eur J Pub Health. 2016;26:628–34.

45. Szostak-Węgierek D, Cichocka A. Żywienie kobiet w ciąży. Wydawnictwo Lekarskie PZWL, Warszawa 2012, (in polish).

46. Suliga E. Nutritional behaviours of pregnant women in rural and urban environments. Ann Agric Environ Med. 2015;22:513–7.

47. Suliga E, Adamczyk-Gruszka O. Birth weight of newborns and health behaviours and haematological parameters of pregnant women – results of preliminary studies. Pediatr Endocrinol Diabetes Metab. 2015;23:6–14.

48. Lai JS, Soh SE, Loy SL, Colega M, Kramer MS, Chan JKY, et al. Macronutrient composition and food groups associated with gestational weight gain: the GUSTO study. Eur J Nutr. 2018;13. https://doi.org/10.1007/s00394-018-1623-3.

49. Stuebe AM, Oken E, Gillman MW. Associations of diet and physical activity during pregnancy with risk for excessive gestational weight gain. Am J Obstet Gynecol. 2009;201:e1–8.

50. Hillesund ER, Bere E, Haufen M, Øverby NC. Development of a new Nordic diet score and its association with gestational weight gain and fetal growth - a study performed in the Norwegian mother and child cohort study (MoBa). Public Health Nutr. 2014;17:1909–18.

51. Wrottesley SV, Pisa PT, Norris SA. The influence of maternal dietary patterns on body mass index and gestational weight gain in urban black south African women. Nutrients. 2017;9:732.

52. Chuang CH, Stengel MR, Hwang SW, Velott D, Kjerulff KH, Kraschniewski JL. Behaviours of overweight and obese women during pregnancy who achieve and exceed recommended gestational weight gain. Obes Res Clin Pract. 2014;8:e577–83.

53. Quinlivan JA, Julania S, Lam L. Antenatal dietary interventions in obese pregnant women to restrict gestational weight gain to Institute of Medicine recommendations: a meta-analysis. Obstet Gynecol. 2011;118:1395–401.

54. Uusitalo U, Arkkola T, Ovaskainen M-L, Kronberg-Kippilä C, Kenward MG, Veijola R, et al. Unhealthy dietary patterns are associated with weight gain during pregnancy among Finnish women. Public Health Nutr. 2009;12:2392–9.

55. Fontaine P, Hellerstedt W, Dayman C, Wall M, Sherwood N. Evaluating body mass index specific trimester weight gain recommendations: differences between black and white women. J Midwifery Womens Health. 2012;57:327–35.

56. Heerman WJ, Bian A, Shintani A, Barkin SL. Interaction between maternal prepregnancy body mass index and gestational weight gain shapes infant growth. Acad Pediatr. 2014;14:463–70.

57. Favaretto AL, Duncan BB, Mengue SS, Nucci LB, Barros EF, Kroeff LR, et al. Prenatal weight gain following smoking cessation. Eur J Obstet Gynecol Reprod Biol. 2007;135:149 53.

58. Levine MD, Cheng Y, Cluss PA Marcus MD, Kalarchian MA. Prenatal smoking cessation intervention and gestational weight gain. Womens Health Issues. 2013;23:e389–93.

59. Hulman A, Lutsiv O, Park CK, Krebs L, Beyene J, McDonald SD. Are women who quit smoking at high risk of excess weight gain throughout pregnancy? BMC Pregnancy Childbirth. 2016;16:263.

60. Veldheer S, Yingst J, Zhu J, Foulds J. Ten-year weight gain in smokers who quit, smokers who continued smoking and never smokers in the United States, NHANES 2003-2012. Int J Obes. 2015;39:1727–32.

61. Bush T, Lovejoy JC, Deprey M. The effect of tobacco cessation on weight gain, obesity and diabetes risk. Obesity (Silver Spring). 2016;24:1834–41.

62. Lan-Pidhainy X, Nohr EA, Rasmussen KM. Comparison of gestational weight gain-related pregnancy outcomes in American primiparous and multiparous women. Am J Clin Nutr. 2013;97:1100–6.

63. Hill B, Bergmeier H, McPhie S, Fuller-Tyszkiewicz M, Teede H, Forster D, et al. Is parity a risk factor for excessive weight gain during pregnancy and postpartum weight retention? A systematic review and meta-analysis. Obes Rev. 2017;18:755–64.

64. Weisman CS, Hillemeier MM, Downs DS, Chuang CH, Dyer AM. Preconception predictors of weight gain during pregnancy: Prospective Findings from the Central Pennsylvania Women's Health Study. Womens Health Issues. 2010;20:126–32.

65. Rosal MC, Wang ML, Moore Simas TA, Bodenlos JS, Crawford SL, Leung K, et al. Predictors of gestational weight gain among white and Latina women and associations with birth weight. J Pregnancy. 2016;2016:8984928.

66. Papazian T, Abi Tayeh G, Sibai D, Hout H, Melki I, Rabbaa Khabbaz L. Impact of maternal body mass index and gestational weight gain on neonatal outcomes among healthy middle-eastern females. PLoS One. 2017;12:e0181255.

67. Restall A, Taylor RS, Thompson JMD, Flower D, Dekker GA, Kenny LC, et al. Risk factors for excessive gestational weight gain in a healthy, nulliparous cohort. J Obes. 2014;2014:148391.

68. Holowko N, Mishra G, Koupil I. Social inequality in excessive gestational weight gain. Int J Obes. 2014;38:91–6.

69. Campbell EE, Dworatzek PDN, Penava D, de Vrijer B, Gilliland J, Matthews JI, et al. Factors that influence excessive gestational weight gain: moving beyond assessment and counselling. J Matern Fetal Neonatal Med 2016;29:3527–31.

70. Guilloty NI, Soto R, Anzalota L, Rosario Z, Cordero JF, Palacios C. Diet, pre-pregnancy BMI, and gestational weight gain in Puerto Rican women. Matern Child Health J. 2016;19:2453–61.

71. O'Brien EC, Alberdi G, McAuliffe FM. The influence of socioeconomic status on gestational weight gain: a systematic review. J Public Health (Oxf). 2017;7:1–15.

72. Holowko N, Chaparro MP, Nilsson K, Ivarsson A, Mishra G, Koupil I, et al. Social inequality in pre-pregnancy BMI and gestational weight gain in the first and second pregnancy among women in Sweden. J Epidemiol Community Health. 2015;69:1154–61.

73. Wronka I, Suliga E, Pawlińska-Chmara R. Socioeconomic determinants of underweight and overweight in female polish students in 2009. Anthrop Anz – J Biol Clinic Anthrop. 2012;(1):85–96.

15

Effects of early pregnancy BMI, mid-gestational weight gain, glucose and lipid levels in pregnancy on offspring's birth weight and subcutaneous fat: a population-based cohort study

Christine Sommer[1,2]*, Line Sletner[3], Kjersti Mørkrid[1,2], Anne Karen Jenum[4,5] and Kåre Inge Birkeland[1,2]

Abstract

Background: Maternal glucose and lipid levels are associated with neonatal anthropometry of the offspring, also independently of maternal body mass index (BMI). Gestational weight gain, however, is often not accounted for. The objective was to explore whether the effects of maternal glucose and lipid levels on offspring's birth weight and subcutaneous fat were independent of early pregnancy BMI and mid-gestational weight gain.

Methods: In a population-based, multi-ethnic, prospective cohort of 699 women and their offspring, maternal anthropometrics were collected in gestational week 15 and 28. Maternal fasting plasma lipids, fasting and 2-hour glucose post 75 g glucose load, were collected in gestational week 28. Maternal risk factors were standardized using z-scores. Outcomes were neonatal birth weight and sum of skinfolds in four different regions.

Results: Mean (standard deviation) birth weight was 3491 ± 498 g and mean sum of skinfolds was 18.2 ± 3.9 mm. Maternal fasting glucose and HDL-cholesterol were predictors of birth weight, and fasting and 2-hour glucose were predictors of neonatal sum of skinfolds, independently of weight gain as well as early pregnancy BMI, gestational week at inclusion, maternal age, parity, smoking status, ethnic origin, gestational age and offspring's sex. However, weight gain was the strongest independent predictor of both birth weight and neonatal sum of skinfolds, with a 0.21 kg/week increased weight gain giving a 110.7 (95% confidence interval 76.6-144.9) g heavier neonate, and with 0.72 (0.38-1.06) mm larger sum of skinfolds. The effect size of mother's early pregnancy BMI on birth weight was higher in non-Europeans than in Europeans.

Conclusions: Maternal fasting glucose and HDL-cholesterol were predictors of offspring's birth weight, and fasting and 2-hour glucose were predictors of neonatal sum of skinfolds, independently of weight gain. Mid-gestational weight gain was a stronger predictor of both birth weight and neonatal sum of skinfolds than early pregnancy BMI, maternal glucose and lipid levels.

Keywords: Maternal glucose, Maternal lipids, Mid-gestational weight gain, Birth weight, Neonatal adiposity, Subcutaneous fat, Skinfolds, Body composition, Newborn, Multi-ethnic

* Correspondence: christine.sommer@medisin.uio.no
[1]Department of Endocrinology, Morbid Obesity and Preventive Medicine, Oslo University Hospital, Postbox 4959 Nydalen, N-0424 Oslo, Norway
[2]Institute of Clinical Medicine, Faculty of Medicine, University of Oslo, Oslo, Norway
Full list of author information is available at the end of the article

Background

Delivery of macrosomic babies is associated with pregnancy complications such as shoulder dystocia in the offspring [1], cesarean delivery and injuries to the birth canal [2]. Both high and low birth weights have been associated with adverse health outcomes for the child in later life, such as obesity [3] and type 2 diabetes [4]. Although easy to measure, birth weight is generally considered a rough indicator of fetal growth, as the differences in birth weight may be attributed both to differences in fat and lean mass [5]. Fat mass is considered a sensitive marker of the fetal environment and high amounts of fat in the newborn may predispose to obesity and its metabolic complications in later life [6].

In the Hyperglycemia and Adverse Pregnancy Outcome (HAPO) study, a continuous relationship between maternal glucose levels and birth weight was demonstrated, indicating that even moderately elevated glucose levels may increase risk of fetal overgrowth [7]. Pedersen [8] suggested already in 1952 that maternal hyperglycemia transmits to the fetus and induce fetal hyperinsulinemia that stimulates growth and leads to increased birth weight and excessive body fat in the offspring [8]. In concordance with the Pedersen hypothesis, maternal glucose is associated with birth weight [9-11]. Also, studies have found associations between maternal lipids and fetal growth, especially triglycerides and HDL-cholesterol, and one study recently found total cholesterol to be of similar importance as maternal glucose for birth weight [12]. However, high maternal prepregnancy weight and gestational weight gain may result in higher risk of increased birth weight and adverse outcomes than gestational diabetes per se [10,13,14]. Prepregnant BMI is readily accounted for in studies of associations between maternal glucose and offspring's birth weight. Gestational weight gain, however, is often not accounted for [10], although excessive gestational weight gain has been associated with both gestational diabetes [15,16] and infants born large for gestational age [10,14].

The HAPO study found an association between maternal glucose and neonatal fat mass [7]. However, whether the association between maternal glucose and neonatal fat mass is independent of weight gain in pregnancy, has to our knowledge not been explored. Maternal glucose and lipid levels and their associations with neonatal anthropometrics could therefore be influenced by maternal weight gain in pregnancy.

The objective was to explore whether the effects of maternal glucose and lipid levels on offspring's birth weight and subcutaneous fat were independent of early pregnancy BMI and mid-gestational weight gain.

Methods

The details of the STORK Groruddalen study have been described previously [17]. In short, it is a population-based cohort study of healthy pregnant women attending Child Health Clinics for antenatal care in three administrative city districts in Oslo, Norway, May 2008-May 2010. Women were eligible if they: 1) lived in the study districts; 2) planned to give birth at one of two study hospitals; 3) were < 20 weeks pregnant; 4) could communicate in Norwegian or any of the eight translated languages; and 5) were able to give a written consent to participate. To allow for as complete sampling as possible, a minor number of women were included later than 20 weeks: 77 (9.4%) women were included from gestational week 20 to 24, while 11 (1.3%) women were included after gestational week 24. Women with pregestational diabetes or in need of intensive hospital follow-up during pregnancy were excluded. The women were included in gestational week 15 (Visit 1). Measurements were repeated in gestational week 28 (Visit 2), when also an oral glucose tolerance test was performed.

The study was approved by the Norwegian "Regional Committee for Medical and Health Research Ethics South East" and "The Norwegian Data Inspectorate", and a written consent was obtained for all participants.

Questionnaire data

Maternal age, parity, smoking status and ethnic origin were collected through interviewer-administered questionnaires at Visit 1. Maternal age was calculated based on date of birth. Parity was dichotomized into nulliparous and parous. Smoking status was collected through two questions: 1) smoker for the last three months prior to pregnancy and 2) smoker during pregnancy. As only 28 women smoked occasionally or daily during pregnancy, we collapsed the two questions before entering it as a dummy variable into the regression analysis. Ethnic origin was defined as country of birth or participant's mother's country of birth if the participant's mother was born outside of Europe or North America, and divided into Europe, South Asia, Middle East, East Asia and South or Central Africa. Three women originating from North America were placed in the Europe category.

Maternal early pregnancy BMI and mid-gestational weight gain

Height was measured to the nearest 0.1 cm with a fixed stadiometer at Visit 1. Body weight was measured with a calibrated digital scale (Tanita-BC 418 MA, Tanita Corporation, Tokyo, Japan) at Visit 1 and Visit 2. BMI in early pregnancy was calculated from weight and height measured at Visit 1. Pre-pregnancy BMI was calculated from self-reported body weight reported at Visit 1 and height measured at Visit 1. Mid-gestational weight gain was defined as the difference in body weight between Visit 1 and Visit 2, divided by the number of weeks between the two visits for each individual.

Maternal glucose and lipids

Maternal glucose and lipid levels were measured at Visit 2. Fasting and 2-hour glucose post 75 g glucose load, and fasting total-, HDL- and LDL-cholesterol and triglycerides were measured from venous blood with a colorimetric method (Vitros 5.1 FS, Ortho clinical diagnostics) at the central laboratory. A minority of participants (4.4% for fasting glucose, 7.2% for 2-hour glucose) lacked valid glucose values from the central laboratory. We supplemented missing values with values obtained with a point of care testing device calibrated for plasma (HemoCue 201+, Angelholm, Sweden) (for fasting glucose: n = 20, 2.9%; for 2-hour glucose: n = 38, 5.5%), or if point of care values were missing as well, we used values collected from medical records (for fasting glucose n = 11, 1.6%; for 2-hour glucose n = 12, 1.7%). Women diagnosed with gestational diabetes by the World Health Organization (WHO) 1999 criteria (fasting plasma glucose ≥ 7.0 mmol/L or 2-hour glucose ≥ 7.8 mmol/L) at Visit 2 received lifestyle advice and were referred to their General Practitioner for follow-up if 2-hour glucose was <9.0 mmol/L or to hospital care if 2-hour glucose was ≥ 9.0 mmol/L [18].

Neonatal variables

To be able to compare our results with similar studies, gestational week was calculated from the first day of the woman's last menstrual period (LMP) and term was calculated as date of LMP +282 days (standard in Norway). Ultrasound term (from routine scan) was used for 24 (3.4%) women where the LMP date was missing or differed ≥ 14 days from ultrasound term [19]. The outcome birth weight was measured with calibrated electronic scales immediately after birth [17]. To assess neonatal subcutaneous fat, we measured skinfolds to the nearest 0.2 mm, with a skinfold caliper (Holtain T/W Skinfold Caliper, Holtain Ltd., Crymych, UK) at subscapular, suprailiac, thigh and triceps sites within 72 hours after birth. We measured all skinfolds twice and used the average. The outcome sum of skinfolds, was calculated by summarizing the four skinfold sites. Inter-rater variability (measured as % Technical Error of Measurement) for the skinfold measurements ranged from 8-13%, while intra-rater variability was less than 5% in all measurements [19].

Statistical analysis

We used maternal early pregnancy BMI from Visit 1, maternal weight gain from Visit 1 to Visit 2, and maternal glucose and lipid level measured at Visit 2 to meet with assumptions of temporality (Figure 1). All maternal risk factor variables were standardized using z-score to ease comparison of their effects on the outcomes. We performed simple univariate linear regression analyses (Model 0) to explore associations between maternal risk

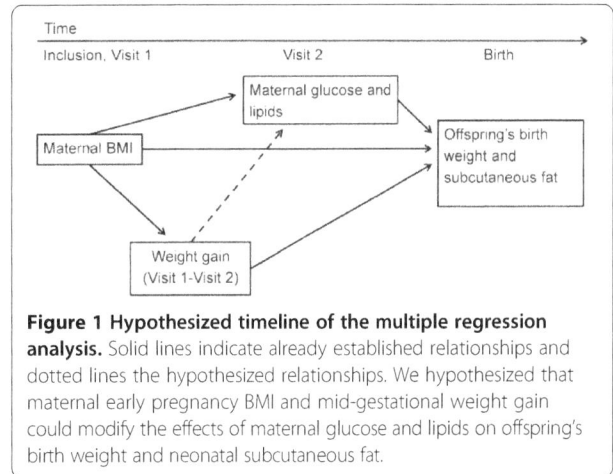

Figure 1 Hypothesized timeline of the multiple regression analysis. Solid lines indicate already established relationships and dotted lines the hypothesized relationships. We hypothesized that maternal early pregnancy BMI and mid-gestational weight gain could modify the effects of maternal glucose and lipids on offspring's birth weight and neonatal subcutaneous fat.

factor variables and the outcomes birth weight and sum of skinfolds. We performed multiple linear regressions separately for the outcomes birth weight and sum of skinfolds to explore independent effects of maternal risk factor variables. In Model 1, maternal glucose and lipid variables that correlated with the respective outcomes with a P-value < 0.2 in Model 0, were entered simultaneously into a multiple regression and adjusted for gestational week at inclusion, maternal age, parity, smoking status, ethnic origin gestational age and offspring's sex. To see if BMI or weight gain influenced the effect of maternal glucose and lipid levels on the outcomes, we additionally adjusted for early pregnancy BMI in Model 2, and additionally for mid-gestational weight gain in Model 3. We explored possible interactions between the maternal risk factor variables and ethnic origin, and between the maternal risk factor variables and offspring's sex, by including interaction terms into the multiple regressions for both outcomes. We performed sensitivity analyses by repeating the multiple regression analysis after excluding 83 women who were diagnosed with gestational diabetes; by using pre-pregnancy (self-reported) weight gain to gestational week 28 and; by analyzing normal weight and overweight women separately, according to classifications by the WHO. All statistical analyses were performed using IBM SPSS Statistics 21. We used the lincom command in StataIC 12 to calculate predicted birth weight and sum of skinfolds for the sole and combined effects of significant risk factor variables, based on Model 3 of the multiple regression analysis separately for each outcome. To estimate an "optimal" birth weight and sum of skinfolds in the offspring, we defined an optimal early pregnancy BMI as 23 kg/m^2 and an optimal weight gain was defined as 0.42 kg/week in accordance with recommendations from the Institute of Medicine [20]. To estimate high or low maternal glucose and lipid levels we used cut offs at the 90th or the 10th percentile.

Flow of the cohort

The participation rate was 74%, varying from 63.9 to 82.6 across ethnic groups [17]. Age did not differ between the 823 who participated and the 291 who chose not to participate. South Asians who did not participate were more parous than those who participated, while there was no difference within the remaining ethnic groups [17]. The study cohort was representative for the main ethnic groups, and there were no ethnic differences in reasons for exclusion [17,21].

Of the 823 women originally included in the study, 751 mothers of singleton neonates met at Visit 2 (Figure 2). We excluded 37 women with preterm births (gestational week < 37), six who were included after gestational week 24 and nine with a South American origin due to heterogeneity, leaving us with a sample of 699 women and their offspring. We found no difference between the 124 excluded women and the 699 included women in age, parity, education level or duration of residence in Norway for immigrants. A higher proportion of the excluded women were single (8.9% vs 3.0%, p = 0.037) and originated from South or Central Africa (14.5% vs 6.3%, p = <0.001). Neonatal skinfold measurements were missing for 187 offspring mainly due to study staff not being notified of the birth within 72 hours [19]. With sum of skinfolds as the outcome, our sample therefore comprised 512 women and their offspring (Figure 2). We did not find any differences in the characteristics listed in Table 1 between mother-offspring pairs with and without neonatal skinfold measurements.

Results

The mean maternal age was 29.3 ± 4.9 years, 45.6% (n = 319) were nulliparous and 47.9% (n = 335) had a European ethnic origin (Table 1). Mean self-reported prepregnancy BMI was 24.6 ± 4.8 kg/m^2, early pregnancy BMI at Visit 1 was 25.3 ± 4.8 and mean mid-gestational weight gain between Visit 1 and Visit 2 was 0.51 ± 0.21 kg/week (Table 1). The women were included in gestational week 15 ± 3, while maternal glucose and lipids were measured in gestational week 29 ± 1. The mean gestational age of the neonates was 281 ± 9 days, birth weight was 3491 ± 498 g and mean sum of skinfolds was 18.2 ± 3.9 mm (Table 1). Girls had lower birth weight (3420 ± 491 vs. 3559 ± 491 g) and had a larger sum of skinfold than boys (18.6 ± 4.0 mm vs. 17.8 ± 3.8 mm).

Predictors of offspring's birth weight and sum of skinfolds

In univariate simple regression analyses (Table 2, Model 1), maternal fasting glucose, early pregnancy BMI, and mid-gestational weight gain were all associated to offspring's birth weight (all P < 0.001), while the associations with HDL-cholesterol (P = 0.023), 2-h glucose (P = 0.069) and triglyceride level (P = 0.105) were non-significant. With sum of skinfolds as the outcome, both fasting and 2-h glucose (both P < 0.001), early pregnancy BMI (P < 0.001) and mid-gestational weight gain (P = 0.006) were associated, while the effect sizes of triglycerides (P = 0.025) and HDL-cholesterol (P = 0.199) on sum of skinfolds were weaker.

In the multiple regression analyses adjusted for relevant covariates (Table 2, Model 1) fasting glucose was a significant predictor of birth weight and both fasting and 2-h glucose were significant predictors of sum of skinfolds. Early pregnancy BMI was a significant and independent predictor of offspring's birth weight, but not for sum of skinfolds (Table 2, Model 2). After adjusting for early pregnancy BMI (Table 2, Model 2) the effect of

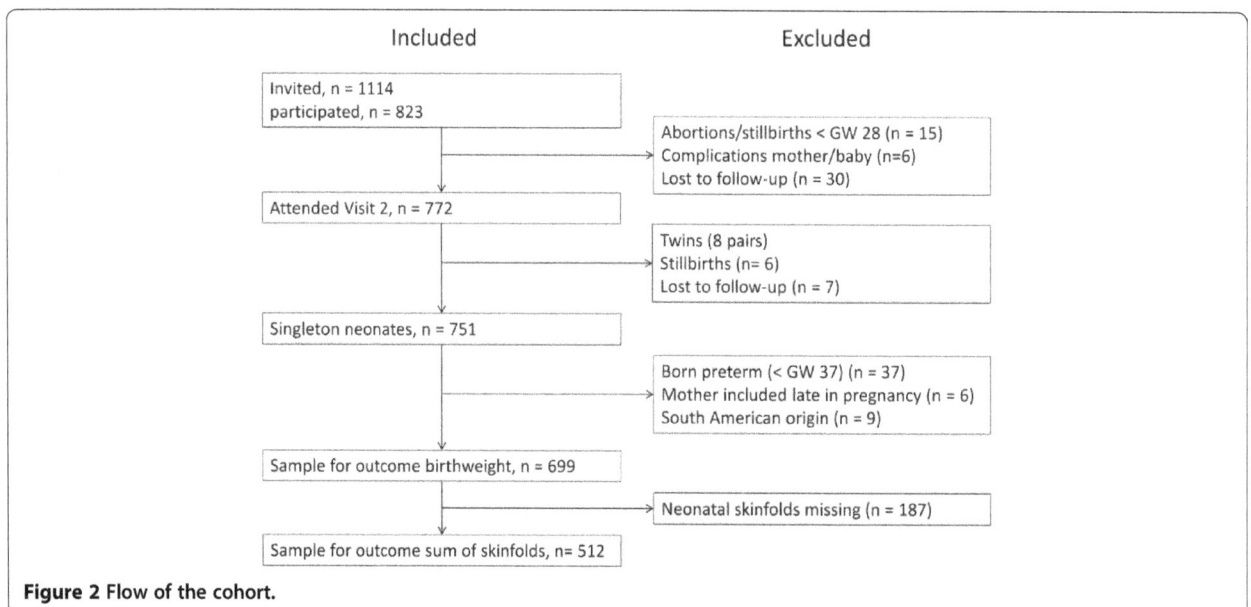

Figure 2 Flow of the cohort.

Table 1 Characteristics of the sample

	Sample (n = 699)
Maternal characteristics	
Age (years)	29.3 ± 4.8
Nulliparous	319 (45.6)
Ethnic origin	
Europe	335 (47.9)
South Asia	173 (24.7)
Middle East	112 (16.0)
East Asia	35 (5.0)
South or Central Africa	44 (6.3)
Prepregnancy BMI (kg/m^2)	24.6 ± 4.8
Early pregnancy BMI, Visit 1 (kg/m^2)	25.3 ± 4.8
Weight gain, Visit 1-2 (kg/week)	0.51 ± 0.21
Visit 1 (gestational week)	15 ± 3
Visit 2 (gestational week)	29 ± 1
Smoked 3 months prior to pregnancy	123 (17.6)
Smoked during pregnancy	28 (4.0)
Neonatal characteristics	
Gestational age at birth (days)	281 ± 9
Female sex	337 (49.7)
Birth weight (g)	3491 ± 498
Neonatal sum of skinfolds (mm) [a]	18.2 ± 3.9
Mean skinfold triceps (mm) [a]	4.4 ± 1.0
Mean skinfold thigh (mm) [a]	5.9 ± 1.4
Mean skinfold suprailiac crest (mm) [a]	3.5 ± 0.9
Mean skinfold subscapular (mm) [a]	4.4 ± 1.1
Maternal glucose and lipids	
Glucose	
Fasting glucose (mmol/L)	
Visit 1	4.4 ± 0.4
Visit 2	4.4 ± 0.5
2-hour glucose (mmol/L)	
Visit 2	5.8 ± 1.5
Gestational diabetes	84 (12.2)
Lipids	
Total cholesterol (mmol/L)	
Visit 1	5.0 ± 0.9
Visit 2	6.2 ± 1.1
HDL-cholesterol (mmol/L)	
Visit 1	1.73 ± 0.39
Visit 2	1.93 ± 0.45
LDL-cholesterol (mmol/L)	
Visit 1	2.71 ± 0.73
Visit 2	3.44 ± 0.99

Table 1 Characteristics of the sample *(Continued)*

Triglycerides (mmol/L)	
Visit 1	1.31 ± 0.55
Visit 2	1.98 ± 0.69

Data are mean ± standard deviation or n (%).
[a] n = 512.

fasting glucose on birth weight decreased, while the effects of fasting and 2-hour glucose on sum of skinfolds were unchanged. Mid-gestational weight gain was a significant and independent predictor of both offspring's birth weight and sum of skinfolds (Table 2, Model 3). After adjusting for weight gain, the effect of fasting glucose on both birth weight and sum of skinfolds decreased, but remained an independent predictor of both outcomes, while the effect of 2-hour glucose on sum of skinfolds was slightly increased and thereby remained an independent predictor (Table 2). HDL-cholesterol was not an independent predictor of birth weight until weight gain was adjusted for, while 2-hour glucose and triglycerides were not independently associated with birth weight (Table 2). None of the lipid parameters were independent predictors of sum of skinfolds (Table 2).

As women who were diagnosed with gestational diabetes received lifestyle advice at time of diagnose, we repeated the analysis without these 83 women. The effects of the risk factor variables were unchanged except for the effect of triglycerides on neonatal sum of skinfolds, where the effect size increased and the association became significant (β =0.45 (95% confidence interval 0.04-0.85). Using weight gain from pre-pregnancy (self-reported) to gestational week 28 did not change the effect estimates of the independent predictors for neither outcome (data not shown). Analyzing normal weight and overweight women separately, using model 3 of the regression, did not change the effect estimates of the independent predictors for neither outcome (data not shown).

Impact of ethnic origin

Compared to offspring of European mothers, the mean birth weight was 325 (408-243) g lower in offspring of South Asian mothers, 168 (263-73) g lower in offspring of Middle Eastern mothers, 239 (389-89) g lower in offspring of East Asian mothers and 161 (303-19) g lower in offspring of African mothers. The mean sum of skinfolds was significantly lower by 1.7 (2.5-0.9) mm in offspring of South Asian mothers and by 1.2 (2.2-0.2) mm in offspring of Middle Eastern mothers than in offspring of European mothers.

We found no interactions between ethnic origin and the risk factor variables with sum of skinfolds as the outcome. With birth weight as the outcome, there was a significant interaction between ethnic origin and maternal early

Table 2 Univariate simple and multiple linear regressions of maternal risk factor variables (z-score) on offspring's birth weight (g) and sum of skinfolds (mm)

	Model 0		Model 1		Model 2		Model 3		Model 4	
	Simple		Adjusted		Model 1 + BMI		Model 2 + Weight gain		Model 3 + interaction term	
	β	P	β	(95% CI)	β	(95% CI)	β	(95% CI)	β	(95% CI)
Birth weight (g)										
Fasting glucose	**83.5**	<0.001	79,5	(42.5 to 115.1)	**64,9**	(26.5 to 103.3)	**43,2**	(5.4 to 81.1)	**43,7**	(5.9 to 81.5)
2-hour glucose	34.7	0.069	11,4	(-24.7 to 47.5)	9,7	(-26.2 to 45.7)	15,9	(-19.1 to 50.8)	16,6	(-18.3 to 51.5)
HDL-cholesterol	**−43.3**	0.023	−28,1	(-63.1 to 6.9)	−27,2	(-62.0 to 7.6)	**−41,6**	(-75.6 to -7.5)	**−44,5**	(-78.6 to -10.4)
Triglycerides	30,8	0.105	32,5	(-4.2 to 69.2)	27,8	(-8.7 to 64.5)	35,0	(-0.7 to 70.6)	34,9	(-0.6 to 70.5)
BMI in early pregnancy	**127.2**	<0.001			**49,5**	(12.6 to 86.4)	**68,3**	(32.0 to 104.5)		
BMI in Europeans									**33,5**	(17.1 to 50.0)
BMI in non-Europeans									**103,7**	(54.7 to 152.7)
Weight gain [a]	**79.5**	<0.001					**110,7**	(76.6 to 144.9)	**111,3**	(77.2 to 145.3)
Sum of skinfolds (mm)										
Fasting glucose	**0.92**	<0.001	**0,75**	(0.39 to 1.12)	**0,73**	(0.36 to 1.11)	**0,57**	(0.19 to 0.95)	**0,58**	(0.20 to 0.96)
2-hour glucose	**0.73**	<0.001	**0,40**	(0.05 to 0.75)	**0,40**	(0.05 to 0.75)	**0,44**	(0.09 to 0.78)	**0,44**	(0.09 to 0.78)
HDL-cholesterol	−0,22	0.199	−0,09	(-0.43 to 0.25)	−0,09	(-0.43 to 0.26)	−0,18	(-0.52 to 0.16)	−0,19	(-0.54 to 0.15)
Triglycerides	**0.39**	0.025	0,21	(-0.15 to 0.57)	0,20	(-0.15 to 0.56)	0,24	(-0.11 to 0.60)	0,25	(-0.11 to 0.60)
BMI in early pregnancy	**0.77**	<0.001			0,08	(-0.30 to 0.47)	0,25	(-0.13 to 0.64)		
BMI in Europeans									0,10	(-0.08 to 0.28)
BMI in non-Europeans									0,41	(-0.11 to 0.92)
Weight gain [a]	**0.48**	0.006					**0,72**	(0.38 to 1.06)		(0.38 to 1.06)

Maternal risk factor variables are expressed as standard deviations (SDs). Values are β and P-value in Model 0, and in the remaining models; β (95% CI), with 1SD increase in maternal risk factor variables representing a unit change in birth weight (g) or sum of skinfolds (mm).
Model 0 are simple regression analyses, listed variables analyzed separately.
Model 1 is a multiple regression of the risk factor variables entered simultaneously, adjusted for gestational week at inclusion, maternal age, parity, smoking status, ethnic origin, offspring's sex and gestational age.
Model 2 = model 1+ early pregnancy BMI.
Model 3 = model 2 + weight gain.
Model 4 = model 3 + interaction term, BMI X European ethnic origin. β's for BMI are presented separately for Europeans and non-Europeans in Model 4.
Bold β value indicates P < 0.05.
[a] Weight gain from Visit 1 (gestational week 15) to Visit 2 (gestational week 28).

pregnancy BMI (Table 2, Model 4). Among Europeans, a 4.8 kg/m² higher BMI resulted in a 33.5 (17.1-50.0) g heavier offspring, while for non-Europeans it resulted in a 103.7 (54.7-152.7) g heavier offspring (Table 2, Model 4). The effect size of BMI on birth weight was higher in all ethnic minority sub-groups (data not shown). Adding the interaction term to the final model of the multiple regression analysis did not substantially change the effect estimates for the other risk factor variables (Table 2, Model 4).

Combined effects

Mid-gestational weight gain was the strongest independent predictor of both birth weight and sum of skinfolds (Table 2), while the other maternal predictors had more similar effects on the outcomes. As maternal fasting glucose, HDL-cholesterol, BMI and weight gain were all independent predictors of birth weight, high levels of fasting glucose, BMI and weight gain and low levels of

HDL-cholesterol combined (Figure 3, diamond to the right) gave a heavier neonate than if all factors were absent (Figure 3, diamond to the left). Likewise, since fasting glucose, 2-hour glucose and weight gain were all independent predictors of neonatal sum of skinfolds, estimations based on a combination of high levels of these maternal factors (Figure 4, diamond to the right) gave a higher amount of subcutaneous fat in the neonate than if all factors were absent (Figure 4, diamond to the left).

Discussion

In this multiethnic, population-based cohort of pregnant women, we found maternal fasting glucose and HDL-cholesterol in gestational week 28 to be important predictors of birth weight, independently of the mother's early pregnancy BMI and mid-gestational weight gain. Maternal fasting and 2-hour glucose in gestational week 28 were predictors of neonatal sum of skinfolds, independently of BMI and mid-gestational weight gain.

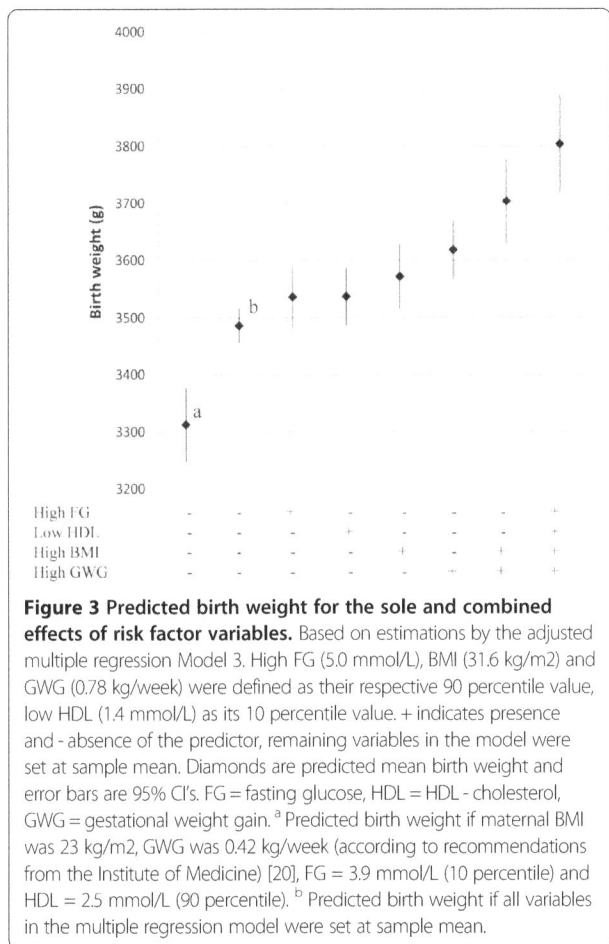

Figure 3 Predicted birth weight for the sole and combined effects of risk factor variables. Based on estimations by the adjusted multiple regression Model 3. High FG (5.0 mmol/L), BMI (31.6 kg/m2) and GWG (0.78 kg/week) were defined as their respective 90 percentile value, low HDL (1.4 mmol/L) as its 10 percentile value. + indicates presence and - absence of the predictor, remaining variables in the model were set at sample mean. Diamonds are predicted mean birth weight and error bars are 95% CI's. FG = fasting glucose, HDL = HDL - cholesterol, GWG = gestational weight gain. [a] Predicted birth weight if maternal BMI was 23 kg/m2, GWG was 0.42 kg/week (according to recommendations from the Institute of Medicine) [20], FG = 3.9 mmol/L (10 percentile) and HDL = 2.5 mmol/L (90 percentile). [b] Predicted birth weight if all variables in the multiple regression model were set at sample mean.

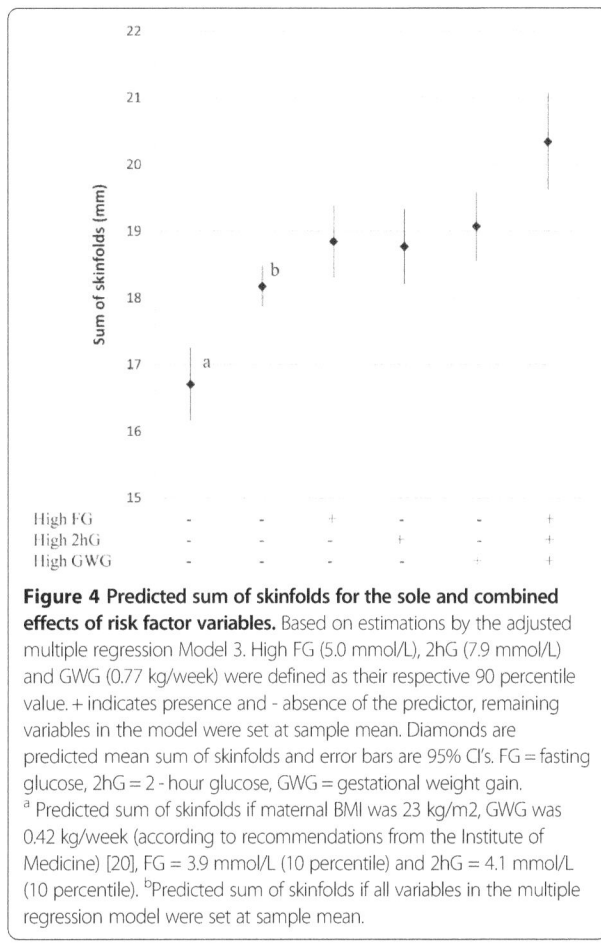

Figure 4 Predicted sum of skinfolds for the sole and combined effects of risk factor variables. Based on estimations by the adjusted multiple regression Model 3. High FG (5.0 mmol/L), 2hG (7.9 mmol/L) and GWG (0.77 kg/week) were defined as their respective 90 percentile value. + indicates presence and - absence of the predictor, remaining variables in the model were set at sample mean. Diamonds are predicted mean sum of skinfolds and error bars are 95% CI's. FG = fasting glucose, 2hG = 2 - hour glucose, GWG = gestational weight gain. [a] Predicted sum of skinfolds if maternal BMI was 23 kg/m2, GWG was 0.42 kg/week (according to recommendations from the Institute of Medicine) [20], FG = 3.9 mmol/L (10 percentile) and 2hG = 4.1 mmol/L (10 percentile). [b]Predicted sum of skinfolds if all variables in the multiple regression model were set at sample mean.

However, mid-gestational weight gain was a stronger independent predictor than maternal glucose, lipids and early pregnancy BMI, for both birth weight and sum of skinfolds in the offspring. Mid-gestational weight gain and fasting glucose were the only risk factor variables that were independent predictors for both outcomes. Furthermore, the effect size of mother's early pregnancy BMI on birth weight was higher in non-Europeans than in Europeans.

Despite a strong focus on maternal glycemia after the HAPO study and the proposed new criteria for gestational diabetes [22], few studies have explored the effects of glucose and lipid levels on the newborn's anthropometrics independently of gestational weight gain. Retnakaran and coworkers [14] also found that weight gain and BMI were the most important determinants of birth weight and large for gestational age offspring, independently of maternal glucose intolerance and lipid levels.

Consistent with our findings, several studies have found a relationship between maternal fasting glucose and offspring's birth weight [12,23,24], and both maternal fasting glucose [7] and 2-hour glucose [25] have been associated with neonatal adiposity. In our study, 2-hour glucose was

independently associated with offspring's subcutaneous fat, but not birth weight.

As found in other studies [26-28], HDL-cholesterol was inversely related to birth weight in our study. One study [27] found an inverse association between HDL-cholesterol and birth weight only in overweight and obese women and suggested that the effect of HDL-cholesterol was modified by BMI. However, we found the same effect of HDL on birth weight in normal weight women as in overweight women. A study of underweight and nutrient deficient women [12] did not find an association between HDL-cholesterol and birth weight, but this study did not adjust for weight gain and had a very different study population.

One of the few studies who adjusted for weight gain in pregnancy [14] did not find any effect of HDL-cholesterol, LDL-cholesterol or triglycerides on birth weight, while others have found a positive association between triglycerides and birth weight [29,30]. It is possible that the effect of triglycerides was neutralized by the glucose variables in our multiple regression, as triglyceride levels will increase when high insulin levels are present (e.g. in an insulin resistant state). However, the unadjusted effect of triglycerides on birth weight was relatively weak in our study.

We found no independent effect of BMI on neonatal sum of skinfolds, while other studies have found an association between maternal BMI and neonatal adiposity [9,31]. In our sample, the association between BMI and neonatal sum of skinfolds disappeared when fasting glucose was adjusted for, also when we excluded women who were diagnosed with gestational diabetes. BMI reflects maternal body size, such as muscle mass, skeletal size and body-build in general, and not merely maternal adiposity. Maternal body size may affect the size of the offspring due to genetic traits, but also, a small maternal body size may constrain the size of the offspring [32]. Our finding that BMI had a different effect on birth weight in non-Europeans than in Europeans, is supported by other studies who also found interactions between ethnicity and BMI in relation to prevalence of diabetes [18], gestational diabetes [33] as well as the risk of offspring born large for gestational age in women with gestational diabetes [34]. The fact that this interaction between BMI and ethnic origin is found in relation to several outcomes could mean that non-Europeans have a lower tolerance of adiposity [18], or that BMI is a poor measure of adiposity across ethnic groups, or possibly a combination of both. This is especially concerning considering the higher prevalence of gestational diabetes and pre-pregnant BMI found in non-European ethnic groups in the STORK Groruddalen study [15,21].

Major strengths of the study are the high participation rate and the inclusion of ethnic minority groups. Our study sample is considered representative for the major ethnic groups of pregnant women living in Norway [17]. To our knowledge, this is the first study to show that the association between maternal glucose and neonatal skinfolds is independent not only of BMI, but also of weight gain in pregnancy.

A limitation to our study is that the observational design cannot prove a causal effect between the maternal factors and offspring's anthropometry. Another limitation is the lack of control with the different components of the weight gain. However, weight gain is easy to measure, reflects fat gain, and is not likely to cause bias. Further, the relative weight of the fetus will not be as pronounced in gestational week 28 as compared to later in pregnancy. Using weight gain up to measurement of maternal glucose and lipid levels allowed us to comply with assumptions of temporality. BMI is generally thought to reflect adiposity and disease risk differently in Asians [35]. However, we found the same interaction in all ethnic minority sub groups, indicating that the interaction we found was not a result of the problem with using BMI in Asians. In addition, the interaction between BMI and

ethnic origin found in our sample did not change the effect of fasting glucose, HDL-cholesterol or weight gain on birth weight.

Conclusions

Our results suggest that mid-gestational weight gain could be more important than hyperglycemia in gestational week 28 in relation to offspring's birth weight and subcutaneous fat. However, maternal prepregnancy BMI, weight gain, glucose and lipid levels are all factors that might benefit from lifestyle advice directed at a healthy diet and increased physical activity, and hence these should, ideally, be optimized before conception. However, since health care workers often meet women when they are already pregnant, promoting an adequate weight gain during pregnancy may be one of the most important modifiable factors of birth weight and subcutaneous fat of the newborn. Future research should explore the long term effects of maternal glucose and lipids in pregnancy, prepregnant obesity and gestational weight gain on the offspring's health in childhood and adult life.

Abbreviations

BMI: Body mass index; HAPO: Hyperglycemia and Adverse Pregnancy Outcome; LMP: Last menstrual period.

Competing interests

The authors declare that they have no competing interest.

Authors' contributions

CS designed the sub study, performed all statistical analyses, drafted and edited the manuscript. LS participated in data acquisition and prepared the offspring data for analysis. KM participated in data acquisition and prepared the glucose data for analysis. AKJ initiated and was the project leader of the STORK Groruddalen study. KIB designed the sub study, contributed to conception and design of the study and is the leader of the study's steering committee. All authors contributed to interpretation of the data, discussions, critical revision of the manuscript and have read and approved the final version.

Acknowledgements

The authors thank the midwives and research staff at Grorud, Bjerke and Stovner child health clinics and the women who participated in the STORK Groruddalen study, and Leiv Sandvik (Oslo University Hospital, Department of Biostatistics and Epidemiology) for statistical guidance.

Author details

[1]Department of Endocrinology, Morbid Obesity and Preventive Medicine, Oslo University Hospital, Postbox 4959 Nydalen, N-0424 Oslo, Norway. Institute of Clinical Medicine, Faculty of Medicine, University of Oslo, Oslo, Norway. [3]Department of Child and Adolescents Medicine, Akershus University Hospital, Lørenskog, Norway. [4]Institute of Health and Society, Department of General Practice, Faculty of Medicine, University of Oslo, Oslo, Norway. [5]Faculty of Health Sciences, Oslo and Akershus University College of Applied Sciences, Oslo, Norway.

References

1. Benedetti TJ, Gabbe SG. Shoulder dystocia A complication of fetal macrosomia and prolonged second stage of labor with midpelvic delivery. Obstet Gynecol. 1978;52(5):526–9.

2. Fuchs F, Bouyer J, Rozenberg P, Senat MV. Adverse maternal outcomes associated with fetal macrosomia: what are the risk factors beyond birthweight? BMC Pregnancy Childbirth. 2013;13:90.

3. Schellong K, Schulz S, Harder T, Plagemann A. Birth weight and long-term overweight risk: systematic review and a meta-analysis including 643,902 persons from 66 studies and 26 countries globally. PLoS One. 2012;7(10):e47776.

4. Harder T, Rodekamp E, Schellong K, Dudenhausen JW, Plagemann A. Birth weight and subsequent risk of type 2 diabetes: a meta-analysis. Am J Epidemiol. 2007;165(8):849–57.

5. Hediger ML, Overpeck MD, Kuczmarski RJ, McGlynn A, Maurer KR, Davis WW. Muscularity and fatness of infants and young children born small- or large-for-gestational-age. Pediatrics. 1998;102(5):E60.

6. Catalano PM, Thomas A, Huston-Presley L, Amini SB. Increased fetal adiposity: a very sensitive marker of abnormal in utero development. Am J Obstet Gynecol. 2003;189(6):1698–704.

7. Hyperglycemia and Adverse Pregnancy Outcome (HAPO) Study. Associations with neonatal anthropometrics. Diabetes. 2009;58(2):453–9.

8. Pedersen J. Diabetes and Pregnancy. Blood Sugar of Newborn Infants. PhD Thesis. Copenhagen: Danish Science Press; 1952.

9. Catalano PM, McIntyre HD, Cruickshank JK, McCance DR, Dyer AR, Metzger BE, et al. The hyperglycemia and adverse pregnancy outcome study: associations of GDM and obesity with pregnancy outcomes. Diabetes Care. 2012;35(4):780–6.

10. Black MH, Sacks DA, Xiang AH, Lawrence JM. The relative contribution of prepregnancy overweight and obesity, gestational weight gain, and IADPSG-defined gestational diabetes mellitus to fetal overgrowth. Diabetes Care. 2013;36(1):56–62.

11. Kim SY, Sharma AJ, Sappenfield W, Wilson HG, Salihu HM. Association of maternal body mass index, excessive weight gain, and gestational diabetes mellitus with large-for-gestational-age births. Obstet Gynecol. 2014;123(4):737–44.

12. Kulkarni SR, Kumaran K, Rao SR, Chougule SD, Deokar TM, Bhalerao AJ, et al. Maternal lipids are as important as glucose for fetal growth: findings from the Pune Maternal Nutrition Study. Diabetes Care. 2013;36(9):2706–13.

13. Hartling L, Dryden DM, Guthrie A, Muise M, Vandermeer B, Donovan L. Benefits and harms of treating gestational diabetes mellitus: a systematic review and meta-analysis for the U.S. Preventive Services Task Force and the National Institutes of Health Office of Medical Applications of Research. Ann Intern Med. 2013;159(2):123–9.

14. Retnakaran R, Ye C, Hanley AJ, Connelly PW, Sermer M, Zinman B, et al. Effect of maternal weight, adipokines, glucose intolerance and lipids on infant birth weight among women without gestational diabetes mellitus. CMAJ. 2012;184(12):1353–60.

15. Sommer C, Mørkrid K, Jenum AK, Sletner L, Mosdøl A, Birkeland KI. Weight gain, total fat gain and regional fat gain during pregnancy and the association with gestational diabetes: a population-based cohort study. Int J Obesity (2005). 2014;38(1):76–81.

16. Hedderson MM, Gunderson EP, Ferrara A. Gestational weight gain and risk of gestational diabetes mellitus. Obstet Gynecol. 2010;115(3):597–604.

17. Jenum AK, Sletner L, Voldner N, Vangen S, Mørkrid K, Andersen LF, et al. The STORK Groruddalen research programme: A population-based cohort study of gestational diabetes, physical activity, and obesity in pregnancy in a multiethnic population. Rationale, methods, study population, and participation rates. Scand J Public Healt. 2010;38:60–70.

18. Jenum AK, Diep LM, Holmboe-Ottesen G, Holme IM, Kumar BN, Birkeland KI. Diabetes susceptibility in ethnic minority groups from Turkey, Vietnam Sri Lanka and Pakistan compared with Norwegians - the association with adiposity is strongest for ethnic minority women. BMC Public Health. 2012;12:150.

19. Sletner L, Nakstad B, Yajnik CS, Morkrid K, Vangen S, Vardal MH, et al. Ethnic differences in neonatal body composition in a multi-ethnic population and the impact of parental factors: a population-based cohort study. PLoS One. 2013;8(8):e73058.

20. IOM. Weight Gain During Pregnancy: Reexamining the Guidelines. Washington DC: National Academy of Sciences; 2009.

21. Jenum AK, Mørkrid K, Sletner L, Vangen S, Torper JL, Nakstad B, et al. Impact of ethnicity on gestational diabetes identified with the WHO and the modified International Association of Diabetes and Pregnancy Study Groups criteria: a population-based cohort study. Eur J Endocrinol. 2012;166(2):317–24.

22. Metzger BE, Gabbe SG, Persson B, Buchanan TA, Catalano PA, Damm P, et al. International association of diabetes and pregnancy study groups recommendations on the diagnosis and classification of hyperglycemia in pregnancy. Diabetes Care. 2010;33(3):676–82.

23. Lowe LP, Metzger BE, Dyer AR, Lowe J, McCance DR, Lappin TR, et al. Hyperglycemia and Adverse Pregnancy Outcome (HAPO) Study: associations of maternal A1C and glucose with pregnancy outcomes. Diabetes Care. 2012;35(3):574–80.

24. Dong L, Liu E, Guo J, Pan L, Li B, Leng J, et al. Relationship between maternal fasting glucose levels at 4-12 gestational weeks and offspring growth and development in early infancy. Diabetes Res Clin Pract. 2013;102(3):210–7.

25. Aris IM, Soh SE, Tint MT, Liang S, Chinnadurai A, Saw SM, et al. Effect of maternal glycemia on neonatal adiposity in a multiethnic Asian birth cohort. J Clin Endocrinol Metab. 2014;99(1):240–7.

26. Clausen T, Burski TK, Oyen N, Godang K, Bollerslev J, Henriksen T. Maternal anthropometric and metabolic factors in the first half of pregnancy and risk of neonatal macrosomia in term pregnancies A prospective study. Eur J Endocrinol. 2005;153(6):887–94.

27. Misra VK, Trudeau S, Perni U. Maternal serum lipids during pregnancy and infant birth weight: the influence of prepregnancy BMI. Obesity (Silver Spring, Md). 2011;19(7):1476–81.

28. Friis CM, Qvigstad E, Paasche Roland MC, Godang K, Voldner N, Bollerslev J, et al. Newborn body fat: associations with maternal metabolic state and placental size. PLoS One. 2013;8(2):e57467.

29. Di Cianni G, Miccoli R, Volpe L, Lencioni C, Ghio A, Giovannitti MG, et al. Maternal triglyceride levels and newborn weight in pregnant women with normal glucose tolerance. Diabet Med. 2005;22(1):21–5.

30. Kitajima M, Oka S, Yasuhi I, Fukuda M, Rii Y, Ishimaru T. Maternal serum triglyceride at 24–32 weeks' gestation and newborn weight in nondiabetic women with positive diabetic screens. Obstet Gynecol. 2001;97(5 Pt 1):776–80.

31. Stuebe AM, Landon MB, Lai Y, Spong CY, Carpenter MW, Ramin SM, et al. Maternal BMI, glucose tolerance, and adverse pregnancy outcomes. Am J Obstet Gynecol. 2012;207(1):62–e61-67.

32. Gluckman PD, Hanson MA. Maternal constraint of fetal growth and its consequences. Semin Fetal Neonatal Med. 2004;9(5):419–25.

33. Hedderson M, Ehrlich S, Sridhar S, Darbinian J, Moore S, Ferrara A. Racial/ethnic disparities in the prevalence of gestational diabetes mellitus by BMI. Diabetes Care. 2012;35(7):1492–8.

34. Sridhar SB, Ferrara A, Ehrlich SF, Brown SD, Hedderson MM. Risk of large-for-gestational-age newborns in women with gestational diabetes by race and ethnicity and body mass index categories. Obstet Gynecol. 2013;121(6):1255–62.

35. Deurenberg P, Deurenberg-Yap M, Guricci S. Asians are different from Caucasians and from each other in their body mass index/body fat per cent relationship. Obes Rev. 2002;3(3):141–6.

Adopting a healthy lifestyle when pregnant and obese

Anna Dencker[1,2*], Åsa Premberg[1,2,5], Ellinor K. Olander[3], Christine McCourt[3], Karin Haby[4], Sofie Dencker[1,2], Anna Glantz[5] and Marie Berg[1,2]

Abstract

Background: Obesity during pregnancy is increasing and is related to life-threatening and ill-health conditions in both mother and child. Initiating and maintaining a healthy lifestyle when pregnant with body mass index (BMI) $\geq$ 30 kg/m^2 can improve health and decrease risks during pregnancy and of long-term illness for the mother and the child. To minimise gestational weight gain women with BMI $\geq$ 30 kg/m^2 in early pregnancy were invited to a lifestyle intervention including advice and support on diet and physical activity in Gothenburg, Sweden.
The aim of this study was to explore the experiences of women with BMI $\geq$ 30 kg/m^2 regarding minimising their gestational weight gain, and to assess how health professionals' care approaches are reflected in the women's narratives.

Methods: Semi-structured interviews were conducted with 17 women who had participated in a lifestyle intervention for women with BMI $\geq$ 30 kg/m^2 during pregnancy 3 years earlier. The interviews were digitally recorded and transcribed in full. Thematic analysis was used.

Results: The meaning of changing lifestyle for minimising weight gain and of the professional's care approaches is described in four themes: the child as the main motivation for making healthy changes; a need to be seen and supported on own terms to establish healthy routines; being able to manage healthy activities and own weight; and need for additional support to maintain a healthy lifestyle.

Conclusions: To support women with BMI $\geq$ 30 kg/m^2 to make healthy lifestyle changes and limit weight gain during pregnancy antenatal health care providers should 1) address women's weight in a non-judgmental way using BMI, and provide accurate and appropriate information about the benefits of limited gestational weight gain; 2) support the woman on her own terms in a collaborative relationship with the midwife; 3) work in partnership to give the woman the tools to self-manage healthy activities and 4) give continued personal support and monitoring to maintain healthy eating and regular physical activity habits after childbirth involving also the partner and family.

Keywords: Body mass index, Obesity, Gestational weight gain, Lifestyle intervention, Antenatal health care, Interview study

* Correspondence: anna.dencker@gu.se
[1]Centre for Person-Centred Care (GPCC), University of Gothenburg, Gothenburg, Sweden
[2]Institute of Health and Care Sciences, Sahlgrenska Academy, University of Gothenburg, Gothenburg, Sweden
Full list of author information is available at the end of the article

Background

Maternal obesity, defined as body mass index (BMI) ≥ 30 kg/m^2, during pregnancy is increasing and related to life-threatening and ill-health conditions in both mother and child. It involves risks of morbidity for the mother and for the fetus to develop birth defects, premature birth, perinatal asphyxia and stillbirth [1]. Furthermore, pregnancy involves a risk for excess weight gain especially for women already overweight or obese [2]. If limited weight gain during pregnancy can be achieved, health outcomes for the mother can improve with lower risk of obstetric complications without elevated risks for the fetus [3]. Initiating and maintaining a healthy lifestyle during pregnancy (i.e. keep active and eat healthily) will improve health and decrease risks of long-term illness in mother, child and whole family [4–8]. The goal during pregnancy, according to the American Institute of Medicine (IOM) recommendations, is for the woman to achieve weight control [9–11]. For this purpose, effective and well-designed interventions directed to pregnant women with BMI ≥ 30 kg/m^2 concerning lifestyle change are still needed [12–14].

Pregnant women with BMI ≥ 30 kg/m^2 have described negative experiences of the professional care they have received during pregnancy and childbirth [15–17]. A negative experience of encounters with health care providers, including stigmatisation and a patronising approach can be a barrier for engaging with lifestyle support [17]. Behavioural change can be difficult to initiate, as deeply rooted lifestyle patterns can be highly resistant to change [18, 19]. However, pregnancy is in itself a crucial period for potential change to a healthier lifestyle due to maternal concerns for the expected child [20]. The support and the motivation that will work for each woman with obesity is unique so to find out what is suitable for her it is necessary to start from her personal circumstances and needs [21, 22].

To date there have been few published accounts of how pregnant women with high BMI experience weight management care pathways and interventions. These have mostly been conducted in the UK [23–25] but also in Sweden [22]. Collectively this research suggests that women who have chosen to take part in a weight management service view this as a positive experience [22, 24, 25] and that it has helped them with physical activity and healthy eating behaviour change [22, 24]. In Gothenburg, Sweden, the project 'Mighty Mums' [26] offering support for pregnant women with BMI ≥ 30 kg/m^2 to adopt a healthy lifestyle was initiated in 2011, including both additional visits to the midwife as well as opportunity to meet a dietician, something previous interventions have lacked [26]. Compared to matched controls the women in the Mighty Mums intervention group had a significantly lower gestational weight gain and lower weight retention postpartum [26].

Furthermore, the results from the project show that care could be provided with only a small additional cost and guidelines built on the project have now been implemented as standard care in the region for women with a BMI ≥ 25 kg/m^2 at antenatal health care enrolment. It has not yet been explored whether the programme affects the women in the long term and what the women experience as helping or hindering factors in the pregnancy care to maintain a healthier lifestyle. Therefore, the aim of this study was to explore the experiences of women with BMI ≥ 30 kg/m^2 regarding minimising their gestational weight gain, and to assess how health professionals' care approaches are reflected in the women's narratives.

Methods

Participants and setting

This study was carried out in Gothenburg, Sweden. All interviewees had participated in an antenatal health care lifestyle intervention called 'Mighty Mums' aiming at a healthy amount of weight gain (below 7 kg) in pregnant women with BMI ≥ 30 kg/m^2 30 in the beginning of pregnancy three years earlier. The women were informed about the benefits, for themselves and the baby, of a gestational weight gain below 7 kg, and that the intervention could be helpful to reach this goal. The intervention comprised of regular weighing, two extra scheduled visits with the antenatal health care midwife, 5 min of advice and support of regular physical activity and healthy nutrition on regular follow-up visits, including exercise on prescription, pedometers, walking poles, aqua aerobics, individually adapted food plans and group or individual sessions with a dietician - all voluntary and free of charge [26]. The women were also informed about ongoing activities offered by community health centres and were actively encouraged to participate in these by the midwife.

Before the start of the project, all midwives in antenatal health care were offered education about obesity in pregnancy in general, and more specifically about nutrition and physical activity in pregnancies with maternal BMI ≥ 30. They also obtained training in motivational interviewing. During the project, the midwife could find information on a website for self-education, as well as pedagogical tools to work with and leaflets to give to the participating women. The women's regular midwives were engaged in the project, and the project leader - a dietician - was available if there were questions on the procedure or on how to work with a logbook (a documentation of how and on what level the woman chose to participate and how the project proceeded on an individual basis). The 'Mighty Mums' project is described in more detail elsewhere [26].

Interviewees were contacted by telephone in connection with or after a follow-up meeting 2½-3 years after they participated in the 'Mighty Mums' project. They received oral and written information and were asked to participate in an interview and all gave written consent. Of a total of 45 eligible women who had participated in the study follow-up at 2½ years after childbirth, 19 women were approached and 17 agreed to participate. Purposive sampling was used to allow a mix of primi- and multiparous women of different age and country of birth. Characteristics of interviewees are shown in Table 1.

Data collection

The interviewees were encouraged to give detailed narratives of their experiences, and a semi-structured interview guide was used to cover all fields of interest. The women were asked about their experience of participating in the lifestyle intervention during pregnancy 3 years earlier [26], whether they received the help and support concerning healthy eating and physical activity they needed during pregnancy, how the planning to achieve a healthy lifestyle was made, whether they had maintained the healthy habits after childbirth and to reflect on what further assistance they would have needed to maintain healthy habits in the long term. The interviews were performed by SD ($n = 16$) and AD ($n = 1$) from July 2014 to April 2015. The interviews took place in a location the interviewees chose ($n = 7$) or were conducted as telephone interviews ($n = 10$). They all lasted between 25 and 75 min, were conducted in Swedish and digitally recorded.

Data analysis

All interviews were transcribed verbatim and analysed using thematic analysis [27]. The analysis was data-driven and performed inductively rather than driven by prior theoretical assumptions and was made separately by three researchers (AD, MB and ÅP) on the basis of the Swedish transcriptions. One researcher (ÅP) was

Table 1 Characteristics of study participants, $n = 17$

Age, median (range), years	35 (28–45)
Nulliparous/multiparous during project	12/5
Age of child in project at time for interview, years	2½-3½
Number of children, range	1-6
Had another child after project	4 women
Pregnant at time for interview	2 women
Born outside Europe	2 women
Gastric by-pass operation before project	3 women
BMI in early pregnancy, median (range), kg/m^2	33.6 (30.1–41.1)
BMI at postpartum check-up, median (range), kg/m^2, 2 missing	33.3 (28.8–40.9)
Self-reported BMI 2½ years postpartum, median (range), kg/m^2, 1 missing	31.7 (27.5–38.5)

familiar with the 'Mighty Mums' project and the two others (AD and MB) are midwives researching obesity in relation to childbearing. First, the text from all interviews was read in full to become familiar with the data. The first author (AD) used NVivo Version 10 to identify, condense and initially code all text features with a meaning. MB and ÅP did these steps manually. Next, using NVivo, codes were sorted into candidate themes in relation to the research question. The candidate themes were refined and adjusted to cover all meaning patterns in the text and to be coherent, enough distinct from other themes, and internally consistent. In the next step, these three researchers (AD, MB and ÅP) reviewed the potential themes in relation to the whole data set and adjustments were made. Last, final themes were defined and named to correspond to the essential meaning in each theme. The first author (AD) wrote the analysis text and chose the quotes. In a final phase the whole findings section was reviewed by the whole research group including midwives, a dietician, a gynaecologist/ obstetrician, a health psychology researcher and a bachelor in global studies. The main data collector (SD) was not familiar with the 'Mighty Mums' project. In the final stage the findings text including quotes, was translated into English by two authors (SD and EKO).

Findings

The meaning of changing lifestyle for minimising weight gain and of the professional's care approaches is described in four themes: the child is the main motivation for making healthy changes; need to be seen and supported on own terms to establish healthy routines; being able to manage healthy activities and own weight; need for additional support to maintain a healthy lifestyle. Quotes are displayed in italics from the interviewees, called IP1-17.

The child is the main motivation for making healthy changes

The expected child was described as the main motivation for a healthy lifestyle, both in terms of healthy eating and physical activity. The women saw their weight as their responsibility, if not caused by a disease, e.g. hypothyreosis. The women's own health, which may have been neglected before, became more significant during pregnancy, due to the direct effect it had on the unborn baby. The women felt that the concern to provide the child with the best conditions possible helped to refrain from unhealthy food.

When I got a craving for sweets or chocolate I said to myself "no, I won't eat it" and that was for the sake of the baby growing inside me. It wasn't for me. I tried to lose weight before but it didn't work. So, now it wasn't for me but for the baby inside me, and that was a much greater motivation. IP5

Living with a high BMI was described by some women as a trauma and taboo including feelings of being judged by an unsympathetic environment. A stressful lifestyle and a demanding work environment stood as obstacles to prioritise own health. Low self-confidence and reluctance to show their body was described as barriers for exercising, and past failures to reduce weight hindered further attempts. Sometimes there was a lack of confidence in their own ability and circumstances to make lifestyle changes.

It (being overweight) is still considered something shameful and most people think that you just have to stop eating and everything will be all right. IP1

Despite awareness of the unhealthy habits, and what a healthy diet includes, it had been difficult to change to healthy habits before the pregnancy. A great awareness was present that the high BMI involved risks and the women were willing to accept help in order to minimise the gestational weight gain and make healthy lifestyle changes.

Something got me motivated to change my diet very-very-very much. And it made me a mother who could cope. IP17

During pregnancy the excess weight caused concern for the women related to the negative impact it might have on the parturition and the expected child. Even though the information concerning increased risks for the baby related to high BMI usually was a motivation for lifestyle change, it could also be perceived as frightening and make the woman feel that she risked the health of her unborn child.

Yeah, I was a bit shocked by it all, that I carried so much extra weight, when we did the weighing. I didn't really know... it was a bit overwhelming. That it was a danger to me and a danger to my child... "Huh!" stressful... I never needed much healthcare before and... now I was a concern, a possible danger to myself and my child. I felt like I was being labelled. IP2

Several narratives of the women revealed a long history of overweight, sometimes since childhood. Others had gained major weight during a previous pregnancy. Some women believed that their genetic predisposition prevented weight loss, and had had gastric surgery or planned to have it. Changing for the baby was a strong

motivation, superseding the previously perceived barriers and demotivating factors.

I know that I have a predisposition to carry extra weight, and I do not want my children to end up in the same situation. If I can influence them to make healthy choices, so that they live well and healthily, I will of course do that. IP8

Need to be seen and supported on own terms to establish healthy routines

To build a trusting relationship with the midwife, the women argued that the midwife must show that she is interested, ask questions in an active way and listen to the woman. Such midwifery involvement made the woman feel secure and confident talking about what was important to her, where weight was one of many topics. The women often met the same midwife at each visit which provided continuity of care and facilitated the communication.

You could say that you gain weight in a controlled way (in the Mighty Mums project). So that you don't gain too much really fast. To share thoughts and ideas; what should I eat? How should I think? Am I eating wrong now? IP8

Frequent visits where the midwife suggested and the women chose activities helped the women modify their weight management through healthy eating and physical activity during pregnancy. The women wanted to demonstrate good results on the planned lifestyle changes in the individual meetings with the midwife and get encouragement and positive feedback in return.

To begin with I was supposed to get a routine for eating breakfast. And get routine eating properly in the first place. And to have set hours... managing it bit by bit. Starting by getting a routine for this and then for that. And that's really good, rather than doing everything at once. IP11

The commitment from the midwife could be limited by stress and lack of time and the visits sometimes felt time pressured for the woman without enough time for consultation, due to limited time for the visit. Some women felt pressure to contribute to get good results at the clinic and perceived the set weight goal (below 7 kg of maternal weight gain) as too difficult to achieve. Focus was then not primarily on the woman's health, but to achieve good results within set healthcare targets.

I think that my midwife was quite stressed and wanted good results to show; therefore she got a bit stressed when I continued to gain weight, although a lot of it was water... I felt pressure, a lot of pressure from outside... it wasn't a lot of: "how are you?" IP2

There were limitations to what kind of support that was possible to get, and some women said that they did not ask for support that they thought was not available. Some women followed the set plan and still gained weight, but there was not always interest to understand why and the women had to seek help elsewhere. The women who were not sufficiently listened to lost confidence in the health care providers and felt that they were badly treated.

They didn't take any tests, instead they assumed that... just assumed that I exercised too little and ate too much, but that wasn't the case. IP10

There was a need for the women to discuss weight with their healthcare provider in a non-judgmental manner. Training for healthcare professionals regarding how to initiate weight discussions was requested. Some women had had bad experiences of not being treated with respect by healthcare staff, with offensive comments about their appearance.

She's beating around the bush for like ten minutes and then it comes: "yeah, well you have to start thinking about what you eat, you're pretty big" instead of, perhaps, talk about BMI and treat it like something normal. It is kind of a delicate issue... and pregnant people are not exactly known for being the most non-sensitive humans in the world (laughing). You are kind of sensitive. IP1

The discussions during pregnancy focused on the women's weight but not what caused this weight, which to some women was very important to discuss. Some women said that the healthy routines were likely to be temporary if you failed addressing the underlying problems and argued that there was a lack of both knowledge and commitment for discussing weight issues within the current healthcare system.

Maybe you need to get to the core of the problem, why the situation looks like it does, and then you can start making changes... because nothing says, when the pregnancy is over, that you will continue if your mind-set hasn't changed... for me it was about so much more than just getting started with exercise. It was about how I looked at myself and

the way I valued myself and how I punished myself – or not punished myself – through food... It was about something much deeper than just working out. This is how I feel about it. IP3

Being able to manage healthy activities and own weight
Different tools and strategies introduced by the midwife helped the women control their weight during pregnancy. The tools referred to by the interviewees consisted of walking poles, pedometers, aqua aerobics, exercise on prescription, food diary, dietary advice, extra visits to the midwife and individual or group sessions with a dietician. At the antenatal visits they were able to discuss their lifestyle and reflect together with the midwife. Measuring own weight with a weighing scale was also used as a tool to gain control. To get a sense of control of the weight management led to more awareness, pride and joy for the women.

When we had the follow-up in the project I felt that it was fun to do the weighing. If it went well it was fun but if you didn't have a good result then it wasn't fun either. But the thing is that you all the time, like... because the main thing is still not to gain too much weight and we saw that on the weighing scale when we did the weighing. IP8

The group meetings with the dietician provided useful tips on regular meals and healthy snacks during pregnancy. There was also need for individual nutrition counselling on how an individual diet could be designed, and when experiencing difficulties relating to how to eat during pregnancy. To meet and discuss with others in the same situation gave a feeling of community.

It was important to discuss with the other mums... the fact that you are not alone but there are others who experience the same thing. IP12

Everyday exercise (for example walking or climbing stairs) in combination with - or instead of - group activities, was used and the women could discover small activities that fit into their own life leading on to more physical activity. The aqua aerobics was considered a fun and gentle exercise where the body felt almost weightless and a good activity when suffering pelvic girdle pain or body aches and which also contained exercises that were preparatory for childbirth.

I have never met a leader who was as committed as her (the aqua aerobics leader). And that was quite wonderful to see because there were a few mums that where quite heavily pregnant, if you say so. The largest bellies I've ever seen that bounced around in the water. It was a lovely... you got a huge energy boost out of it, which lasted longer than for just that moment when you where there. IP9

Some women experienced that there was an uncertainty in planning and goalsetting and had wished for a more strict approach to weight management. Some women chose instead to manage the planning of their lifestyle change at home with the support of their partner.

Especially when it came to physical activity he (partner) was very important. Because I'd asked him to encourage me and to be positive and to set up and prepare my exercise machine so that when I got home I couldn't dodge it (laughing). IP6

Need for additional support to maintain a healthy lifestyle

The extra support during pregnancy ended when the women needed it the most. The follow-up after child-birth was limited or absent and the healthcare focus shifted to the child. The women experienced that they were not prepared to face new situations with the child and how to handle food after they stopped breastfeeding. Coping with own work situation, stress, keeping busy with child care and the relationship with the partner were other barriers for keeping healthy habits in the long term. The strong motivation gained during pregnancy decreased when the woman no longer was directly connected to her child.

Suddenly, it was about taking care of myself for my own sake ... so then it was like sweets and less healthy food, not as much salad, I mean, the bad things came back in a way. IP7

Some women were disappointed with their own effort and thought that they could have asked for more specific help during pregnancy, and now they find themselves back in the same situation as before the lifestyle intervention. As the women sometimes assumed that the health care providers would know what was needed, they accepted the offer given without further reflection, suppressing own opinions and personal beliefs. Sometimes the project was perceived as a fixed concept not adaptable to individual needs.

In the beginning you could get some talks and the opportunity to adjust to the situation. I mean get the person on track instead of run into action right away, so to speak. To get the chance to come to terms with the whole thing and also to be a bit more flexible: "what may work for you?" IP2

Nonetheless, for some women the healthy eating habits during pregnancy and the everyday exercise stood as a beginning of a maintained lifestyle change. The women tried to find other alternatives to food that could serve as reward and strategies to make time for physical activity, putting the knowledge of healthy habits into practice.

What was best for me anyway was that you recognise and become aware of the importance of getting started with the little things, so to speak, to keep the body in motion. It doesn't have to be workout in the sense of going to the gym or so; but daily physical movement, that you implement this more and more. IP13

Health was described as an active choice where it was more important to achieve a weight that was healthy than being skinny. The women had joined the lifestyle project without hesitation because they felt that they did not have anything to lose and because they were prepared to change their lifestyle. Some of the women had already begun losing weight before pregnancy and for those women the intervention worked as support to continue on this path.

To stay healthy is work. You have to do exercise and... I mean it's not that motivating to go to the gym every day... it takes an effort. Staying at home watching soaps and play with your bellybutton, that's more comfortable, it's not that big of an effort, but it is more harmful. It is a choice you do, an active choice. IP7

To maintain a healthy lifestyle became more difficult in the long run and the women missed having someone who was there to do follow-ups, to motivate and provide feedback in lifestyle issues, on how to maintain good eating habits and strategies for exercise. There were insights regarding the necessity of finding balance in order to maintain a healthy weight and that has to be a long-term goal because it takes time to change thoughts and behaviour.

I'm thinking like this that maybe you could have, through your medical centre, an appointment once a month. Because then you would know that you were going to be checked on and then perhaps you would have had a bit better focus on how to take care of yourself ... I function like that, when I have some work assignment for which I have the responsibility, then that requires all my brain capacity and then it won't leave much time or planning for taking care of yourself. IP6

Discussion

The results show in four themes how women with BMI ≥ 30 kg/m^2 experience participation in a lifestyle intervention during pregnancy and how they reflect on how this participation affected them three years later. The main motivation for attendance in the lifestyle intervention was to provide good conditions for the child, both in the womb, and with healthy habits in the family. The women had been living with a high weight before pregnancy and sometimes since childhood. Although they had knowledge of how to eat healthily the expected child became the main motivation for changing lifestyle. The women needed to get personal support from the health care providers and receive help to be able to control the selection and implementation of healthy activities. Extra support during pregnancy helped temporarily but there was still a need of support to maintain a healthy lifestyle in the long run, suggesting pregnancy is not necessarily a 'window of opportunity' for long-term, but rather for short-term behaviour change. Pregnancy as a window of opportunity is naturally used for motivation [28], but can provocatively be seen as an automatic mantra of the health care professionals without long-term meaning. Some, not all, women clearly expressed that they felt abandoned postpartum, although for others this window of opportunity seems to have worked for the long run.

In contrast to previous research [19, 25] the interviewees in this study had received information and were aware about the risks with the high BMI for themselves and their unborn babies. Due to this knowledge, the women could feel anxious and have feelings of being a danger to the child even though the information and awareness of the risks was a motivating factor. The women wanted clear and factual information and help to adopt a healthier lifestyle for the sake of the baby, corresponding to earlier research where motivation for lifestyle change during pregnancy are described [23, 29]. Women with BMI ≥ 30 kg/m^2 often report a long struggle with their weight and difficulties to lose extra weight after an earlier pregnancy [30], which also applies to the women in this study. Living with a high BMI was experienced negatively, similar to descriptions in other studies [31]. Contrasting with some earlier research [29] our interviewees considered pregnancy as an opportunity to avoid excessive weight gain. The reason for this fact could be due to the design of the intervention project where the women were informed of health benefits of limited gestational weight gain for own health, lower risk facing the birth and better outcomes for the baby [26]. This approach is more motivating in a positive sense rather than an intervention where people are simply given risk information to frighten them into change.

The theme of managing weight for the sake of the baby suggests, however, that even if the women are given the information about health benefits to themselves they may not experience this as motivating in the same manner. This is in line with a range of sociological literature that has discussed the moral burden on mothers, in which the need to fulfil the role of a good

mother is stronger than the perceived need to protect one's own health. Social and cultural attitudes towards motherhood, in addition to gender constructs, mean that women perceive a strong need to present themselves as good mothers and experience considerable stigma if they are socially perceived as not fulfilling such a role – such as by having a normal weight or by adopting normative choices in pregnancy, around birth and in their mothering [32].

Central in the women's stories was the need to get personal attention and support on their own terms. They wished that the issue of weight was discussed in a straightforward and non-judgmental way by health professionals because it is a sensitive issue [16, 24, 33, 34]. The women preferred professionals to refer to BMI when discussing weight [23] and the interviewees also requested training of health care providers in how to approach the subject and counsel them, which is consistent with previous qualitative studies showing that health care staff face difficulties in communication about weight and weight management during pregnancy with women with high BMI [14]. Furthermore, our results underpin earlier findings of the stigmatisation of obesity where attitudes among health care providers, guidelines, written information and how weight discussions are initiated and performed need scrutinising not to include hidden stigma messages [35].

Some of the interviewed women reported that the health care providers lacked interest in their personal well-being. Instead they could feel being reduced to a weight issue with the purpose of getting good results at the antenatal care clinic. This approach is opposite to the one described by Ekman et al. as person-centred care (PCC) [36] where PCC reduces the risk of depersonalisation. Instead, the core elements in person-centred care include listening to the person's narrative, working in partnership and safeguarding the partnership through documentation [36]. Our results confirm earlier studies showing that women with a high BMI may feel badly treated in health care [31] and support previous arguments for PCC in antenatal care of women with BMI ≥ 30 kg/m^2 [21, 37]. The current study finding that the women wanted to be listened to and be met with respect in a personal relationship with the midwife corresponds to initiating the partnership in person-centred care [36]. Furthermore, focusing solely on the importance of weight in itself could pose a risk for people who have obesity to neglect health exams or screenings due to the stigmatisation [17]. For health care it is therefore important to emphasise increased health, instead of merely weight management, to provide good help and support to suit the individual woman [25, 31]. In addition, this may help to improve the focus on the women's positive health gains, given that the theme of motivation for the sake of the unborn child may not encourage *long-term* weight management and health benefits for the women.

Help and support to be able to choose healthy activities was described as important. An approach that suited the women well was when in discussions with the midwife, she suggested options, and the woman decided which to aim for. This compares well with the routine of working the partnership in PCC [36]. This partnership is described in these interviews as discussing together what is desirable and at the same time realistic and in collaboration making a plan that takes into account the woman's own situation. Working in partnership then means that the women receive knowledge and help to manage information to be able to make informed decisions and find activities that promote health and that suit their own situation. This gives the woman the tools to manage her situation of her own accord and being less subjected to conflicting advice and general prescriptions about pregnancy [14, 18, 21, 37].

Our results indicate that follow-up appointments are needed to maintain healthy routines over time. This is consistent with previous research that has shown that the effect decreases when the intervention ends [23, 25]. Continued health care support for the woman after pregnancy can give positive health effects for her and her family. Lifestyle interventions during pregnancy is most often targeting the pregnant woman only and not her partner or family who have a great influence over her habits [14, 29]. To be truly meaningful the help and support to the woman should give her the tools to self-manage her situation and also involve her partner and family. In the lifestyle intervention described here the women completed food diaries and the midwife made notes about the lifestyle activities in a logbook [26]. Our interviewees did not talk specifically about documentation but about the importance of follow-up meetings. Therefore, safeguarding the partnership according to PCC [36] can be understood as providing continued support to maintain a healthy lifestyle after childbirth in the care of women with BMI $\geq$ 30 kg/m^2.

The woman and her family are living in a context that cannot be separated from the individual, with opportunities to consume food and beverages at convenience and inexpensively. In the modern society it is easy to obtain a lot of energy with little of nutritional value [38] and therefore approaches that simply target individual behaviour without recognising the social context may not be as effective as they optimally could have been. There are also barriers to physical activity, and some of them reported by women are scarcity of time and lack of energy [38]. Furthermore, a longer distance to open green space areas, which is often the case in a city, will render it more difficult taking walks [39]. The driving force for the increasing prevalence of overweight and obesity is the obesogenic environment, and it is important to have this in mind when dealing with individuals with difficulties to keep their weight within healthy limits [40]. It would be of advantage for the woman and her family if the society was more oriented towards health, and more helpful when it comes to making healthy everyday choices, e.g. marketing of healthy/unhealthy food and supporting healthy alternatives, decreasing servings and package sizes, facilitating safe walking in green areas close to home, promoting architecture that makes it easier to take the stairs, and similar measures. A clear stance for health on the whole life span is of uttermost importance, and women need to universally be reached by the same health message – in health care, school, work, media and public places.

Strengths and limitations

Women who declined to participate in the lifestyle intervention are not accounted for, which is a limitation since interviewing pregnant women about why they chose to decline weight management support can help improve said intervention [41, 42]. Another limitation of this study is that the small sample size (17 women) may limit the applicability of these results. Two approached women declined to participate and may have had other views. Professional background of researchers may influence data interpretation. This risk of bias was reduced by a mixture of professions in the group, with experience both within and outside the health care system. The interviewees were encouraged to speak freely in a place of their own choice and the interviewers were not involved in delivering the intervention. This together with the length of the interviews was considered to reduce the risk of social desirability. Almost all of the contacted women agreed to be interviewed (17/19). Likewise, the first author had no experience of the intervention and therefore less risk of influencing the results. Strengths also include that the interviews were performed three years after the intervention and the women could reflect upon how their day-to-day behaviour was affected after these years. The purposive sampling of participants allowed a mix of primi- and multiparous women of different age and countries of birth and therefore the results may be representative for Swedish women.

Conclusions

Our findings have implications for how services are organised to support women with BMI $\geq$ 30 kg/m^2 to gain a healthy lifestyle during pregnancy and postpartum. First, the health care providers should address women's weight in a non-judgmental way using BMI, not make assumptions about their diet and activity levels or their motivations and difficulties and give accurate information about the benefits of a limited gestational weight gain and the risks of obesity in accurate and manageable manner. Second, that the women want support on their own terms in a personal relationship with the health care provider (midwife). Third, working in a partnership regarding lifestyle changes during pregnancy gives the woman the tools to manage choosing and performing healthy activities. Support is also needed postpartum to aid long-term behaviour change. Furthermore, these results contribute to the understanding of what is important for women's lifestyle in the long term, i.e. that the strong motivation to change for the sake of the child may subside after childbirth, and the need of continued personal support and monitoring to maintain healthy eating and exercise habits. Therefore, the help and support of the woman should also involve her partner and family and optimally include referral to community health centres or lifestyle receptions at primary care level.

Abbreviations
BMI, body mass index

Acknowledgement
We would like to express our gratitude to all women who participated in the interviews and shared their experiences.

Funding
This study was funded by the University of Gothenburg Centre for Person-Centred Care (GPCC).

Authors' contributions
AD, MB, EKO and CMcC planned the study. SD and AD performed the interviews. AD, ÅP and MB made separate analyses of the data. AD drafted the manuscript. SD and EKO translated the findings. All authors (AD, ÅP, EKO, CMcC, KH, SD, AG and MB) contributed to the writing of the manuscript. All authors read and approved the final manuscript.

Competing interests
The authors declare that they have no competing interests.

Author details
[1]Centre for Person-Centred Care (GPCC), University of Gothenburg, Gothenburg, Sweden. [2]Institute of Health and Care Sciences, Sahlgrenska Academy, University of Gothenburg, Gothenburg, Sweden. [3]Centre for Maternal and Child Health Research, City University London, London, UK. [4]Antenatal Health Care, Primary Health Care, Research and Development Unit, Närhälsan, Gothenburg, Sweden. [5]Primary Health Care, Närhälsan, Gothenburg, Sweden.

References
1. Marchi J, Berg M, Dencker A, Olander EK, Begley C. Risks associated with obesity in pregnancy, for the mother and baby: a systematic review of reviews. Obes Rev. 2015;16(8):621–38.
2. Lof M, Hilakivi-Clarke L, Sandin S, Weiderpass E. Effects of pre-pregnancy physical activity and maternal BMI on gestational weight gain and birth weight. Acta Obstet Gynecol Scand. 2008;87(5):524–30.
3. Blomberg M. Maternal and neonatal outcomes among obese women with weight gain below the new institute of medicine recommendations. Obstet Gynecol. 2011;117(5):1065–70.
4. Heslehurst N. Identifying   at risk' women and the impact of maternal obesity on National Health Service maternity services. Proc Nutr Soc. 2011;70(4):439–49.
5. Claesson IM, Sydsjo G, Brynhildsen J, Blomberg M, Jeppsson A, Sydsjo A, Josefsson A. Weight after childbirth: a 2-year follow-up of obese women in a weight-gain restriction program. Acta Obstet Gynecol Scand. 2011;90(1):103–10.
6. Cedergren MI. Optimal gestational weight gain for body mass index categories. Obstet Gynecol. 2007;110(4):759–64.
7. Thangaratinam S, Rogozinska E, Jolly K, Glinkowski S, Roseboom T, Tomlinson JW, Kunz R, Mol BW, Coomarasamy A, Khan KS. Effects of interventions in pregnancy on maternal weight and obstetric outcomes: meta-analysis of randomised evidence. BMJ (Clinical research ed). 2012;344:e2088.
8. Mourtakos SP, Tambalis KD, Panagiotakos DB, Antonogeorgos G, Arnaoutis G, Karteroliotis K, Sidossis LS. Maternal lifestyle characteristics during pregnancy, and the risk of obesity in the offspring: a study of 5,125 children. BMC Pregnancy Childbirth. 2015;15:66.
9. IOM: Weight Gain During Pregnancy: Reexamining the Guidelines. National Academy Press, Washington. In.; 2009.
10. Rasmussen KM, Abrams B, Bodnar LM, Butte NF, Catalano PM, Maria Siega-Riz A. Recommendations for weight gain during pregnancy in the context of the obesity epidemic. Obstet Gynecol. 2010;116(5):1191–5.
11. Quinlivan JA, Julania S, Lam L. Antenatal dietary interventions in obese pregnant women to restrict gestational weight gain to Institute of Medicine recommendations: a meta-analysis. Obstet Gynecol. 2011;118(6):1395–401.
12. Oteng-Ntim E, Varma R, Croker H, Poston L, Doyle P. Lifestyle interventions for overweight and obese pregnant women to improve pregnancy outcome: systematic review and meta-analysis. BMC Med. 2012;10:47.
13. Heslehurst N, Newham J, Maniatopoulos G, Fleetwood C, Robalino S, Rankin J. Implementation of pregnancy weight management and obesity guidelines: a meta-synthesis of healthcare professionals' barriers and facilitators using the theoretical domains framework. Obes Rev. 2014;15(6):462–86.
14. Campbell F, Johnson M, Messina J, Guillaume L, Goyder E. Behavioural interventions for weight management in pregnancy: a systematic review of quantitative and qualitative data. BMC Public Health. 2011;11:491.
15. Nyman VM, Prebensen AK, Flensner GE. Obese women's experiences of encounters with midwives and physicians during pregnancy and childbirth. Midwifery. 2010;26(4):424–9.
16. Furber CM, McGowan L. A qualitative study of the experiences of women who are obese and pregnant in the UK. Midwifery. 2011;27(4):437–44.
17. Puhl RM, Heuer CA. The stigma of obesity: a review and update. Obesity (Silver Spring). 2009;17(5):941–64.
18. Olander EK, Fletcher H, Williams S, Atkinson L, Turner A, French DP. What are the most effective techniques in changing obese individuals' physical activity self-efficacy and behaviour: a systematic review and meta-analysis. Int J Behav Nutr Phys Act. 2013;10:29.
19. Olander EK, Atkinson L, Edmunds JK, French DP. The views of pre- and post-natal women and health professionals regarding gestational weight gain: an exploratory study. Sex Reprod Healthc. 2011;2(1):43–8.
20. Heslehurst N, Moore H, Rankin J, Ells LJ, Wilkinson JR, Summerbell CD. How can maternity services be developed to effectively address maternal obesity? A qualitative study. Midwifery. 2011;27(5):e170–177.
21. Olander EK, Berg M, McCourt C, Carlstrom E, Dencker A. Person-centred care in interventions to limit weight gain in pregnant women with obesity - a systematic review. BMC Pregnancy Childbirth. 2015;15:50.
22. Claesson I-M, Josefsson A, Cedergren M, Brynhildsen J, Jeppsson A, Nyström F, Sydsjö A, Sydsjö G. Consumer satisfaction with a weight-gain intervention programme for obese pregnant women. Midwifery. 2008;24(2):163–7.
23. Jewell K, Avery A, Barber J, Simpson DS. The healthy eating and lifestyle in pregnancy (HELP) feasibility study. Br J Midwifery. 2014;22(10):727–36.
24. Atkinson L, Olander EK, French DP. Acceptability of a weight management intervention for pregnant and postpartum women with BMI >/=30 kg/m2: a qualitative evaluation of an individualized, home-based service. Matern Child Health J. 2016;20(1):88–96.
25. Heslehurst N, Dinsdale S, Sedgewick G, Simpson H, Sen S, Summerbell CD,

Rankin J. An evaluation of the implementation of maternal obesity pathways of care: a mixed methods study with data integration. PLoS One. 2015;10(5), e0127122.

26. Haby K, Glantz A, Hanas R, Premberg A. Mighty mums - an antenatal health care intervention can reduce gestational weight gain in women with obesity. Midwifery. 2015;31(7):685–92.

27. Braun V, Clarke V. Using thematic analysis in psychology. Qual Res Psychol. 2006;3(2):77–101.

28. Olander EK, Darwin ZJ, Atkinson L, Smith DM, Gardner B. Beyond the 'teachable moment' - A conceptual analysis of women's perinatal behaviour change. Women Birth. 2016;29(3):e67–71.

29. Sui Z, Turnbull D, Dodd J. Enablers of and barriers to making healthy change during pregnancy in overweight and obese women. Australasian Med J. 2013;6(11):565–77.

30. Amorim Adegboye AR, Linne YM. Diet or exercise, or both, for weight reduction in women after childbirth. Cochrane Database Syst Rev. 2013;7, CD005627.

31. Arden MA, Duxbury AM, Soltani H. Responses to gestational weight management guidance: a thematic analysis of comments made by women in online parenting forums. BMC Pregnancy Childbirth. 2014;14:216.

32. Harman V, Cappellini B. Mothers on display: lunchboxes. Social Class and Moral Accountability Sociology. 2015;49(4):764–81.

33. Furness PJ, McSeveny K, Arden MA, Garland C, Dearden AM, Soltani H. Maternal obesity support services: a qualitative study of the perspectives of women and midwives. BMC Pregnancy Childbirth. 2011;11:69.

34. Merrill E, Grassley J. Women's stories of their experiences as overweight patients. J Adv Nurs. 2008;64(2):139–46.

35. Puhl RM, Heuer CA. Obesity stigma: important considerations for public health. Am J Public Health. 2010;100(6):1019–28.

36. Ekman I, Swedberg K, Taft C, Lindseth A, Norberg A, Brink E, Carlsson J, Dahlin-Ivanoff S, Johansson IL, Kjellgren K, et al. Person-centered care–ready for prime time. Eur J Cardiovasc Nurs. 2011;10(4):248–51.

37. National Institute for Health and Clinical Excellence. NICE Clinical guideline 62. Antentatal care: Routine care for the healthy pregnant woman. London: National Institute for Health and Clinical Excellence 2008(modified: December 2014): 4-58

38. Popkin BM, Adair LS, Ng SW. Global nutrition transition and the pandemic of obesity in developing countries. Nutr Rev. 2012;70(1):3–21.

39. Grahn P, Stigsdotter UA. Landscape planning and stress. Urban For Urban Green. 2003;2(1):1–18.

40. Egger G, Swinburn B. An "ecological" approach to the obesity pandemic. BMJ (Clinical research ed). 1997;315(7106):477–80.

41. Atkinson L, Olander EK, French DP. Why don't many obese pregnant and post-natal women engage with a weight management service? J Reproductive Infant Psychol. 2013;31(3):245–56.

42. Olander EK, Atkinson L. Obese women's reasons for not attending a weight management service during pregnancy. Acta Obstet Gynecol Scand. 2013;92(10):1227–30.

Higher maternal leptin levels at second trimester are associated with subsequent greater gestational weight gain in late pregnancy

Marilyn Lacroix[1], Marie-Claude Battista[1], Myriam Doyon[2], Julie Moreau[2], Julie Patenaude[1], Laetitia Guillemette[1], Julie Ménard[2], Jean-Luc Ardilouze[1,2], Patrice Perron[1,2] and Marie-France Hivert[1,2,3,4*]

Abstract

Background: Excessive gestational weight gain (GWG) is associated with adverse pregnancy outcomes. In non-pregnant populations, low leptin levels stimulate positive energy balance. In pregnancy, both the placenta and adipose tissue contribute to circulating leptin levels. We tested whether maternal leptin levels are associated with subsequent GWG and whether this association varies depending on stage of pregnancy and on maternal body mass index (BMI).

Methods: This prospective cohort study included 675 pregnant women followed from 1st trimester until delivery. We collected anthropometric measurements, blood samples at 1st and 2nd trimester, and clinical data until delivery. Maternal leptin was measured by ELISA (Luminex technology). We classified women by BMI measured at 1st trimester: BMI < 25 kg/m^2 = normal weight; 25 ≤ BMI < 30 kg/m^2 = overweight; and BMI ≥ 30 kg/m^2 = obese.

Results: Women gained a mean of 6.7 ± 3.0 kg between 1st and 2nd trimester (mid pregnancy GWG) and 5.6 ± 2.5 kg between 2nd and the end of 3rd trimester (late pregnancy GWG). Higher 1st trimester leptin levels were associated with lower mid pregnancy GWG, but the association was no longer significant after adjusting for % body fat (%BF; β = 0.38 kg per log-leptin; SE = 0.52; P = 0.46). Higher 2nd trimester leptin levels were associated with greater late pregnancy GWG and this association remained significant after adjustment for BMI (β = 2.35; SE = 0.41; P < 0.0001) or %BF (β = 2.01; SE = 0.42; P < 0.0001). In BMI stratified analyses, higher 2nd trimester leptin levels were associated with greater late pregnancy GWG in normal weight women (β = 1.33; SE = 0.42; P = 0.002), and this association was stronger in overweight women (β = 2.85; SE = 0.94; P = 0.003 – P for interaction = 0.05).

Conclusions: Our results suggest that leptin may regulate weight gain differentially at 1st versus 2nd trimester of pregnancy: at 2nd trimester, higher leptin levels were associated with greater subsequent weight gain – the opposite of its physiologic regulation in non-pregnancy – and this association was stronger in overweight women. We suspect the existence of a feed-forward signal from leptin in second half of pregnancy, stimulating a positive energy balance and leading to greater weight gain.

Keywords: Leptin, Pregnancy, Weight gain, Body mass index

* Correspondence: marie-france_hivert@harvardpilgrim.org
[1]Department of Medicine, Université de Sherbrooke, 3001 12th Avenue North, Sherbrooke, Québec, Canada
[2]Centre de recherche du Centre Hospitalier Universitaire de Sherbrooke, 3001 12th Avenue North, wing 9, door 6, Sherbrooke, Québec, Canada
Full list of author information is available at the end of the article

Background

Excessive gestational weight gain (GWG) and pre-pregnancy obesity are associated with higher risk of adverse pregnancy outcomes, such as macrosomia, gestational diabetes mellitus (GDM), preeclampsia, and caesarean delivery [1]. Several factors influence GWG, including quality of diet, physical activity levels, pre-pregnancy body mass index (BMI), maternal age and parity [2, 3]. The physiologic regulation of GWG is highly variable from one woman to another [4]; a few pregnancy-related hormones such as progesterone have been suggested to participate in GWG regulation [5] but most endogenous regulators are still unknown.

Leptin is an adipokine secreted mainly from adipocytes that circulates in proportion to white adipose tissue mass in non-pregnant individuals [6], reflecting energy stores in adipose tissue. Leptin is known for its role in energy homeostasis: monogenic leptin deficiency is associated with hyperphagia and morbid obesity in both animals and humans [7–9]. However, leptin resistance also appears to exist in obese individuals since higher endogenic leptin levels or exogenic leptin administration does not reduce weight in humans [10, 11]. In a physiologic framework, lower leptin levels are associated with increased weight gain in normal-weight young adults [12] and with greater weight regain after weight loss in obese individuals [13].

In pregnancy, the placenta is a substantial source of circulating leptin and levels increase throughout pregnancy [14, 15]. This seems counter-intuitive to leptin's classic physiological role, as pregnancy should be a state where the energy signalling pathways favour a positive balance by increasing food intake. While we know that adiposity accumulation leads to higher leptin levels [15–19], how leptin may conversely act as regulator of subsequent weight gain in pregnancy is less understood. Current literature on this topic is sparse and inconclusive because of inconsistencies in study design – leptin levels measured before, during or after weight gain assessment – and incomplete adjustment for potential confounders [19–21]. Thus, we present here our prospective study designed to assess the associations between baseline leptin levels and subsequent GWG in a large population-based cohort of pregnant women, taking into account maternal adiposity status and period of the pregnancy.

Methods

We recruited pregnant women at 1st trimester (5–16 weeks) of pregnancy and followed them until delivery in the prospective cohort study Glycemic regulation in Gestation and Growth (Gen3G). Pregnant women arriving for their 1st trimester blood sample visit between January 2010 and July 2013 were invited to participate in our study if they expected to deliver at the Centre Hospitalier Universitaire de Sherbrooke (CHUS). We excluded women who had any of the following criteria: age <18 years old, multiple pregnancy, pregestational diabetes (type 1 or 2) or diabetes discovered at 1st trimester (criteria based on 2008 Canadian Diabetes Association guidelines [22]), drugs and/or alcohol abuse, uncontrolled endocrine disease, or other major medical conditions (for attrition and further details, see [23]). The CHUS human-research ethics committee approved the project and all women gave written informed consent before they were included in the study, in accordance with the Declaration of Helsinki.

During their 1st visit, we collected demographics and baseline characteristics of participants, including maternal age, ethnic background, gestational age (confirmed by echography), parity, and personal and familial medical history. In order to collect data on lifestyle, we used validated questionnaires concerning nutrition and physical activity adapted from the Canadian Community Health Survey [24]. Anthropometric measurements including weight (kg; by a calibrated electronic scale, bare feet, in light clothing), height (m), BMI (kg/m^2), % body fat (%BF; estimated by electrical bioimpedance using a standing foot-to-foot scale) and systolic and diastolic blood pressures were performed according to standardized procedures as described previously [25]. The majority of women (97%) also performed a 50g glucose challenge test with glucose levels measured 1-h after glucose ingestion, for early screening of GDM. We collected random non-fasting blood samples in the remaining participants.

At 2nd trimester (23–30 weeks), all women performed a 75g oral glucose tolerance test (OGTT) under fasting state for routine GDM diagnosis based on International Association of Diabetes and Pregnancy Study Groups criteria [26]. We collected extra fasting blood samples and at 1-h and 2-h during the OGTT for further analyses. Measures of glucose and insulin over the course of the OGTT allowed determination of dynamic indices of insulin sensitivity and secretion, respectively; Matsuda index (validated in pregnancy [27]), 10,000/ [square root (fasting glucose × fasting insulin) × (mean glucose × mean insulin)] [28]; and total area under the curve (AUC)$_{insulin/glucose}$ was calculated using the trapezoidal rule applied to the insulin and glucose curves during the OGTT. We collected data concerning any medical updates since the last visit and repeated the nutrition and physical activity questionnaires. Once again, we measured anthropometry, according to the same standardized procedures. We calculated maternal GWG (kg) between 1st and 2nd trimester (mid pregnancy GWG) by subtracting 1st trimester from 2nd trimester maternal measured weights.

At the end of the 3rd trimester, we collected maternal weight (kg) based on the last prenatal visit (34–42 weeks of gestation) available in our electronic medical records (EMR). From the EMR, we additionally collected medical events from 2nd trimester to delivery for any additional major complications (premature deliveries, GDM, and pre-eclampsia) and placental and birth weights recorded by clinical staff at delivery. Women lost to follow-up did not differ from the ones followed until delivery [23]. We calculated maternal weight gain between 2nd and 3rd trimester (late pregnancy GWG) by subtracting 2nd trimester from 3rd trimester maternal weights.

Laboratory measurements

All blood samples collected at 1st and 2nd trimester were maintained at 4°C and centrifuged. Plasma was distributed in aliquots and stored at –80°C until measurements. Plasma leptin and insulin levels were measured by enzyme-linked immunosorbent assay (ELISA Luminex technology; Millipore Corp, Billerica, MA, USA). Plasma glucose levels were measured by glucose hexokinase (Roche Diagnostics, Indianapolis, IN, USA). Intra- and inter-assays coefficients of variation for leptin levels were respectively of 3 and 4%.

Statistical analyses

From all women followed until delivery, we excluded pregnancies with major complications (prematurity <37 weeks, pre-eclampsia) and missing data for weight or leptin levels at any of the time points. Participants excluded for complications, missing data or lost to follow-up ($n = 288$) were similar to women remaining in our dataset ($n = 736$) in terms of maternal age, ethnicity and pre-pregnancy BMI (all $P > 0.05$). We further excluded women diagnosed with GDM ($n = 61$) for this analysis because diagnosis and treatment of GDM greatly influence GWG. This report included 675 normoglycemic pregnant women who had a complete dataset from 1st trimester to delivery, including all necessary maternal weight and leptin levels.

Characteristics of participants are presented as means ± standard deviations if normally distributed or as median and interquartile ranges otherwise; categorical variables are presented as percentage. Continuous variables not normally distributed were log-transformed and we used log-transformed variables for correlations and linear regression models when appropriate; leptin levels were normally distributed after log-transformation. We performed correlation analyses (Pearson and Spearman as appropriate) to assess variables associated cross-sectionally with leptin levels and to evaluate potential confounders. We conducted linear regression analyses to assess associations between leptin levels (per one log increase) and subsequent GWG (using kg/week to standardize for different follow-up time), taking into account potential confounding factors. We first adjusted for gestational weeks and BMI (model 2a) measured cross-sectionally with leptin levels of

interest at each time period assessed: for example the model testing the association between leptin at 1st trimester and subsequent GWG was adjusted for gestational age and BMI measured at 1st trimester. We then adjusted for %BF instead of BMI to account for adiposity per se (model 3a). We additionally adjusted for systolic and diastolic blood pressures, physical activity, quantity of fruits and vegetables consumed per day and frequency of restaurant meals per week to account for potential confounders including life-style (models 2b and 3b) using characteristics measured cross-sectionally with leptin levels for each respective model. We also performed linear regression analyses according to initial 1st trimester BMI categories as internationally defined (BMI <25 kg/m^2 = normal weight; 25 ≤ BMI <30 kg/m^2 = overweight; or BMI ≥30 kg/m^2 = obese) to assess associations between leptin levels (per one log increase) and subsequent GWG (kg/week) per clinically defined BMI status. In addition to linear regression analyses assessing GWG per week (in tables), we performed subsidiary linear regression analyses with weight gain expressed as GWG between 1st and 2nd trimester (mid pregnancy GWG) and GWG between 2nd and 3rd trimester (late pregnancy GWG) for easier interpretation. We also conducted sensitivity analyses: 1- excluding underweight women defined as 1st trimester BMI <18.5 kg/m^2 ($n = 17$); 2- excluding morbidly obese women defined as 1st trimester BMI >40 kg/m^2 ($n = 9$); and by adding an additional variable in adjusted models, namely: 3- placental weight (available in 529 deliveries); 4- Matsuda index (insulin sensitivity index); or 5- AUC$_{insulin/glucose}$ (insulin secretion index). $P < 0.05$ was considered statistically significant. All the analyses were performed using version 18 of Statistical Package for the Social Sciences (SPSS) for Windows.

Results

Characteristics of the 675 pregnant women included in the present study are presented in Table 1. Participants were 28.2 ± 4.3 years old and 97.2% were of European descent, similar to the general population of pregnant women receiving care at our institution [23].

Adiposity and weight gain

At 1st trimester, participants had a median BMI of 23.9[21.5–27.3] kg/m^2 and a mean %BF equal to 31.3 ± 8.0 % (see Table 1). At 2nd trimester, median BMI was 26.6[24.1–29.8] kg/m^2 and mean %BF was 35.4 ± 6.4 %. Women gained a mean of 6.7 ± 3.0 kg between 1st and 2nd trimester (weekly GWG = 0.40 ± 0.18 kg/week), and a mean of 5.6 ± 2.5 kg between 2nd trimester and late 3rd trimester (weekly GWG = 0.54 ± 0.23 kg/week) for a global mean GWG of 12.2 ± 4.4 kg between the 1st and the end of the 3rd trimester. Maternal factors at 1st trimester associated with larger subsequent GWG were lower adiposity levels (lower BMI and %BF) and being

Table 1 Characteristics of 675 pregnant women included in Gen3G at 1st and 2nd trimesters

Characteristics	1st trimester	2nd trimester
	Mean ± SD or median [IQR] or %	Mean ± SD or median [IQR] or %
Age (years)	28.2 ± 4.3	—
Ethnic background	97.2	—
(% European descent)		
Parity (% primiparous)	52.0	—
Gestational weeks	9.4 ± 2.0	26.4 ± 1.0
Body mass index (kg/m^2)	23.9 [21.5–27.3]	26.6 [24.1–29.8]
% body fat	31.3 ± 8.0	35.4 ± 6.4
Systolic blood pressure (mmHg)	110.5 ± 9.8	107.3 ± 8.9
Diastolic blood pressure (mmHg)	68.9 ± 6.9	67.4 ± 6.6
Physical activity (kcal/kg/day)	1.1 [0.5–1.9]	0.9 [0.4–1.5]
Nutrition		
Fruits & vegetables (per day)	5.6 ± 2.4	6.1 ± 2.5
Restaurant meals (per week)	1.0 [0.5–2.0]	1.0 [0.5–2.0]
Leptin levels non fasting (ng/ml)	8.0 [4.5–13.0]	—
Leptin levels during OGTT (ng/ml)		
Fasting	—	13.3 [8.3–20.6]
1-h post OGTT	—	10.3 [6.1–16.0]
2-h post OGTT	—	9.6 [5.3–15.3]

Data are presented as mean ± standard deviation (SD) or median (interquartile range). Variables not normally distributed were log-transformed. At 1st trimester, ranges of leptin levels were 0.9 to 59.7 ng/ml. At 2nd trimester, ranges of leptin were 1.1 to 85.8 ng/ml fasting, 0.9 to 56.2 ng/ml 1-h post OGTT, and 0.8 to 53.2 ng/ml 2-h post OGTT. For ethnic background and % body fat at 1st trimester: $n = 671$. For gestational weeks at 2nd trimester and body mass index at 2nd trimester: $n = 674$. For parity and systolic and diastolic blood pressures at 2nd trimester: $n = 673$. For waist circumference at 1st trimester: $n = 662$. For physical activity at 1st trimester: $n = 666$. For nutrition: $641 \leq n \leq 667$. For % body fat at 2nd trimester and physical activity at 2nd trimester: $n = 669$

assessed at an earlier point of the pregnancy (as represented by gestational weeks). Other factors measured at 1st or 2nd trimester were weakly or non-significantly associated with subsequent GWG (see Additional file 1: Table S1). At delivery, birth weight was 3.408 ± 0.461 kg and placental weight was 557.4 ± 133.4 g in average. Most maternal weight and adiposity variables at 1st and 2nd trimester were positively correlated with birth weight and placental weight; the strongest associations were observed between maternal weight or %BF and either birth outcomes (see Additional file 2: Table S2).

Leptin levels

Leptin levels increased from 1st (8.0[4.5–13.0] ng/ml) to 2nd trimester (10.3[6.1–16.0] ng/ml 1-h post OGTT; see Table 1), with a increase between 1st and 2nd trimester of 2.1[−0.5–5.3] ng/ml. Maternal factors positively asso-ciated cross–sectionally with leptin levels at 1st and 2nd trimester were adiposity levels (BMI and %BF) and blood pressures, while other factors were weakly or non-

significantly associated with leptin levels (see Table 2 and Additional file 3: Table S3). Birth weight and placental weight were also weakly associated with maternal leptin levels at 1st and 2nd trimester (see Additional file 2: Table S2); these associations were substantially reduced and none of them remained significant after adjustments for maternal BMI.

Leptin levels and subsequent weight gain

Table 3 presents linear regression analyses testing the associations between leptin levels and subsequent GWG. In unadjusted analyses, higher 1st trimester leptin levels were associated with lower mid pregnancy GWG ($\beta = -1.68$, meaning a decrease of 1.68 kg per increase of one log-leptin at 1st trimester; standard error (SE) = 0.35; $P < 0.0001$). After adjusting for 1st trimester gestational weeks and BMI (model 2a), the direction of effect was re-versed, meaning that higher leptin levels were associated with greater GWG ($\beta = 1.32$; SE = 0.49; $P = 0.007$).

Table 2 Cross-sectional correlations between women's characteristics and leptin levels measured at 1st and 2nd trimester

Characteristics at 1st trimester	Correlations^a with leptin levels at 1st trimester	
	r	P value
Age (years)	0.04	0.31
Gestational weeks	0.12	0.002
Body mass index (kg/m^2)	0.73	<0.0001
% body fat	0.74	<0.0001
Systolic blood pressure (mmHg)	0.21	<0.0001
Diastolic blood pressure (mmHg)	0.25	<0.0001
Physical activity (kcal/kg/day)	−0.11	0.005
Nutrition		
Fruits & vegetables (per day)	−0.09	0.02
Restaurant meals (per week)	0.10	0.01
Characteristics at 2nd trimester	Correlations^a with leptin levels 1-h post OGTTat 2nd trimester	
	r	P value
Gestational weeks	−0.04	0.25
Body mass index (kg/m^2)	0.67	<0.0001
% body fat	0.69	<0.0001
Systolic blood pressure (mmHg)	0.23	<0.0001
Diastolic blood pressure (mmHg)	0.31	<0.0001
Physical activity (kcal/kg/day)	−0.07	0.08
Nutrition		
Fruits & vegetables (per day)	−0.09	0.02
Restaurant meals (per week)	0.09	0.02

^{a}These are all Pearson correlations, except for correlations with physical activity at 1st and 2nd trimester that are Spearman correlations

Table 3 Associations between 1st or 2nd trimester leptin levels and subsequent mid or late pregnancy GWG[a]

Models	Associations: 1st trimester leptin levels and mid pregnancy GWG		Associations: 2nd trimester leptin levels 1-h post OGTT and late pregnancy GWG	
	$\beta \pm SE$	P value	$\beta \pm SE$	P value
Model 1: unadjusted	-0.08 ± 0.02	<0.0001	0.11 ± 0.03	0.0001
Model 2a: adjusted for BMI and gestational weeks	0.07 ± 0.03	0.01	0.24 ± 0.04	<0.0001
Model 2b: BMI-fully adjusted[1]	0.07 ± 0.03	0.02	0.21 ± 0.04	<0.0001
Model 3a: adjusted for %BF and gestational weeks	0.01 ± 0.03	0.64	0.20 ± 0.04	<0.0001
Model 3b: %BF-fully adjusted[1]	0.01 ± 0.03	0.74	0.18 ± 0.04	<0.0001

[a]All β represent the change in weight gain (kg) per week associated to a change of 1 log of leptin levels. GWG: gestational weight gain. BMI: body mass index. %BF: percent body fat. OGTT: oral glucose tolerance test. All models were adjusted with variables measured cross-sectionally with leptin levels of interest. For example in model 2a, model testing association between leptin levels measured at 1st trimester and mid pregnancy GWG is adjusted for BMI at 1st trimester and the number of weeks of gestation at the moment of assessment. [1]Adjusted for further potential confounders (always measured cross-sectionally to leptin levels respectively to trimester): systolic and diastolic blood pressures (1st or 2nd trimester), physical activity (1st or 2nd trimester), fruits and vegetables per day (1st or 2nd trimester) and restaurant meals per week (1st or 2nd trimester)

Replacing BMI by %BF at 1st trimester (model 3a) showed flattening of the association and leptin levels were no longer associated with mid pregnancy GWG ($\beta = 0.38$; SE $= 0.52$; $P = 0.46$). Further adjustments for blood pressure, physical activity, fruit and vegetable portions per day and restaurant meals per week did not modify associations in BMI of %BF adjusted models.

Higher 2nd trimester leptin levels were associated with greater late pregnancy GWG ($\beta = 1.17$; SE $= 0.31$; $P = 0.0002$ for 1-h post OGTT leptin levels). Associations were strengthened by adjustment for 2nd trimester gestational weeks and BMI with effect sizes almost doubling ($\beta = 2.35$; SE $= 0.41$; $P < 0.0001$ again for 1-h post OGTT leptin levels). Replacing BMI by %BF did not modify results in size or direction of effect. All associations remained statistically significant after further adjustment for blood pressure, physical activity, fruit and vegetable portions per day and restaurant meals per week, all measured at 2nd trimester ($\beta = 2.15$; SE $= 0.42$; $P < 0.0001$ for 1-h post OGTT leptin levels). Excluding underweight women (BMI <18.5 kg/m²) or morbidly obese women (BMI >40 kg/m²), or adding placental weight as an additional co-variable did not modify the results in sensitivity analyses. Our sensitivity analyses including insulin sensitivity or insulin secretion indices did not modify the associations.

Linear regression analyses concerning late pregnancy GWG and 2nd trimester leptin levels measured fasting and 2-h post OGTT showed similar associations than those observed with 2nd trimester 1-h post OGTT leptin levels (see Additional file 4: Table S4).

Leptin levels and subsequent weight gain stratified by maternal weight status

In order to further investigate the role of initial adiposity in the association between leptin levels and subsequent GWG, we performed our analyses stratified by maternal weight status defined by BMI measured at 1st trimester (see Table 4). We found no association between 1st trimester leptin levels and mid pregnancy GWG in any BMI strata, neither in unadjusted nor in multivariate models (all $P > 0.05$).

Higher 2nd trimester leptin levels were associated with greater late pregnancy GWG in normal weight women (unadjusted $\beta = 1.66$, kg per log-leptin levels at 1h-OGTT; SE $= 0.41$; $P < 0.0001$). Associations between leptin levels and late GWG appeared stronger among overweight women with effect sizes almost twice the ones observed in normal weight women (unadjusted $\beta = 3.60$; SE $= 0.88$; $P < 0.0001$ – $P = 0.05$ for interaction between normal weight and overweight strata). Strength of associations

Table 4 Associations between 1st or 2nd trimester leptin and subsequent GWG[a] stratified by 1st trimester BMI

Models		BMI < 25 kg/m²(n = 406)		25 ≤ BMI < 30 kg/m²(n = 159)		BMI ≥ 30 kg/m²(n = 110)	
		$\beta \pm SE$	P value	$\beta \pm SE$	P value	$\beta \pm SE$	P value
1st trimester leptin levels and mid pregnancy GWG	Unadjusted	0.02 ± 0.03	0.46	0.10 ± 0.08	0.23	0.01 ± 0.09	0.92
	Adjusted[1]	0.01 ± 0.03	0.60	0.01 ± 0.08	0.88	-0.01 ± 0.10	0.92
2nd trimester leptin levels 1-h post OGTT and late pregnancy GWG	Unadjusted	0.17 ± 0.04	<0.0001	0.33 ± 0.08	<0.0001	0.12 ± 0.12	0.33
	Adjusted[1]	0.15 ± 0.04	0.0001	0.26 ± 0.09	0.004	0.13 ± 0.12	0.29

[a]All β represent the change in weight gain (kg) per week associated to a change of 1 log of leptin levels. [1] Adjusted for variables measured cross-sectionally to leptin levels of interest respectively to trimester: the number of weeks of gestation at the moment of assessment, systolic and diastolic blood pressures (1st or 2nd trimester), physical activity (1st or 2nd trimester), fruits and vegetables per day (1st or 2nd trimester) and restaurant meals per week (1st or 2nd trimester). BMI: body mass index. GWG: gestational weight gain. OGTT: oral glucose tolerance test

was slightly reduced by adding potential confounders in fully adjusted models for normal weight and overweight women, mainly driven by presence of blood pressure and consumption of fruits/vegetables in the models. We observed no significant associations between 2nd trimester leptin levels and late pregnancy GWG in obese women (unadjusted $\beta = 0.85$; SE = 1.29; $P = 0.51$ for 1-h post OGTT leptin levels) in either unadjusted or adjusted analyses. After removing women with BMI >40 kg/m^2 from the obese group, we observed that the effect size was slightly greater (unadjusted $\beta = 1.66$; SE = 1.38; $P = 0.23$ for 1-h post OGTT leptin levels; $n = 101$ women) but this remained non-significant. Our sensitivity analyses excluding underweight women (BMI <18.5 kg/m^2) or including either placental weight, insulin sensitivity index or insulin secretion index as co-variables did not modify the results. Linear regression analyses using 2nd trimester leptin levels measured fasting and 2-h post OGTT showed similar associations than those observed with 1-h post OGTT leptin levels (see Additional file 5: Table S5).

Discussion

We demonstrated that higher 2nd trimester leptin levels were associated with greater subsequent GWG in pregnant women from a general population cohort, independent of maternal adiposity and other confounders. This positive association is the opposite of the expected physiologic regulation observed in non-pregnant individuals. Interestingly, this positive association was particularly observable and stronger in women classified as overweight at the beginning of pregnancy than in normal weight women.

Only a few studies have reported associations between baseline maternal leptin levels – measured at the beginning of the weight gain period – and subsequent GWG [19–21]. Our findings at 1st trimester are in line with previous findings from Walsh et al. and Kim et al., where 1st trimester leptin levels do not show a significant association with subsequent GWG after adjustments for %BF and other confounders [19, 21]. Thus, based on our results and those of others, lower 1st trimester leptin levels represent lower adiposity, signaling the need to increase positive energy balance and leading to greater weight gain early in pregnancy – similar to non-pregnant leptin's role into central nervous system (CNS) signaling.

Our study adds to the current literature by investigating leptin levels measured at 24–28 weeks and subsequent GWG in a wide range of maternal BMI status. In contrast to our results, Kim et al. did not show associations between leptin levels measured at 24 weeks and any weight variables, including GWG. Difference in populations or limited power due to a smaller sample size ($n = 75$) may explain different findings from Kim et al. [21]. Walsh et al. measured leptin at 28 weeks, but assessed association with overall GWG throughout pregnancy – i.e. spanning a time

period before and after our leptin measurement, and thus, we cannot compare their results to ours [19]. In line with our results in normal weight pregnant women, Stein et al. reported that higher leptin levels measured at 17 weeks of gestation were associated with a higher measured rate of weight gain between 20 and 36 gestational weeks in women with a pregravid BMI from 19.8 to 26.0 kg/m^2 [20]. Our results expand current knowledge and suggest that this positive association is more prominent in overweight women. This is highly intriguing, as we know that clinically, overweight women are more likely to gain excessive GWG compared to normal weight and obese women.

The physiologic role of leptin during pregnancy is still obscure, but our results suggest that leptin promotes weight gain in a feed-forward mechanism during the second half of pregnancy. The placenta produces leptin in high quantity and contributes to maternal circulating levels throughout pregnancy, but why the placenta produces such a high quantity of leptin remains in question. Our results showing larger effect size in overweight women argue for the existence of this feed-forward regulation, as overweight women presented higher levels of leptin throughout pregnancy: if a pregnancy-specific CNS signal emerges as pregnancy advances, rising placental-derived leptin, in addition to high leptin from pre-pregnancy overweight status, might enhanced this positive feed-forward loop. Our findings of reduced associations in obese women could be explained by a state of central leptin resistance when levels reach the extreme upper range; but they could also reflect obese women self-regulating their energy balance based on clinical recommendations. It is also possible that leptin resistance occurring at the placenta level contributes to the absence of this feed-forward mechanism in obese women [29, 30]. However, the reduced effect sizes we observed in obese women should be interpreted with caution, given large confidence intervals and our smaller sample in this stratum.

Animal studies have supported the existence of a pregnancy-induced leptin resistance status [31–34]. For example, Ladyman et al. observed that intraperitoneal injections of leptin did not suppress food intake in pregnant mice compared to its observed effect of food intake reduction in non-pregnant mice [31]. The same report also demonstrated that the ventromedial hypothalamus and the paraventricular nucleus of pregnant mice showed a decrease in leptin sensitivity compared to non-pregnant mice [31]. Based on animal models, other potential mechanisms that could contribute to leptin resistance during pregnancy include an increase in circulating leptin binding protein, an impairment in leptin transport through the blood brain barrier, a decrease in Ob-Rb (isoform b of leptin's receptor) mRNA (messenger ribonucleic acid) levels in the hypothalamus, and/or an impairment in the intracellular signalization induced by the binding of leptin to Ob-Rb [32–34]. In term human placenta tissue sections from obese pregnancies, it has also been shown that Ob-Rb is down regulated in comparison to lean pregnancies, raising the possibility of placental leptin resistance [29, 30]. Our results add to the current knowledge in suggesting that a state of leptin resistance also exists in human pregnancy, though the exact mechanisms leading to pregnancy-induced leptin resistance and a possible feed-forward loop in humans remain to be investigated. It did not seem that insulin resistance or insulin secretion influenced our observations, but other factors such as specific pregnancy hormones may be implicated and merit future investigations.

Strengths and limitations
A major strength of our study is the design, as participants were followed prospectively and represent the general population of pregnant women receiving care at our hospital [35]. Strengths of this study also include our large sample size, exclusion of diabetes at 1st and 2nd trimester, and use of standardized procedures with high reliability for all laboratory and clinical measures, including anthropometry.

The main limitation of our study is the observational study design; consequently, we cannot conclude about causality or any mechanistic pathways. Despite being validated in pregnancy [36], measurement of %BF by bioimpedance could be influenced differently at 2nd trimester by the presence of larger amount of body water, the placenta and the fetus. We used validated questionnaires for self-report of physical activity and nutrition, but direct measurements of energy intake and expenditure would have provided greater precision. Our population is mainly of European descent, so our results might not apply to other ethnicities.

Conclusions
In summary, our results suggest that body weight regulation by leptin during the second half of pregnancy does not follow the physiologic role as an adipostat with negative feedback to CNS that is classically attributed to leptin. We revealed a positive association between higher 2nd trimester leptin levels and greater subsequent GWG in normal weight women, and this association was stronger in overweight women. Our findings suggest a potential feed forward mechanism where higher leptin levels could signal the need to increase food intake and lead to greater weight gain. Feed forward loops are rare in human physiology, but are well known in the reproductive endocrine system – such as the menstrual cycle [37]. Mechanistic studies will be necessary to test this hypothesis and elucidate these mechanisms at the CNS and peripheral levels.

Ethics approval and consent to participate
The Centre Hospitalier Universitaire de Sherbrooke human-research ethics committee approved the project and all women gave a written informed consent before they were included in the study, in accordance with the Declaration of Helsinki.

Consent for publication
Not applicable.

Additional files

Additional file 1: Table S1. Correlations between women's characteristics and subsequent GWG (expressed per week) in mid and late pregnancy.

Additional file 2: Table S2. Birth and placenta weights correlations with maternal weight-related variables and maternal leptin levels during pregnancy.

Additional file 3: Table S3. Correlations between women's characteristics and leptin levels measured at 2nd trimester.

Additional file 4: Table S4. Correlations between 2nd trimester leptin levels and subsequent GWG (expressed per week)*.

Additional file 5: Table S5. Correlations between 2nd trimester leptin levels and subsequent GWG* stratified by 1st trimester BMI.

Abbreviations
%BF: percent body fat; AUC: area under the curve; BMI: body mass index; CHUS: Centre Hospitalier Universitaire de Sherbrooke; CNS: central nervous system; ELISA: enzyme-linked immunosorbent assay; EMR: electronic medical records; GDM: gestational diabetes mellitus; GWG: gestational weight gain; mRNA: messenger ribonucleic acid; Ob-Rb: isoform b of leptin's receptor; OGTT: oral glucose tolerance test; SD: standard deviation; SE: standard error; SPSS: Statistical Package for the Social Sciences.

Competing interests
The authors declare that they have no competing interests.

Authors' contributions
ML performed data collection, data analysis/interpretation, and wrote the manuscript. MFH conceived the study design, provided assistance with the statistical analysis, and actively participated in data interpretation and the writing of the manuscript. MCB, MD, JMoreau and JMénard participated in recruitment and data collection. JP and LG participated in data collection. PP and JLA participated in study design conception. All authors revised the manuscript critically and gave their final approval of the submitted and published versions.

Acknowledgements
The authors wish to acknowledge the Blood Sampling in Pregnancy clinic at the Research Center of the Centre Hospitalier Universitaire de Sherbrooke (CR-CHUS; a Fonds de Recherche du Québec - Santé (FRQ-S) supported research center); the assistance of clinical research nurses (Maude Gérard, Marie-Josée Gosselin, Suzan Hayes, Georgette Proulx) and research assistants (Pascal Brassard, Caroline Rousseau) for recruitment and obtainment of consent from participants (all staff were employees of the CR-CHUS or the University of Sherbrooke); and the CHUS Biochemistry laboratory for performing blood glucose measurements.

Funding

The study was supported by a Fonds de Recherche du Québec - Santé (FRQ-S) Operating Grant (MF Hivert), Diabète Québec (P Perron) and a Canadian Diabetes Association Operating Grant (JL Ardilouze). MF Hivert was a FRQ-S research scholar and the recipient of a Clinical Scientist Award from the Canadian Diabetes Association (CDA) and the Maud Menten Award from the Institute of Genetics (IG) - Canadian Institute of Health Research (CIHR); MF Hivert is now the recipient of an ADA Accelerator Award #1-15-ACE-26. JL Ardilouze is a FRQ-S Junior 2 scholar. M Lacroix was supported by the FRQ-S, Diabète Québec, the Centre de recherche Mère-Enfant of Sherbrooke's University, and the Foundation of Stars.

Author details

[1]Department of Medicine, Université de Sherbrooke, 3001 12th Avenue North, Sherbrooke, Québec, Canada. [2]Centre de recherche du Centre Hospitalier Universitaire de Sherbrooke, 3001 12th Avenue North, wing 9, door 6, Sherbrooke, Québec, Canada. [3]Diabetes Center, Massachusetts General Hospital, 50 Staniford Street, Boston, MA, USA. [4]Department of Population Medicine, Harvard Medical School, Harvard Pilgrim Health Care Institute, 401 Park Drive, suite 401, Boston, MA, USA.

References

1. Smith SA, Hulsey T, Goodnight W. Effects of obesity on pregnancy. J Obstet Gynecol Neonatal Nurs. 2008;37:176–84.
2. Wells CS, Schwalberg R, Noonan G, Gabor V. Factors influencing inadequate and excessive weight gain in pregnancy: Colorado, 2000-2002. Matern Child Health J. 2006;10:55–62.
3. Gardner B, Wardle J, Poston L, Croker H. Changing diet and physical activity to reduce gestational weight gain: a meta-analysis. Obes Rev. 2011;12:e602–20.
4. Dawes MG, Grudzinskas JG. Patterns of maternal weight gain in pregnancy. Br J Obstet Gynaecol. 1991;98:195–201.
5. Wuu J, Hellerstein S, Lipworth L, Wide L, Xu B, Yu GP, Kuper H, Lagiou P, Hankinson SE, Ekbom A, Carlstrom K, Trichopoulos D, Adami HO, Hsieh CC. Correlates of pregnancy oestrogen, progesterone and sex hormone-binding globulin in the USA and China. Eur J Cancer Prev. 2002;11:283–93.
6. Considine RV, Sinha MK, Heiman ML, Kriauciunas A, Stephens TW, Nyce MR, Ohannesian JP, Marco CC, McKee LJ, Bauer TL. Serum immunoreactive-leptin concentrations in normal-weight and obese humans. N Engl J Med. 1996;334:292–5.
7. Hwa JJ, Ghibaudi L, Compton D, Fawzi AB, Strader CD. Intracerebroventricular injection of leptin increases thermogenesis and mobilizes fat metabolism in ob/ob mice. Horm Metab Res. 1996;28:659–63.
8. Farooqi IS, Matarese G, Lord GM, Keogh JM, Lawrence E, Agwu C, Sanna V, Jebb SA, Perna F, Fontana S, Lechler RI, DePaoli AM, O'Rahilly S. Beneficial effects of leptin on obesity, T cell hyporesponsiveness, and neuroendocrine/metabolic dysfunction of human congenital leptin deficiency. J Clin Invest. 2002;110:1093–103.
9. Gibson WT, Farooqi IS, Moreau M, DePaoli AM, Lawrence E, O'Rahilly S, Trussell RA. Congenital leptin deficiency due to homozygosity for the Delta133G mutation: report of another case and evaluation of response to four years of leptin therapy. J Clin Endocrinol Metab. 2004;89:4821–6.
10. Hukshorn CJ, Saris WH, Westerterp-Plantenga MS, Farid AR, Smith FJ, Campfield LA. Weekly subcutaneous pegylated recombinant native human leptin (PEG-OB) administration in obese men. J Clin Endocrinol Metab. 2000;85:4003–9.
11. Zelissen PM, Stenlof K, Lean ME, Fogteloo J, Keulen ET, Wilding J, Finer N, Rossner S, Lawrence E, Fletcher C, McCamish M, Group A. Effect of three treatment schedules of recombinant methionyl human leptin on body weight in obese adults: a randomized, placebo-controlled trial. Diabetes Obes Metab. 2005;7:755–61.
12. Allard C, Doyon M, Brown C, Carpentier AC, Langlois MF, Hivert MF. Lower leptin levels are associated with higher risk of weight gain over 2 years in healthy young adults. Appl Physiol Nutr Metab. 2013;38:280–5.
13. Holm JC, Gamborg M, Ward L, Ibsen KK, Gammeltoft S, Sorensen TI, Heitmann BL. Longitudinal analysis of leptin variation during weight regain after weight loss in obese children. Obes Facts. 2009;2:243–8.
14. Masuzaki H, Ogawa Y, Sagawa N, Hosoda K, Matsumoto T, Mise H, Nishimura H, Yoshimasa Y, Tanaka I, Mori T, Nakao K. Nonadipose tissue production of leptin: leptin as a novel placenta-derived hormone in humans. Nat Med. 1997;3:1029–33.
15. Misra VK, Trudeau S. The influence of overweight and obesity on longitudinal trends in maternal serum leptin levels during pregnancy. Obesity (Silver Spring). 2011;19:416–21.
16. Wolff S, Legarth J, Vangsgaard K, Toubro S, Astrup A. A randomized trial of the effects of dietary counseling on gestational weight gain and glucose metabolism in obese pregnant women. Int J Obes (Lond). 2008;32:495–501.
17. Ferraro ZM, Qiu Q, Gruslin A, Adamo KB. Excessive gestational weight gain and obesity contribute to altered expression of maternal insulin-like growth factor binding protein-3. Int J Womens Health. 2013;5:657–65.
18. Castellano Filho DS, do Amaral Correa JO, Dos Santos Ramos P, de Oliveira Montessi M, Aarestrup BJ, Aarestrup FM. Body weight gain and serum leptin levels of non-overweight and overweight/obese pregnant women. Med Sci Monit. 2013;19:1043–9.
19. Walsh JM, McGowan CA, Mahony RM, Foley ME, McAuliffe FM. Obstetric and metabolic implications of excessive gestational weight gain in pregnancy. Obesity (Silver Spring). 2014;22:1594–600.
20. Stein TP, Scholl TO, Schluter MD, Schroeder CM. Plasma leptin influences gestational weight gain and postpartum weight retention. Am J Clin Nutr. 1998;68:1236–40.
21. Kim KH, Kim YJ, Lee S, Oh SW, Lee K, Park Y, Kim HJ, Kwak H. Evaluation of plasma leptin levels & BMI as predictor of postpartum weight retention. Indian J Med Res. 2008;128:595–600.
22. Canadian Journal of Diabetes. [http://archive.diabetes.ca/files/cpg2008/cpg-2008.pdf]. Accessed 8 March 2016.
23. Guillemette L, Allard C, Lacroix M, Patenaude J, Battista M-C, Doyon M, Moreau J, Ménard J, Bouchard L, Ardilouze J-L, Perron P, Hivert M-F. Cohort profile: Genetics of Glucose regulation in Gestation and Growth (Gen3G) – a prospective pre-birth cohort of mother-child pairs in Sherbrooke, Canada. BMJ Open. 2016;6(2):e010031. doi:10.1136/bmjopen-2015-010031.
24. Canadian Community Health Survey, Cycle 2.2, Nutrition (2004)A Guide to Accessing and Interpreting the Data. [http://www.hc-sc.gc.ca/fn-an/alt_formats/hpfb-dgpsa/pdf/surveill/cchs-guide-escc-eng.pdf]. Accessed 8 March 2016.
25. Lacroix M, Battista MC, Doyon M, Menard J, Ardilouze JL, Perron P, Hivert MF. Lower adiponectin levels at first trimester of pregnancy are associated with increased insulin resistance and higher risk of developing gestational diabetes mellitus. Diabetes Care. 2013;36:1577–83.
26. Panel IA of D and PSGC, Metzger BE, Gabbe SG, Persson B, Buchanan TA, Catalano PA, Damm P, Dyer AR, Leiva A, Hod M, Kitzmiler JL, Lowe LP, McIntyre HD, Oats JJ, Omori Y, Schmidt MI. International association of diabetes and pregnancy study groups recommendations on the diagnosis and classification of hyperglycemia in pregnancy. Diabetes Care. 2010;33:676–82.
27. Kirwan JP, Huston-Presley L, Kalhan SC, Catalano PM. Clinically useful estimates of insulin sensitivity during pregnancy: validation studies in women with normal glucose tolerance and gestational diabetes mellitus. Diabetes Care. 2001;24:1602–7.
28. Matsuda M, DeFronzo RA. Insulin sensitivity indices obtained from oral glucose tolerance testing: comparison with the euglycemic insulin clamp. Diabetes Care. 1999;22:1462–70.
29. Farley DM, Choi J, Dudley DJ, Li C, Jenkins SL, Myatt L, Nathanielsz PW. Placental amino acid transport and placental leptin resistance in pregnancies complicated by maternal obesity. Placenta. 2010;31:718–24.
30. Tessier DR, Ferraro ZM, Gruslin A. Role of leptin in pregnancy: consequences of maternal obesity. Placenta. 2013;34:205–11.
31. Ladyman SR, Fieldwick DM, Grattan DR. Suppression of leptin-induced hypothalamic JAK/STAT signalling and feeding response during pregnancy in the mouse. Reproduction. 2012;144:83–90.
32. Ladyman SR, Grattan DR. Suppression of leptin receptor messenger ribonucleic acid and leptin responsiveness in the ventromedial nucleus of the hypothalamus during pregnancy in the rat. Endocrinology. 2005;146:3868–74.
33. Ladyman SR, Grattan DR. Region-specific reduction in leptin-induced phosphorylation of signal transducer and activator of transcription-3 (STAT3) in the rat hypothalamus is associated with leptin resistance during pregnancy. Endocrinology. 2004;145:3704–11.
34. Trujillo ML, Spuch C, Carro E, Senaris R. Hyperphagia and central mechanisms for leptin resistance during pregnancy. Endocrinology. 2011;152:1355–65.

Maternal super-obesity and perinatal outcomes in Australia

Elizabeth A. Sullivan[1,2*], Jan E. Dickinson[3], Geraldine A Vaughan[1], Michael J. Peek[4,5], David Ellwood[6,7], Caroline SE Homer[1], Marian Knight[8], Claire McLintock[9], Alex Wang[1], Wendy Pollock[10,11], Lisa Jackson Pulver[12], Zhuoyang Li[1], Nasrin Javid[1], Elizabeth Denney-Wilson[1], Leonie Callaway[13,14] and on behalf of the Australasian Maternity Outcomes Surveillance System (AMOSS)

Abstract

Background: Super-obesity is associated with significantly elevated rates of obstetric complications, adverse perinatal outcomes and interventions. The purpose of this study was to determine the prevalence, risk factors, management and perinatal outcomes of super-obese women giving birth in Australia.

Methods: A national population-based cohort study. Super-obese pregnant women (body mass index (BMI) >50 kg/m^2 or weight >140 kg) who gave birth between January 1 and October 31, 2010 and a comparison cohort were identified using the Australasian Maternity Outcomes Surveillance System (AMOSS). Outcomes included maternal and perinatal morbidity and mortality. Prevalence estimates calculated with 95 % confidence intervals (CIs). Adjusted odds ratios (ORs) were calculated using multivariable logistic regression.

Results: 370 super-obese women with a median BMI of 52.8 kg/m^2 (range 40.9–79.9 kg/m^2) and prevalence of 2.1 per 1 000 women giving birth (95 % CI: 1.96–2.40). Super-obese women were significantly more likely to be public patients (96.2 %), smoke (23.8 %) and be socio-economically disadvantaged (36.2 %). Compared with other women, super-obese women had a significantly higher risk for obstetric (adjusted odds ratio (AOR) 2.42, 95 % CI: 1.77–3.29) and medical (AOR: 2.89, 95 % CI: 2.64–4.11) complications during pregnancy, birth by caesarean section (51.6 %) and admission to special care (HDU/ICU) (6.2 %). The 372 babies born to 365 super-obese women with outcomes known had significantly higher rates of birthweight ≥4500 g (AOR 19.94, 95 % CI: 6.81–58.36), hospital transfer (AOR 3.81, 95 % CI: 1.93–7.55) and admission to Neonatal Intensive Care Unit (NICU) (AOR 1.83, 95 % CI: 1.27–2.65) compared to babies of the comparison group, but not prematurity (10.5 % versus 9.2 %) or perinatal mortality (11.0 (95 % CI: 4.3–28.0) versus 6.6 (95 % CI: 2.6- 16.8) per 1 000 singleton births).

Conclusions: Super-obesity in pregnancy in Australia is associated with increased rates of pregnancy and birth complications, and with social disadvantage. There is an urgent need to further address risk factors leading to super-obesity among pregnant women and for maternity services to better address pre-pregnancy and pregnancy care to reduce associated inequalities in perinatal outcomes.

Keywords: Super-obesity, Obesity, Perinatal outcomes, Pregnancy, Maternal socio-economic disadvantage, Obstetric complications

* Correspondence: elizabeth.sullivan@uts.edu.au
[1]Faculty of Health, University of Technology Sydney, PO Box 123, Broadway NSW, 2007 Sydney, Australia
[2]School of Women's and Children's Health, The University of New South Wales, Sydney, Australia
Full list of author information is available at the end of the article

Background

The prevalence of obesity (body mass index (BMI) ≥ 30 kg/m^2) among women of reproductive age continues to rise in developed countries, with Australia at 28.3 % among the highest in the world ahead of United Kingdom [1] and similar to the United States. It is estimated that about one in five women giving birth in Australia are obese [2]. Of increasing concern is the rising rate of so-called super-obesity, defined as a BMI of ≥ 50 kg/m^2 in pregnancy, or women weighing 225 % of ideal body weight [3, 4]. Super-obesity is associated with significantly elevated rates of obstetric complications, adverse perinatal outcomes and interventions including pre-eclampsia, gestational diabetes mellitus (GDM), preterm birth, caesarean section, general anaesthesia, wound infection, intensive care admission, macrosomia, neonatal hypoglycaemia and congenital anomalies [3–6]. However, there has been no national study of super-obesity in Australian women giving birth. A population study from the United Kingdom reported the prevalence of women with BMI ≥50 kg/m2 as 8.7 per 10 000 women giving birth or 0.1 % [7]. In contrast, the prevalence of super-obesity ranged from 1.8 % [4] in a 7-year (2000 to 2006) US retrospective cohort study in Missouri, to 2.2 % for a 12-year (1996 to 2007) case series of 19 700 women giving birth in South Carolina [5]. A retrospective 12-year cohort study of 75 432 women giving birth in a Brisbane hospital (Australia) found a significant increase in the proportion of Class III obesity (≥40 kg/m2) during the course of the study [8]. This suggests that the prevalence of super-obesity among women giving birth is also on the rise in Australia although this has not been previously reported [8].

The objective of this study was to determine the prevalence, risk factors, management and perinatal outcomes of super-obese women giving birth in Australia; and to determine the effect of maternal super-obesity on perinatal outcomes compared with other women. We hypothesized that pregnancy in super-obese women compared with other women is associated with a higher risk of maternal morbidity and adverse perinatal outcomes.

Methods

Study design and population

A national, prospective cohort study was undertaken using the Australasian Maternity Outcomes Surveillance System (AMOSS). The AMOSS methods have been described in detail elsewhere [9]. Women were identified by participating AMOSS sites, responding to a monthly email that included negative reporting of whether a case had been identified between January and October 2010. Hospital (n = 226) sites progressively joined AMOSS on completion of relevant ethics/governance processes and were included for the period they participated in the study. The denominator of 171 289 women giving birth

was calculated using the number of days of participation in the study multiplied by number of births per day for that hospital and gave approximate coverage of 66 % of all women giving birth in Australia. The case definition included any pregnant woman of 20 weeks' gestation or more who, at any point in pregnancy, had a BMI of greater than 50 kg/m^2 or a weight of more than 140 kg. The case definition was clinician informed with a weight of >140 kg at any point in pregnancy considered super-obese irrespective of having a BMI <50 kg/m^2. The comparison group for a series of AMOSS studies were the two women who gave birth immediately before women with placenta accreta and/or women who underwent a peripartum hysterectomy between January 2010 and December 2011 [10]. The comparison group represented the general population of women giving birth in Australia and New Zealand and inclusion criteria did not include BMI, however all comparison women had a BMI ≤50 kg/m^2 or weight ≤140 kg.

A questionnaire completed by AMOSS site coordinators for all eligible women sought information on demographic and pregnancy factors, obstetric interventions and perinatal outcomes as well as models of antenatal care, specified medical and obstetric complications and bariatric equipment (e.g., high-weight capacity bed, operating table, hoist, chair) availability. Free-text responses to questions regarding medical/obstetric morbidity were categorised according to ICD-10 AM codes.

We anticipated identifying 264 super-obese women and 528 comparison women over 12 months, based on the prevalence of the United Kingdom study of 8.7 per 10 000 women giving birth [7]. These numbers give a power of 80 % at the 5 % level of significance to detect difference in proportions of outcomes (gestational diabetes, caesarean section and admission to NICU) by 10 % in study group over a range of incidences from 5 to 30 % in the comparison group.

Other study factors

The woman's age was calculated in completed years at the time of the antenatal care booking visit and classified into four categories: <25, 25–29, 30–34, and ≥ 35 years. Other demographic characteristics such as parity (0, 1–2, and ≥ 3), Indigenous status, marital status, admission as private/public patient, smoking during pregnancy, socio-economic status (Australian socio-economic indices for areas (SEIFA) of relative advantage/disadvantage quintile) [11], previous caesarean section, multiple pregnancy and assisted reproductive technology treatment were recorded.

Outcomes

Models of care, obstetric interventions, and birth outcomes were measured for both groups. Health professional involvement during antenatal care, specific medical and obstetric complications and bariatric equipment availability were recorded for the super-obese women only.

Statistical analysis

Prevalence estimates with 95 % confidence intervals (CIs) were calculated. Distribution of BMI was graphically compared between super-obese women and the comparison group. Chi-square or Fisher's exact test was used to investigate difference in obstetric interventions and birth outcomes of study and comparison groups. Multivariable logistic regression was used to examine the medical and obstetric complications (gestational diabetes, gestational hypertension, pre-eclampsia, etc.), labour characteristics (onset of labour and method of delivery), maternal outcomes (admission to ICU or HDU) and perinatal outcomes (birthweight ≥4 500 g, admission to NICU, and need for transfer). Odds ratio (OR) and adjusted odds ratio (AOR) and 95 % confidence interval (CI) were calculated. Adjustment was made for maternal age, maternal Indigenous status, marital status, admission as private/public patient, smoking status, assisted reproductive technology, parity, multiple gestation and socio-economic status. Any p-values less than 0.05 were considered statistically significant. Data were analysed using the Statistical Package for the Social Sciences software, version 22.0 (IBM Corporation, Somers, NY, USA).

Ethics approval

Ethics approval for AMOSS was granted by NSW Population and Health Services Research Ethics Committee and multiple Human Research Ethics Committees across Australia [12] and the multiregional ethics approval in New Zealand. The AMOSS studies are considered low-risk under (Australian) National Health and Medical Research Council (NHMRC) guidelines. The data collected from case notes by onsite AMOSS data coordinators were de-identified, and no consent was required by participants. Data were reported at an aggregate level only [12].

Results

A total of 370 super-obese pregnant women (297 women had a BMI of greater than 50 kg/m^2 and 73 women had a weight of more than 140 kg) were confirmed as cases with an estimated prevalence of 2.14 per 1000 (95 % CI: 1.96–2.40) women giving birth (Fig. 1). Data were available for 621 women in the comparative group. The median BMI (Fig. 2) of the super-obese women was 52.8 kg/m^2 (range, 40.9–79.9 kg/m^2) compared to 24.8 kg/m^2 (range, 16.3–48.9 kg/m^2) for comparison women. The median weight of super-obese women was 156 kg (range 108–204 kg) which was over twice the median weight for the comparison women of 67 kg (range 42–138 kg). Demographic and pregnancy-related

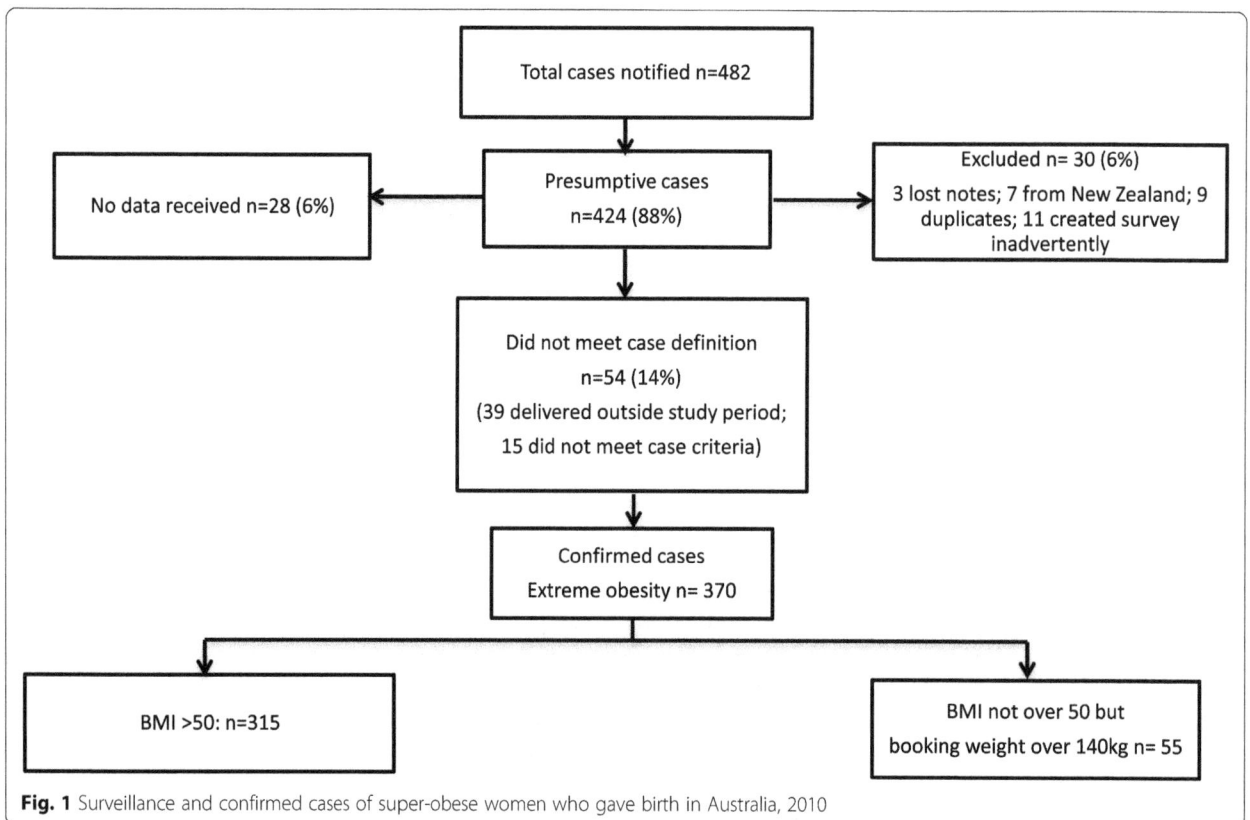

Fig. 1 Surveillance and confirmed cases of super-obese women who gave birth in Australia, 2010

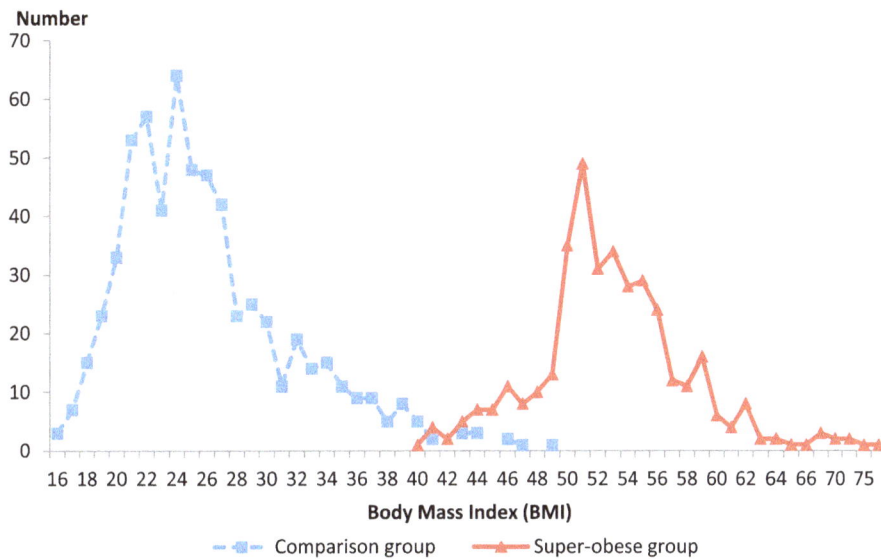

Fig. 2 Distribution of body mass index of super-obese and comparison women who gave birth in Australia, 2010

characteristics of super-obese and comparison groups are shown in Table 1. The super-obese women (cases) were of similar age but of significantly higher parity than the comparison women (parity ≥ 3: 22.2 % versus 9.2 %, $p < 0.01$). They were more likely to smoke (23.8 % versus 16.1 %, $p < 0.01$), to be socio-economically disadvantaged (lowest SEIFA quintile: 17.8 % versus 7.9 %, $p < 0.01$) and be admitted as a public patient (96.2 % versus 76.7 %, $p < 0.01$).

Models of care
The majority of super-obese women had a hospital-based, medical model of care with few under the care of midwives or private obstetricians, which was significantly different from the comparison group (Table 2). Changes in the model of care and rates of transfer between hospitals were higher for the super-obese group compared with comparison women (Table 2). Fewer than half ($n = 173$, 46.8 %) of the super-obese women saw a dietician during pregnancy, while 70.5 % ($n = 261$) consulted obstetric anaesthetists and 17.8 % ($n = 66$) consulted maternal-fetal medicine specialists during pregnancy (data unavailable for comparison group). Multi-disciplinary meetings were held for 12 % of super-obese women during the antenatal period to plan management.

Medical and obstetric complications during pregnancy
Super-obese women had significantly higher rates of obstetric (42.0 % versus 23.2 %; AOR: 2.42, 95 % CI: 1.77–3.29) and medical (33.3 % versus 13.0 %; AOR: 2.89, 95 % CI: 2.64–4.11) complications during pregnancy (Table 3). Super-obese women were significantly more likely to develop gestational diabetes (15.6 % versus 7.2 %; AOR: 2.52, 95 % CI: 1.58–4.65), pre-eclampsia

(8.5 % versus 2.6 %; AOR: 3.43, 95 % CI: 1.72–6.84) or gestational hypertension (12.3 % versus 1.5 %; AOR: 10.24, 95 % CI: 4.67–22.44) than comparison women. Of the 18 (4.9 %) of super-obese women who had antenatal thromboprophylaxis, nine (2.4 %) were given low-molecular weight heparin.

Labour and birth
Compared to the comparison women, the super-obese women were more likely to undergo induction of labour or no labour (Table 4). The likelihood of having caesarean section was significantly higher among super-obese women (51.6 %) than the comparison women (31.7 %) (AOR: 2.73, 95 % CI: 2.02–3.69) with 9.9 % of caesarean section performed under general anaesthesia (Table 3). The most common indications for planned caesarean section were previous CS (72 %, $n = 76$), abnormal fetal presentation (breech, transverse, or unstable lie (18 %, $n = 19$), macrosomia (7 %, $n = 7$) and maternal medical complications (7.5 %, $n = 8$). Shoulder dystocia occurred in 11 (6 %) of super-obese women who gave birth vaginally.

Perinatal outcomes
Birth outcomes were known for 365 (98.6 %) of the super-obese women ($n = 372$ infants, including 7 sets of twins. Super-obese women were significantly more likely to give birth to babies with a birthweight ≥4 500 g (AOR: 19.94, 95 % CI: 6.81–58.36) (Table 4). Thirty-six (9.8 %) of 362 singleton infants born to super-obese women had a birthweight ≥4 500 g, in contrast to 0.8 % ($n = 5/608$) of the singleton infants in the comparison group. Of the 36 singletons with a birthweight ≥4 500 g,

Table 1 Demographic and obstetric characteristics among super-obese and comparison women who gave birth in Australia, 2010

	Super-obese group (N = 370)		Comparison (N = 621)		P value
	No.	%	No.	%	
Age (years)					
< 25	60	16.2	99	15.9	1.00
25–29	109	29.5	185	29.8	
30–34	110	29.7	187	30.1	
≥ 35	91	24.6	150	24.2	
Indigenous status					
No	341	92.2	572	92.1	0.23
Yes	17	4.6	19	3.1	
Not stated	12	3.2	30	4.8	
Marital status					
Single	71	19.2	71	11.4	<0.01
Married/cohabit	277	74.9	508	81.8	
Not stated	22	5.9	42	6.8	
Private health insurance					
No	356	96.2	474	76.3	<0.01
Yes	14	3.8	145	23.3	
Not stated	0	0.0	2	0.3	
Smoking during pregnancy					
No	265	71.6	484	77.9	<0.01
Yes	88	23.8	100	16.1	
Not stated	17	4.6	37	6.0	
Assisted reproductive technology					
No	357	96.5	574	92.4	0.17
Yes	11	3.0	29	4.7	
Not stated	2	0.5	18	2.9	
Parity					
0	115	31.1	251	40.4	<0.01
1–2	173	46.8	313	50.4	
3+	82	22.2	57	9.2	
Multiple gestation pregnancy					
No	362	97.8	608	97.9	0.81
Yes	8	2.2	12	1.9	
Not stated	0	0.0	1	0.2	
Socio-economic status[a]					
Most disadvantage 1	66	17.8	49	7.9	<0.01
2	68	18.4	73	11.8	
3	109	29.5	121	19.5	
4	80	21.6	181	29.1	
Least disadvantage 5	40	10.8	191	30.8	
Not stated	7	1.9	6	1.0	

Table 1 Demographic and obstetric characteristics among super-obese and comparison women who gave birth in Australia, 2010 *(Continued)*

Previous caesarean section (exclude primiparous)					
No	140	54.9	250	67.6	<0.01
Yes	112	43.9	115	31.1	
Not stated	3	1.2	5	1.4	

[a]Socio-Economic Indexes for Areas Index for Relative Socio-economic Disadvantage quintiles assigned to those residents in the most disadvantaged areas to Quintile 1 and those in the least disadvantaged areas to Quintile 5

16.6 % of their mothers had pre-existing diabetes. There was no significant difference in preterm birth between super-obese and comparison women ($n = 39/370$, 10.5 % versus $n = 57/621$, 9.2 %) (Table 4). Of the singletons born to super-obese women, 22.9 % ($n = 83/362$) were admitted to the neonatal intensive care unit (NICU) compared to 13.7 % ($n = 83/608$) of singletons in the comparison group (Table 4). The perinatal mortality rate for the infants born to super-obese women was 11.0 per 1 000 (95 % CI: 4.3–28.0) singleton births which consisted of four stillbirths (one <30 weeks) and no neonatal deaths. There were three stillbirths (2 antepartum and 1 intrapartum) among the infants born in the comparison group (all <30 weeks) and one neonatal death, giving a perinatal mortality rate of 6.6 per 1 000 (95 % CI: 2.6, 16.8) singleton births. Three of the four super-obese

Table 2 Model of care among super-obese and comparison women who gave birth in Australia, 2010

	Super-obese group (N = 370)		Comparison (N = 621)		P value
	No.	%	No.	%	
Lead care provider					
General practitioner	72	19.5	122	19.6	<0.01
Hospital medical	247	66.8	175	28.2	
Hospital midwife	34	9.2	182	29.3	
Private obstetrician	17	4.6	140	22.5	
Not stated	0	0.0	2	0.3	
Changed during pregnancy					
No	312	84.3	566	91.1	<0.01
Yes	56	15.1	55	8.9	
Not stated	2	0.5	0	0.0	
Transfer					
No	326	88.1	596	96.0	<0.01
Yes	44	11.9	25	4.0	
Timing of maternal transfer					
Antepartum	34	77.3	19	76.0	0.77
Intrapartum/Postpartum	9	20.5	6	24.0	
Not stated	1	2.3	1	0.0	

Table 3 Labour and birth characteristics among super-obese and comparison women who gave birth in Australia, 2010

	Super-obese group (N = 370)		Comparison (N = 621)		P value
	No.	%	No.	%	
Multiple births					
Singleton	362	97.8	608	97.9	0.81
Twin	8	2.2	12	1.9	
Not stated	0	0.0	1	0.2	
Labour					
No	125	33.8	139	22.4	<0.01
Yes	241	65.1	482	77.6	
Not stated	4	1.1	0	0.0	
Induction of labour					
No	100	41.5	351	72.8	<0.01
Yes	140	58.1	129	26.8	
Not stated	1	0.4	2	0.4	
Method of birth					
Vaginal birth	176	47.6	424	68.3	<0.01
Caesarean section	191	51.6	197	31.7	
Not stated	3	0.8	0	0.0	
Caesarean section					
Planned	103	53.9	122	61.9	0.1
Unplanned	87	45.5	73	37.1	
Not stated	1	0.5	2	1.0	
Use of general anaesthetic					
No	172	90.1	191	97.0	0.01
Yes	19	9.9	6	3.0	

women who had stillbirths reported gestational hypertension compared to none of the comparison women.

Postpartum maternal complications

Thirteen per cent (49/370) of the super-obese women experienced a postpartum infection; of those, 69 % (n = 34) had undergone a caesarean section. The most common infection was wound infection (n = 25, 51 %) with 12 (24 %) women having multiple complications from infection. Postnatally, 224 (60.5 %) super-obese women received thromboprophylaxis, of these, 78.1 % received low-molecular-weight heparin (LMWH). Postnatal thromboprophylaxis was administered in 29.7 % of super-obese women who gave birth vaginally compared to 90.5 % of super-obese women following caesarean section (p < 0.01). Of the 18 women who did not receive thromboprophylaxis following caesarean section, two women were aged >35 years, six continued to smoke during pregnancy and five had a history of hypertensive disorders (HTD). The median length of stay for super-obese women was 4 days (range 1–32 days). Super-obese women were

significantly more likely to be admitted to a High Dependency Unit (HDU) or Intensive Care Unit (ICU) (6.2 % versus 1.3 %; AOR: 5.67, 95 % CI: 2.31–13.93) compared to the comparison women (Table 4). No maternal deaths were woman reported in either group.

Discussion

Super-obesity was reported in more than 1 in 500 women giving birth in Australia with these women experiencing higher rates of obstetric complications and adverse perinatal outcomes. Compared to other women, the birth experience of super-obese women was characterised by higher rates of caesarean section, general anaesthesia, admission to HDU and ICU and hospital transfer. Fewer than one in 10 super-obese women accessed a midwifery led model of care or private obstetric care with the usual model of care being a hospital-based, medical model. Super-obese women had more than twice the risk of caesarean section (CS) with almost half of the CS unplanned and around 10 % conducted under general anaesthesia. Maternal obesity may be an independent risk factor for CS as it interferes with the progress of labour, specifically the arrest of dilation in active phase labour [13]. The higher rate of CS has been explained in other studies by the association of super-obesity with conditions such as gestational diabetes, gestational hypertension and preeclampsia [14–16], all of which were more prevalent in women in our study. This is consistent with other research including comparison with other obese women (BMI 30.0–49.9 kg/m^2) [5]. Other studies of super-obese women (BMI ≥ 50 kg/m^2) have reported higher rates of both early preeclampsia (AOR: 2.97, 95 % CI: 2.07- 4.26) and late preeclampsia (AOR: 4.79, 95 % CI: 4.26–5.39) compared with normal weight mothers (BMI = 18.5–24.9 kg/m^2) [6]. While clinicians have raised concerns about ability to monitor progress of labour and assess fetal wellbeing in obese women [17], it is argued that there is insufficient evidence to justify a routine policy of CS for all super-obese women solely because of higher recorded rates of complications, but that the mode of birth should be based on a careful assessment of risk factors [18]. Hospital guidelines and other recommendations would suggest thromboprophylaxis for women in the study group who had caesarean sections is warranted. There is, however, little or no differentiation of risk according to degree of obesity [19–21]; although Martin et al. highlights the dose–response of increased risk of thromboembolic events and eclampsia as BMI increases and suggests this can be usefully applied to other pregnancy-related complications [16]. This amplified risk of morbidity according to BMI is consistent with the Mbah study discussed earlier and showed a significantly increased risk of preeclampsia between super-obese women (BMI ≥ 50 kg/m^2

Table 4 Maternal, obstetric and perinatal outcomes among super-obese and comparison women who gave birth in Australia, 2010[a]

	Super-obese group (N = 370) %	Comparison (N = 621) %	OR	AOR[b]
Complications during pregnancy				
Medical problems during pregnancy	33.3	13	3.35 (2.43–4.62)	2.89 (2.64–4.11)
Obstetric problems during pregnancy	42	23.2	2.40 (1.81–3.17)	2.42 (1.77–3.29)
Gestational diabetes	15.6	7.2	2.36 (1.56–3.59)	2.52 (1.58–4.65)
Gestational hypertension	12.3	1.5	9.33 (4.50–19.33)	10.24 (4.67–22.44)
Preeclampsia	8.5	2.6	3.42 (1.85–6.35)	3.43 (1.72–6.84)
Obstetric				
Labour	65.8	77.6	0.55 (0.42–0.74)	0.49 (0.35–0.68)
Induction of labour	58.3	26.9	3.81 (2.75–5.28)	4.33 (3.21–6.24)
Caesarean section	52	31.7	2.33 (1.79–3.65)	2.73 (2.02–3.69)
Perinatal outcomes (singletons only)				
Birthweight ≥4500 g	10.1	0.8	13.44 (5.22–34.57)	19.94 (6.81–58.36)
Admitted to NICU	23.7	13.9	1.93 (1.38–2.71)	1.83 (1.27–2.65)
Need for transfer	8.5	2.7	3.39 (1.82–6.31)	3.81 (1.93–7.55)
Preterm birth <37 weeks	10.1	8.1	1.28 (0.81–2.00)	1.18 (0.72,1.93)
Maternal outcomes				
Admission to ICU	2.2	0.5	4.56 (1.25–17.32)	7.38 (1.52–35.87)
Admission to HDU	4.3	0.8	5.58 (2.43–15.37)	5.40 (1.78–16.38)
Admission to either ICU or HDU	6.2	1.3	5.09 (2.25–11.51)	5.67 (2.31–13.93)

OR odds ratio, AOR adjusted odds ratio, NICU neonatal intensive care unit, ICU intensive care unit, HDU high dependency unit
[a]Table 4 data excludes not stated and this may produce discrepant results to previous tables where not stated is included
[b]Outcomes are adjusted for age, Indigenous status, marital status, private health insurance, smoking during pregnancy, assisted reproductive technology, parity, multiple gestation pregnancy, and Socio-Economic Indexes for Areas Index for Relative Socio-economic Disadvantage

adjusted odds ratio 4.71 [4.20–5.28]) compared to women with Class III obesity (3.75 [3.59–3.92] [6].

The number of infants with birth weight > 4500 g found in our cohort is similar to the UKOSS study of super-obese women that reported a rate of almost nine percent [7]. The long term clinical impact of a high birthweight is unknown. While some studies [22] suggest these infants may have higher rates of obesity and metabolic syndrome in adolescence and adulthood, whether this is a product of the intrauterine environment or of growing up in an environment where children are exposed to sociodemographic factors that promote the development of obesity is uncertain. There were elevated rates of admission of infants to special and intensive care units placing a higher burden on the health system. A perinatal mortality rate of 11.0 per 1000 was not different to that in the comparison group or to national Australian data [23] and was slightly lower than that reported in the UKOSS study on super-obese women (16.0 per 1000) [7]. There was no difference in the rate of preterm birth among super-obese group, so any difference in perinatal outcomes was not related to prematurity.

The rising prevalence of obesity in Australian women of reproductive age suggests that strategies of weight loss, diet, exercise and bariatric surgery have been of limited benefit or that women are not aware of the potential health adverse outcomes associated with obesity in pregnancy. Our study finds that 2.1 per 1000 women giving birth in Australia are super-obese. The Royal Australia and New Zealand College of Obstetricians and Gynaecologists (RANZCOG) recommends pre-conception management of obesity and weight loss through lifestyle approaches of exercise and nutrition, bariatric surgery, nutritional supplementation and psychosocial support. It also recommends that women should have their BMI measures at their first antenatal consultation and, if indicated, multidisciplinary care should be organised to advise and monitor about gestational weight gain, nutritional supplementation, exercise and ensure access to antenatal facilities with appropriate equipment [24].

The National Institute for Health and Clinical Excellence has recommended bariatric surgery as a first-line option for adults with BMI > 50 kg/m[2], instead of lifestyle interventions or drug treatment [25]. Studies have shown that super-obese women who had bariatric surgery prior to pregnancy had lower rates of gestational hypertension, pre-eclampsia, gestational diabetes, and macrosomic infants compared with super-obese women who had not had surgery [26–28]. Nutritional deficiencies during pregnancy have been reported among women following bariatric surgery [29] and nutritional follow-up and careful weight gain management should be provided. A recent systematic review suggests that antenatal interventions targeting diet and/or physical activity have mixed results [30]. Some studies show a reduction in maternal weight gain from antenatal dietary intervention but no effect on maternal or infant morbidity. This may reflect the limitation of intervention being focused on dietary advice alone rather than a more holistic approach which provides support for the woman and her general wellbeing. There are little data on interventions in super obese women. Interventions in the postnatal period should be considered to encourage postpartum weight loss and improve outcomes in subsequent pregnancies [31].

A strength of this study was the use of a comparison group that was representative of the women giving birth in Australia [23]. This allowed investigation of whether there was an increased clinical impact and associated burden on health services for women with super obesity. Martin et al. [16] suggest the need for differential management of super-obese pregnant women compared to the lower range of BMI 40–49.9 kg/m^2, including the need for larger antibiotic dosage for women with BMIs of >50 kg/m^2 to that of women with BMI of >35 kg/m^2, and a need for more research on the specific anticoagulation requirements according to tiered classification of obesity [5, 16]. A limitation of this approach is that it potentially decreases the capacity to detect difference in our study between the super-obese group and the comparison group in maternal and perinatal outcomes due to the inclusion of obese women in the comparison group.

A limitation of the study was that there was no specific question on whether the super-obese women had previous bariatric surgery. There was a question on previous abdominal surgery with a free text response possible. Interestingly, nine super-obese women and one control reported gastric banding suggesting that any further research on super-obese women should include questions on bariatric surgery and laparoscopic-bands. Pre conception options for super-obese women may be the insertion of an adjustable laparoscopic band or gastric sleeve procedure prior to pregnancy. These procedures are associated with fewer nutritional deficiencies than bariatric surgery, and several observational studies have reported encouraging results, including lower incidence of gestational diabetes, pregnancy induced hypertension and lower weight gain during pregnancy. However women with adjustable laparoscopic bands require close monitoring from

a multidisciplinary team and may need the band adjusted during pregnancy, especially in women with frequent vomiting [32]. Adjustable laparoscopic band surgery and or gastric sleeves are rarely available in the public or Medicare funded hospital system in Australia. In our sample of super obese women, only 3.8 % had private health insurance, and over one third were from the two least advantaged quintiles of socio-economic status, suggesting that lap band surgery pre-pregnancy may not be an option for many women.

Measurement error of BMI is another potential limitation of the study. Despite recommendations for maternal BMI to be recorded at the booking visit [24, 33] this was not done at all participating AMOSS sites nor were serial measures of BMI throughout pregnancy available. In a separate survey to participating sites in 2010, BMI at booking was routinely undertaken at 74 % of the 195 sites that responded. There may be some information bias regarding the BMI as weight and/or height could be self-reported or measured depending upon the maternity unit practice. At this level of obesity, some error in the BMI precision is likely to have minimal impact on the generalisability of the results, as alternative measures such as skinfolds are impractical and unreliable in general clinical practice.

A potential limitation of the study was the incremental participation of maternity sites in AMOSS over the course of the study which may have impacted recruitment of cases. Conversely, a strength of the study is that the findings are consistent with routine perinatal data which also demonstrates variation in the prevalence of super-obesity across jurisdictions ranging from 1.8 per 1000 births in NSW [34] to 3.67 per 1000 in Queensland [35] and 4.68 per 1000 births in Western Australia [36]. A second strength was the distribution of participating sites which was representative of Australian maternity services [37].

The increasing prevalence of super-obesity has important implications for maternity services as the evidence suggests current strategies have had limited impact. Super-obesity is associated with and may be a manifestation of complex socio-economic disadvantage and needs innovative interventions and strategies to address underlying health inequity. This study found over a third of super-obese women were in the two most disadvantaged quintiles with only 10.8 % in the least disadvantaged and confirms previous research findings of lower socio-economic status being associated with super-obesity [38–41]. Super obese women risk substantial co-morbidity affecting both them and their offspring. This calls for targeted strategies to address weight gain before, within and between pregnancies, that are appropriate, collaborative and provide training for clinicians within the health services. In the absence of effective interventions to enable women to lose weight (or maintain weight) during pregnancy, super-obese women planning a pregnancy should be supported to make lifestyle changes or consider laparoscopic band, gastric sleeve or bariatric surgery prior to pregnancy.

Conclusions

The findings from our study underline the imperative to prioritise initiatives that address the increased perinatal risks of super-obese women and their babies. The overall resource burden of maternity care for super-obese women was evident with higher rates of obstetric and medical complications, intervention in pregnancy and childbirth, and for infants postnatally. Super-obesity in pregnancy is associated with social disadvantage. There is an urgent need to address pre-pregnancy and pregnancy care and ensure that appropriate initiatives are in place to reduce associated inequalities in perinatal outcomes and future pregnancies of super-obese women.

Competing interests
The authors declare that they have no competing interests.

Authors' contributions
All authors have contributed to the conducting of this study. EAS designed the study, interpreted data and drafted the manuscript. GV participated in the study design, assisted in drafting the manuscript and acquired data. NJ acquired data and assisted in drafting the manuscript. YAW and ZL conducted the data analysis and assisted in drafting the manuscript. JED, MJP, DE, CSEH, MK, WP, LJP, ZL, CM, EDW, and LC have participated in the study design and/or revised the manuscript critically for important intellectual content. The manuscript has been seen and approved by all authors.

Acknowledgements
The National Health and Medical Research Council Project Grant (Application 510298) for funding The Australian Maternity Outcomes Surveillance System: Improving safety and quality of maternity care in Australia (AMOSS) from 2008–2012. We acknowledge the significant support of participating maternity units and AMOSS data collectors in Australia and New Zealand who participated in the study, as well as the AMOSS Associate Investigators and AMOSS Advisory Group. We acknowledge Yelena Fridgant who assisted in data preparation.

Author details
[1]Faculty of Health, University of Technology Sydney, PO Box 123, Broadway NSW, 2007 Sydney, Australia. [2]School of Women's and Children's Health, The University of New South Wales, Sydney, Australia. [3]School of Women's and Infants' Health, The University of Western Australia, Perth, Australia. [4]Department of Obstetrics and Gynaecology Medical School College of Medicine, Biology and Environment, The Australian National University, Canberra, Australia. [5]Obstetrics and Gynaecology, Centenary Hospital for Women and Children, Canberra, Australia. [6]School of Medicine, Griffith University, Queensland, Australia. [7]Gold Coast University Hospital, Queensland, Australia. [8]National Perinatal Epidemiology Unit, University of Oxford, Oxford, United Kingdom. [9]Obstetrics and Gynaecology, National Women's Health, Auckland City Hospital, Auckland, New Zealand. [10]Judith Lumley Centre, La Trobe University, Melbourne, Australia. [11]Department of Nursing, Melbourne School of Health Sciences, The University of Melbourne, Melbourne, Australia. [12]Muru Marri Indigenous Health Unit, School of Public Health and Community Medicine, The University of New South Wales, Sydney, Australia. [13]Royal Brisbane and Women's Hospital, Brisbane, Australia. [14]School of Medicine, The University of Queensland, Brisbane, Australia.

References
1. OECD. Health at a Glance 2013: OECD Indicators. Edited by EOECD. Paris, France: OECD Publishing; 2013.
2. Hilder L, Zhichao Z, Parker M, Jahan S, Chambers G. Australia's mothers and babies 2012. AIHW, editor. Perinatal statistics series no 30. Canberra: AIHW; 2014.
3. Mason EE, Doherty C, Maher JW, Scott DH, Rodriguez EM, Blommers TJ. Super obesity and gastric reduction procedures. Gastroenterol Clin N Am. 1987;16(3):495–502.
4. Marshall NE, Guild C, Cheng YW, Caughey AB, Halloran DR. Maternal superobesity and perinatal outcomes. Am J Obstet Gynecol. 2012;206(5):417. e411–416.
5. Alanis MC, Goodnight WH, Hill EG, Robinson CJ, Villers MS, Johnson DD. Maternal super-obesity (body mass index > or = 50) and adverse pregnancy outcomes. Acta Obstet Gynecol Scand. 2010;89(7):924–30.
6. Mbah A, Kornosky J, Kristensen S, August E, Alio A, Marty P, et al. Super-obesity and risk for early and late pre-eclampsia. Br J Obstet Gynaecol. 2010;117(8):997–1004.
7. Knight M, Kurinczuk J, Spark P, Brocklehurst P, on behalf of the UK Obstetric Surveillance System (UKOSS). Extreme Obesity in Pregnancy in the United Kingdom. Am Coll Obstet Gynecol. 2010;115(5):9.
8. McIntyre HD, Gibbons KS, Flenady VJ, Callaway LK. Overweight and obesity in Australian mothers: epidemic or endemic? Med J Aust. 2012;196(3):184–8.
9. Halliday LE, Peek MJ, Ellwood DA, Homer C, Knight M, McLintock C, et al. The Australasian Maternity Outcomes Surveillance System: An evaluation of stakeholder engagement, usefulness, simplicity, acceptability, data quality and stability. Aust N Z J Obstet Gynaecol. 2012;53(2):152–7.
10. Lindquist A, Noor N, Sullivan E, Knight M. The impact of socioeconomic position on severe maternal morbidity outcomes among women in Australia: a national case–control study. BJOG. 2014. doi:10.1111/1471-0528.13058.
11. ABS. Census of Population and Housing: Socio-Economic Indexes for Areas (SEIFA), Australia, 2011,. In. Edited by ABS. Canberra ACT; 2013.
12. Vaughan G, Pollock W, Peek MJ, Knight M, Ellwood D, Homer CS, et al. Ethical issues: The multi-centre low-risk ethics/governance review process and AMOSS. Aust N Z J Obstet Gynaecol. 2012;52(2):195–203.
13. Verdiales M, Pacheco C, Cohen WR. The effect of maternal obesity on the course of labor. J Perinat Med. 2009;37(6):651–5.
14. Chu S, Kim S, Schmid C, Dietz P, Callaghan W, Lau J, et al. Maternal obesity and risk of cesarean delivery: a meta-analysis. Obesity Reviews. 2007;8(5):385–94.
15. Poobalan A, Aucott L, Gurung T, Smith W, Bhattacharya S. Obesity as an independent risk factor for elective and emergency caesarean delivery in nulliparous women–systematic review and meta-analysis of cohort studies. Obesity Reviews. 2009;10(1):28–35.
16. Martin A, Krishna I, Ellis J, Paccione R, Badell M. Super obesity in pregnancy: difficulties in clinical management. J Perinatol. 2014;34(7):495–502.
17. Schmied VA, Duff M, Dahlen HG, Mills AE, Kolt GS. 'Not waving but drowning': a study of the experiences and concerns of midwives and other health professionals caring for obese childbearing women. Midwifery. 2011;27(4):424–30.
18. Homer CSE, Kurinczuk JJ, Spark P, Brocklehurst P, Knight M. Planned vaginal delivery or planned caesarean delivery in women with extreme obesity. BJOG. 2011;118(4):480–6.
19. McLintock C, Brighton T, Chunilal S, Dekker G, McDonnell N, McRae S, et al. Recommendations for the prevention of pregnancy-associated venous thromboembolism. ANZJOG. 2012;52:3–13.
20. National Health and Medical Research Council: Clinical practice guideline for the prevention of venous thromboembolism (deep vein thrombosis and pulmonary embolism) in patients admitted to Australian hospitals. Melbourne: NHMRC; 2009.
21. The Women's Hospital: Thromboprophylaxis. Caesarean Section. In: Policy, Guideline and Procedure Manual. Melbourne: The Women's Hospital; 2013. p. 4.
22. Catalano PM, Ehrenberg HM. The short- and long-term implications of maternal obesity on the mother and her offspring. BJOG. 2006;113(10):1126–33.
23. Li Z, Zeki R, Hilder L, Sullivan EA. Australia's mothers and babies 2010. In: Perinatal statistics series no 27 Cat no PER 57. Canberra: AIHW National Perinatal Epidemiology and Statistics Unit; 2012.
24. RANZCOG: Management of Obesity in Pregnancy. College statement., vol. C-Obs 49. Melbourne: RANZCOG; 2013: 9.
25. National Institute for Health and Clinical Excellence: Obesity: Guidance on the prevention, identification, assessment and management of overweight

and obesity in adults and children. Edited by National Institute for Health and Clinical Excellence (NIHCE); 2006.

26. Dalfra MG, Busetto L, Chilelli NC, Lapolla A. Pregnancy and foetal outcome after bariatric surgery: a review of recent studies. J Matern Fetal Neonatal Med. 2012;25(9):1537–43.

27. Lapolla A, Marangon M, Dalfra MG, Segato G, De Luca M, Fedele D, et al. Pregnancy outcome in morbidly obese women before and after laparoscopic gastric banding. Obes Surg. 2010;20(9):1251–7.

28. Weintraub AY, Levy A, Levi I, Mazor M, Wiznitzer A, Sheiner E. Effect of bariatric surgery on pregnancy outcome. Int J Gynaecol Obstet. 2008;103(3):246–51.

29. Eerdekens A, Debeer A, Van Hoey G, De Borger C, Sachar V, Guelinckx I, et al. Maternal bariatric surgery: adverse outcomes in neonates. Eur J Pediatr. 2010;169(2):191–6.

30. Dodd J, Grivell R, Crowther C, Robinson J. Antenatal interventions for overweight or obese pregnant women: a systematic review of randomised trials. BJOG. 2010;117:1316–26.

31. van der Pligt P, Willcox J, Hesketh KD, Ball K, Wilkinson S, Crawford D, et al. Systematic review of lifestyle interventions to limit postpartum weight retention: implications for future opportunities to prevent maternal overweight and obesity following childbirth. Obes Rev. 2013;14(10):792–805.

32. Vrebosch L, Bel S, Vansant G, Guelinckx I, Devlieger R. Maternal and neonatal outcome after laparoscopic adjustable gastric banding: a systematic review. Obes Surg. 2012;22(10):1568–79.

33. Callaway LK, Prins JB, Chang AM, McIntyre HD. The prevalence and impact of overweight and obesity in an Australian obstetric population. Med J Aust. 2006;184(2):56–9.

34. NSW Department of Health. ObstetriX Perinatal data collection. Edited by NSW Department of Health. Sydney: NSW Department of Health; 2010.

35. Queensland Health. Perinatal data collection. Edited by Queensland Health. Brisbane: Queensland Health; 2010.

36. Western Australia Department of Health. Perinatal data collection. Edited by WA Department of Health. Perth: Western Australia Department of Health; 2010.

37. Homer CSE, Biggs J, Vaughan G, Sullivan EA. Mapping maternity services in Australia: location, classification and services. Aust. Health Rev. 2011;35(2):222-9

38. Heslehurst N, Ells LJ, Simpson H, Batterham A, Wilkinson J, Summerbell CD. Trends in maternal obesity incidence rates, demographic predictors, and health inequalities in 36 821 women over a 15-year period. BJOG: An International Journal of Obstetrics & Gynaecology. 2007;114(2):187–94.

39. Kim SY, Dietz P, England L, Morrow B, Callaghan WM. Trends in pre-pregnancy obesity in nine states, 1993-2003. Obesity. 2007;15(4):986–93.

40. Nagahawatte NT, Goldenberg RL. Poverty, Maternal Health, and Adverse Pregnancy Outcomes. Annals of the New York Academy of Sciences. 2008;1136(1):80–5.

41. Australian Institute of Health and Welfare. Australia's health 2014. Canberra: AIHW, 2014

Changes in the biochemical and immunological components of serum and colostrum of overweight and obese mothers

Mahmi Fujimori[1], Eduardo L. França[2], Vanessa Fiorin[3], Tassiane C. Morais[1,2], Adenilda C. Honorio-França[2]* and Luiz C. de Abreu[1]

Abstract

Background: Obesity in pregnancy is associated with systemic inflammation, immunological changes and adverse maternal-fetal outcomes. Information on the association between maternal obesity and breast milk composition is scarce. This study describes changes and relationships between biochemical and immunological parameters of colostrum and serum of overweight and obese women.

Methods: Colostrum and blood samples were collected from 25 normal weight, 24 overweight and 19 obese women for determination of glucose, total protein, triglycerides, cholesterol, immunoglobulins, complement proteins (C3 and C4), fat and calorie content and C-reactive protein (CRP).

Results: Glucose was higher in colostrum of obese women ($p = .002$). In normal weight and obese women, total protein content was higher in colostrum than in serum ($p = .001$). Serum triglycerides ($p = .008$) and cholesterol ($p = .010$) concentrations were significantly higher in overweight and obese women than in their normal weight counterparts, but in colostrum their concentrations were similar across the three groups. Secretory IgA (sIgA) in colostrum and IgA in serum concentrations were significantly higher ($p = .001$) in overweight and obese mothers, whereas IgG and IgM concentrations did not vary among the groups ($p = .825$). Serum C3 ($p = .001$) and C4 ($p = .040$) concentrations were higher in obese women. No differences in colostrum complement proteins were detected among the groups. Calorie content ($p = .003$) and fat ($p = .005$) concentrations in colostrum and serum CRP ($p = .002$) were higher in obese women.

Conclusions: The results corroborate the hypothesis that colostrum of overweight and obese women undergoes biochemical and immunological changes that affect its composition, namely increasing glucose concentrations, calorie content, fat and sIgA concentrations.

Keywords: Colostrum, Obesity, Antibody, Complement protein, Fat

Background

Breastfeeding promotion is one of the main strategies for reducing child mortality worldwide [1]. Breast milk contains a balanced content of macro and micronutrients that are essential for infant growth and development, and several immunological components that provide protection to newborns [2–4]. Antibodies, complement proteins, hormones, immunocompetent cells [3, 5–9] cytokines [10–12] and other milk components appear to play a role in the modulation and development of the immune system and inflammatory responses of newborns.

In recent decades, due to changes in lifestyle the incidence of overweight and obesity are increasing among breast-feeding mothers. Obesity and overweight are common metabolic disorders and their growing frequencies worldwide are a major public health concern [13]. Obesity has been shown to increase the expression and secretion of proinflammatory cytokines such as tumor necrosis alpha factor (TNF-α) and interleukin 6 (IL-6) and raises plasma C-reactive protein (CRP) concentrations, leading to the chronic low-grade inflammation that characterizes the disease [14] and appears to play a central role in the

* Correspondence: adenildachf@gmail.com
[2]Institute of Biological and Health Science, Federal University of Mato Grosso, Barra do Garças, MT, Brazil
Full list of author information is available at the end of the article

development of a variety of metabolic disorders and hormonal dysfunctions [15–17]. The fact that obesity affects components of the cellular and humoral immune response may result in a state of immunodeficiency [18]. Epidemiological and clinical findings corroborate this, showing a higher incidence and severity of infectious diseases in the obese [19].

The risks associated with obesity become even more relevant in women of reproductive age [20, 21] because pregnancy is another condition that affects immune response. Moreover, excess weight during pregnancy contributes to increasing perinatal morbidity and mortality, posing risks of long-term consequences for mother and child [22].

Other studies show that chronic inflammation caused by obesity may be related to an exaggerated inflammatory response in the placenta of pregnant women, with an accumulation of macrophages and pro-inflammatory mediators [23]. However, it is unclear whether the effects of obesity in pregnancy are accompanied by changes in colostrum composition in the post partum period.

Changes in maternal metabolism and immunological response may affect the developing immune system of newborns because of the intense interplay between mother and child during pregnancy and breastfeeding. To clarify this issue, the present study investigated the association between maternal weight and immunological, biochemical and nutritional parameters of colostrum.

Methods

This cross-sectional study evaluated 68 mothers (18–36 years of age), divided into three groups according to their prepregnancy body mass index (BMI): normal weight ($n = 25$); overweight ($n = 24$) and obese ($n = 19$). Group definition was based on the World Health Organization [24] criterion, considering normal weight for BMI 18.5–24.9, overweight for BMI 25–29.9, and obesity for BMI of 30 or more. Participants were recruited from the Pregnancy and Obstetric Service of the Maria José dos Santos Stein Hospital, managed by the School of Medicine of ABC, Santo André, SP, Brazil. The volunteers signed an informed consent form before entering the study, which was approved by the local ethics committee of the Faculty of Public Health of the University of São Paulo (Protocol Number CAAE: 05269612.7.0000.5421).

A number of variables were controlled in both groups. These patients were characterized by the age, gestational age at delivery, smoking status, hypertension, body mass indexes before pregnancy, diabetes prior to pregnancy and gestational diabetes.

Inclusion and exclusion criteria

The inclusion criteria were as follows: (a) women with breasts without nipple fissures or mastitis; (b) who were exclusively breastfeeding their babies; and (c) signed a Consent Form. Women with multiple pregnancies, fetal malformations and deliveries before the 37th week of gestation were excluded.

Colostrum sampling

About 48–72 h post-partum, 10 mL colostrum was collected from the volunteers. Supernatant was obtained by colostrum centrifugation at 160 × g for 10 min at 4 °C. The upper fat layer was discarded, and the aqueous supernatant was stored at –80 °C for later biochemical and immunological analyses.

Blood sampling

Samples of 10 mL of blood were collected prior to the beginning of labor from each mother in tubes without anticoagulant and the blood samples were centrifuged at 160 × g for 15 min, until serum separation. Serum samples were stored individually at –80 °C for further glucose, enzyme and protein determination.

Glucose determination

Glucose concentrations of colostrum supernatant and maternal serum were determined by the enzymatic system [25]. Samples of 20 µL colostrum, serum and standard of 100 mg/dL (BioTécnica®, Ref 10.008.00, Brazil) were placed in 2.0 mL phosphate buffer solution (0.05 M, pH7.45, with aminoantipyrine 0.03 mM, 15 mM sodium p-hydroxybenzoate, 12 kU/L glucose oxidase and 0.8 kU/L peroxidase). The suspensions were mixed and incubated for 5 min at 37 °C. The reactions were read on a spectrophotometer at 510 nm.

Total protein determination

Total protein of colostrum supernatant and maternal serum was determined by the Biuret colorimetric method [25]. Samples of 20 µL of colostrum, serum and standard of 4 g/dL (BioTécnica®, Ref 10.009.00, Brazil) were placed in 1.0 mL Biuret reagent (ions of copper in alkaline medium). The suspensions were mixed and incubated for 10 min at 37 °C. The reactions were read on a spectrophotometer at 545 nm.

Cholesterol determination

Cholesterol concentrations of colostrum supernatant and maternal serum were determined by enzymatic colorimetric method [26]. Samples of 10 µL colostrum/ serum and standard of 200 mg/dL BioTécnica®, Ref 10.004.00, Brazil), were placed in 1 mL of buffer solution (100 mmol/L, pH 7.0; Sodium cholate 8 mmol/L; cholesterol esterase 750 U/L; Cholesterol oxidase/200 U/L; Peroxidase > 2000 U/L; 4-aminoantipyrine 0.6 mmol; phenol 20 mmol /L; Sodium azide 0.05 % v/v). The suspensions were mixed and incubated for 10 min at 37 °C. The reactions were read on a spectrophotometer at 505 nm.

Triglycerides determination

Triglycerides concentrations in colostrum supernatant and maternal serum were determined by the enzymatic colorimetric method [26]. Samples of 10 μL of colostrum/serum, standard of 200 mg/dL (BioTécnica®, Ref 10.010.00, Brazil), were placed in 1.0 mL of buffer solution (50 mmol/L pH 7.2 Glicerol kinase/1000 U/L; Peroxidase/1000 U/L; Lipoprotein lipase/2000 U/Ll; Glycerol-3-phosphate oxidase/5000 U/L; 4-chlorophenol 2.7 mmol/L; 4-aminoantipyrine 0.3 mmol/L; ATP - adenosine triphosphate 2.0 mmol/L; Sodium azide 0.01 % v/v). The suspensions were mixed and incubated for 10 min at 37 °C. The reactions were read on a spectrophotometer at 505 nm.

Immunoglobulin, C3 and C4 complement determination

The immunoglobulin (Ig), complement protein (C) 3 and 4 concentrations in colostrum and serum were determined by turbidimetric method [11].

For sIgA in colostrum and IgA in serum determinations, the samples were diluted at 1:5 (v/v) with saline solution (9 g/L), for IgM at 1:11 (v/v) and for IgG at 1:15 (v/v), and the antibody concentrations were determined using IgA (Bioclin®, Brazil, Ref K061), IgM (Bioclin®, Brazil, Ref K063) and IgG antiserum (Bioclin®, Brazil, Ref K062) diluted at 1:12 (v/v). A calibration curve obtained by the Multical (Bioclin®, Brazil, Ref K064) calibrator was used to determine the standard curve for each immunoglobulin. Samples of colostrum, serum, standards, positive and negative control sera were placed in 500 μL of buffer solution (sodium chloride 0.15 moL/L, Tris 50 mmol/L, 6.0000 PEG 50 g/L, sodium azide 15.38 nmol/L). The suspensions were mixed and incubated at 37 °C for 10 min. The reactions were read on a spectrophotometer at 340 nm.

For C3 and C4 concentration determination the samples (colostrum and serum) were diluted at 1:12 (v/v) with saline solution (9 g/L), and the C3 and C4 concentrations in sample supernatants were determined using C3 and C4 antiserum (Bioclin®, Brazil) diluted at 1:12 (v/v). A calibration curve obtained by the Multical (Bioclin®, Brazil), Ref K064) calibrator was used to determine the standard curve. Ten microliter samples of colostrum, serum, standards, positive and negative control sera were placed in 500 μL of buffer solution (sodium chloride 0:15 mol/L, Tris 50 mmol/L, 6.0000 PEG 50 g/L, sodium azide 15:38 nmol/L). The suspensions were mixed and incubated at 37 °C for 15 min. The reactions were read on a spectrophotometer at 340 nm.

Creamatocrit analysis

Colostrum samples were water-bath-heated at 40 °C for 15 min and subjected to vortex mixing. Capillary tubes (2 μL) were filled to approximately three quarters with the samples, sealed with sealing wax and centrifuged for 15 min. Centrifugation separated the samples into cream

and serum [2]. The cream column and the total column were measured, and fat and Kcal content calculated using the following formulae:

$$\text{Fat content} = \% \text{ cream} - 0.59/1.46, \text{ where the } \% \text{ cream}$$
$$= \text{ cream column (mm)}$$
$$\times \ 100 \text{ /total column (mm)};$$

$$\text{Kcal/L} = (68.8 \times \% \text{ cream}) + 290$$

C-Reactive Protein assay

C-Reactive Protein (CRP) concentrations in human colostrum and serum were measured using the PCR Turbilatex Kit (BioTécnica®, Brazil, Catalog 20.015.00) by turbidimetric method [26]. Samples of 5 μL of colostrum, serum and standard were placed in 1000 μL of solution (phosphate Buffer 40 mmol, sodium azide 0.95 g/L, suspension of latex particles sensitized with goat IgG anti Human C-reactive protein). The suspensions were mixed and placed at 37 °C and the reactions were measured immediately and at 120 s. The reactions were read on a spectrophotometer at 540 nm.

Statistical analysis

Two-way Analysis of variance (ANOVA) with calculation of F statistic and Tukey's multiple comparison test were used to evaluate glucose, total protein, cholesterol, triglycerides, antibody concentration, complement protein, CRP, calories and fat considering the BMI status as one factor and the biological materials (colostrum or serum) as the other. Statistical significance was considered when the p-value was less than .05.

Results

Clinical characteristics from all groups are shown in Table 1. Maternal age, gestational age at birth and height before pregnancy were similar among groups. The cesarean birth percentage was higher in overweight and obese groups. Neonates from the groups studied (normal weight, overweight and obese) exhibited similar somatometry at birth (Table 1).

We evaluated biochemical (Table 2) and immunological (Table 3) parameters in the blood and colostrum of mothers with different body mass index (BMI).

Colostrum glucose concentrations were higher in obese (p = .002) than in overweight and normal weight groups. Serum glucose concentrations were higher (p = .001) than colostrum glucose concentrations in overweight mothers (Table 2). Total protein concentrations were similar (p = .758) across the groups. In normal weight and obese groups, total protein concentrations were higher in colostrum (p = .001) than in maternal serum (Table 2).

Table 1 Clinical characteristics of woman included in the study according to pregestacional BMI group (normal, overweight and obese)

Variables	Normal weight (n = 25)	Overweight (n = 24)	Obese (n = 18)
Mothers			
Age (year)	25.0 (18–37)	24.1 (18–37)	26.8 (21–38)
height before pregnancy (cm)	161.0 (150.0-171.0)	162.8 (150.0-172.0)	160.4 (144.0-189.0)
Weight before pregnancy (kg)	56.2 (43.0-68.5)	71.2 (56.5-82.0)	87.3 (66.0-110.0)
BMI before pregnancy (kg/m^2)	21.4 (18.4-24.4)	26.6 (25.2-28.6)	34.7 (30.1-47.9)
Cesarean (%)	6/25 (24.0 %)	11/24 (45.8 %)	10/18 (55.5 %)
Gestational age at delivery (week)	39.7 (37.0-41.3)	39.5 (37.6-41.0)	39.5 (37.0-40.7)
Primipara (%)	13/25 (52.0 %)	11/24 (45.8 %)	8/18 (44.4 %)
Diabetes	0/25 (0.0 %)	0/24 (0.0 %)	0/18 (0.0 %)
Gestational diabetes	0/25 (0.0 %)	0/24 (0.0 %)	2/18 (11.0 %)
Hypertension	1/25 (4.0 %)	1/24 (4.0 %)	2/18 (11.0 %)
Smoking status	4/25 (16.0 %)	2/24 (8.0 %)	2/18 (11.0 %)
Infants			
Infant gender (% female)	12/25 (48.8 %)	10/24 (41.6 %)	8/18 (44.4 %)
Weight (kg)	3.6 (2.40-4.20)	3.2 (2.54-3.91)	3.4 (2.54-4.34)
Height (cm)	48.1 (44.0-52.0)	48.2 (44.5-53.0)	49.2 (46–52)

Data for all mothers included are shown as median, minimum and maximum values or number and percentages (%)

Intergroup colostrum triglyceride concentrations were similar, but in serum they were significantly higher (p = .008) in the obese group. Irrespective of the BMI, triglyceride concentrations were higher (p = .001) in colostrum than in serum (Table 2). No statistical intergroup differences (p > 0.05) in cholesterol concentrations were detected in colostrum. However, obese women exhibited higher cholesterol concentrations in serum (p = .010) than normal weight individuals. In the obese group, cholesterol concentrations were higher in serum (p = .001) than in colostrum (Table 2).

As shown in Fig. 1 and Table 2, fat (p = .005) and calorie (p = .003) content of colostrum was higher in the obese group. Colostrum CRP concentrations were similar among

Table 2 Biochemical parameters in colostrum and serum from normal weight, overweight and obese mothers

Parameter		Normal weight	Overweight	Obese	Statistical
Glucose concentrations (mmol/L)	Colostrum	1.9 (0.7–2.9) [3]	2.6 (2.1–3.1) [1,3]	3.2 (2.0–4.5) [1,2,3]	F = 5.94; p = .002 (comparing the groups)
	Serum	4.3 (4.2–5.1)	4.4 (3.7–5.4)	4.3 (3.7–5.7)	F = 139.15; p = .001 (comparing the colostrum and serum)
Total Protein (g/L)	Colostrum	101.0 (91.0–115.0) [3]	89.0 (76.0–127.0)	86.0 (61.0–157.0) [3]	F = 0.25; p = .758 (comparing the groups)
	Serum	59.0 (57.0–67.0)	62.5 (58.0–83.0)	66.5 (54.0–76.0)	F = 47.53; p = .001 (comparing the colostrum and serum)
Triglyceride concentrations (mmol/L)	Colostrum	5.3 (2.5–6.6) [3]	5.1 (2.5–6.3) [3]	4.6 (2.6–8.0) [3]	F = 10.59; p = .008 (comparing the groups)
	Serum	1.6 (0.8–2.2)	1.9 (0.9–3.3)	2.9 (2.0–5.5) [1]	F = 57.47; p = .001 (comparing the colostrum and serum)
Cholesterol concentrations (mmol/L)	Colostrum	4.3 (2.1–6.2)	4.1 (2.7–5.9)	5.2 (2.9–8.2) [3]	F = 5.05; p = .010 (comparing the groups)
	Serum	5.1 (4.7–5.4)	5.4 (4.6–5.9)	6.0 (5.2–12.3) [1]	F = 11.08; p = .002 (comparing the colostrum and serum)
CRP concentrations (mg/L)	Colostrum	4.0 (0.0–8.0)	5.0 (0.0–11.0)	6.0 (0.0–12.0)	F = 12.30; p = .002 (comparing the groups)
	Serum	9.0 (5.0–28.0)	16.0 (0.0–26.0) [3]	85.0 (17.0–201.0) [1,2,3]	F = 20.71; p = .001 (comparing the colostrum and serum)
Fat (%)	Colostrum	3.3 (0.4–6.7)	3.6 (1.2–9.4)	5.6 (2.0–11.9) [1]	F = 7.27; p = .005 (comparing the groups)
Calories (Kcal)	Colostrum	537.9 (396.7–764.3)	543.6 (396.7–944.6)	688.2 (450.3–1111.6) [1]	F = 6.90; p = .003 (comparing the groups)

Data presented as media, minimum and maximum values
[1] Statistically significant differences in relation to the normal weight category, considering the same sample (colostrum or serum)
[2] Statistically significant differences in relation to the overweight category, considering the same sample (colostrum or serum)
[3] Statistically significant differences between colostrum and serum, considering the same group (normal weight, overweight and obese)

Table 3 Immunoglobulins and complement protein concentrations in colostrum and serum from normal weight, overweight and obese mothers

Parameter		Normal weight	Overweight	Obese	Statistical
IgA (g/L)	Colostrum	3.3 (2.3-5.5) [3]	3.8 (2.1-5.0)	5.1 (3.3-9.6) [1,2,3]	F = 12.44; p = .001 (comparing the groups)
	Serum	2.2 (1.6-3.1)	2.7 (2.2-3.5)	3.9 (2.1-4.7) [1]	F = 21.69; p = .002 (comparing the colostrum and serum)
IgM (g/L)	Colostrum	1.3 (0.85-2.2)	1.2 (0.8-2.1)	1.4 (1.0-3.4)	F = 0.19; p = .825 (comparing the groups)
	Serum	1.3 (1.1-1.8)	1.4 (0.8-2.4)	1.0 (0.8-2.0)	F = 1.84; p = .177 (comparing the colostrum and serum)
IgG (g/L)	Colostrum	0.4 (0.1-0.6) [3]	0.3 (0.2-0.5) [3]	0.4 (0.2-0.6) [3]	F = 0.05; p = .947 (comparing the groups)
	Serum	11.3 (9.2-14.2)	9.3 (8.5-16.7)	10.8 (7.6-18.4)	F = 495.8; p = .001 (comparing the colostrum and serum)
C3 (mg/dL)	Colostrum	91.7 (50.5-110.2) [3]	90.3 (44.1-97.9) [3]	95.7 (41.3-130.9) [3]	F = 14.98; p = .001 (comparing the groups)
	Serum	121.1 (109.5-139.3)	152.4 (90.6-250.0)	249.8 (119.1-312.9) [1,2]	F = 117.30; p = .001 (comparing the colostrum and serum)
C4 (mg/dL)	Colostrum	30.1 (15.6-34.8) [3]	24.2 (19.6-40.7) [3]	28.8 (17.7-40.2)	F = 5.91; p = .040 (comparing the groups)
	Serum	16.4 (9.9-25.6)	17.2 (7.1-25.8)	22.9 (13.3-37.1) [1,2]	F = 20.68; p = .001 (comparing the colostrum and serum)

Data presented as median, minimum and maximum values (within parentheses)
[1] Statistically significant differences in relation to the normal weight category, considering the same sample (colostrum or blood)
[2] Statistically significant differences in relation to the overweight category, considering the same sample (colostrum or blood)
[3] Statistically significant differences between colostrum and serum, considering the same group (normal weight, overweight and obese)

the groups, but in serum, they were significantly higher in the obese group (p = .002) than in the other groups. The highest concentrations of CRP (p = .001) were found in serum (Fig. 2 and Table 2).

The obese group showed significantly higher (p = .001) colostrum sIgA and serum IgA concentrations than normal weight women. IgM concentrations did not vary (p = .825) among the groups and between serum and colostrum samples (p = .177). IgG concentrations were significantly higher in serum (p = .001) than in colostrum (Table 3).

In serum, the concentrations of complement proteins C3 (p = .001) and C4 (p = .040) were significantly higher (p = .010) in the obese group than in normal weight and overweight groups, but in colostrum did not differ among the groups. Irrespective of weight status, C3 concentrations were significantly higher in serum (p = .001) than in colostrum, and in normal weight and overweight groups, C4 concentrations were significantly higher in serum (p = .001) than in colostrum samples (Table 3).

Discussion

The immune protection that breast milk provides and its nutritional importance has been widely described, and the composition of this secretion is known to undergo inter-and intra-individual variations [27]. These variations in breast milk can be affected by several factors, such as maternal diet, nutritional status, smoking, parity and period of the day [2, 28, 29].

Other studies report that maternal anemia, hypertension and diabetes can change nutritional and immunological features of breast milk [11, 30–32]. The present study shows that although serum cholesterol, triglycerides, CRP, C3 and C4 protein concentrations were higher in obese women, their concentrations in colostrum were similar across the groups. On the other hand, although glucose and IgA concentrations were similar among serum samples of the different groups, in colostrum samples sIgA concentrations were significantly higher in obese mothers. An increase in glucose concentrations in the breast milk of diabetic women are associated with

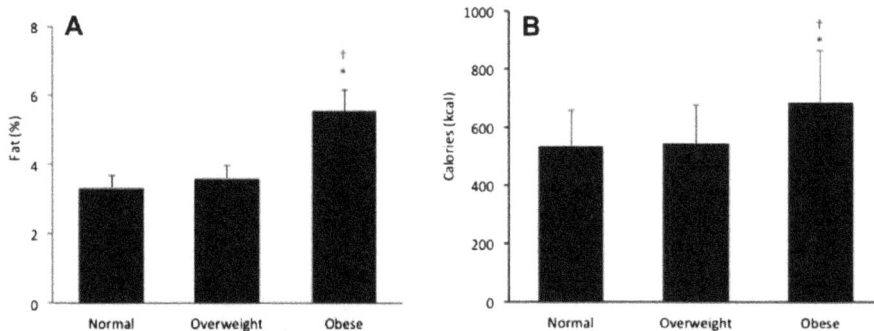

Fig. 1 Fat **a** and calories **b** in the colostrum of normal, overweight and obese mothers. Data presented as mean ± standard error (SE). F(A) = 7.27; p = .005; F(B) = 6.90; p = .003. *Statistically significant differences between normal and obese groups. †Statistically significant differences between overweight and obese groups

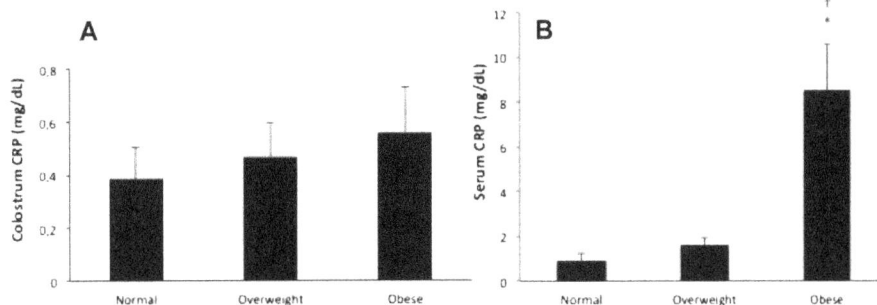

Fig. 2 CRP concentrations in the colostrum **a** and serum **b** of normal, overweight and obese mothers. Data presented as mean ± standard error (SE). F = 12.30; p = .002 comparing the groups; F = 20.71; p = .001 comparing the samples (colostrum and serum). * Statistically significant differences between normal and obese groups. †Statistically significant differences between overweight and obese groups

long-term consequences for their children, such as an increase in weight gain and metabolic changes [33, 34]. This suggests that infants born to and breastfed by women with high prepregnancy BMI may be heavier and predisposed to develop obesity and related disorders in adulthood. Other studies should investigate the effects of maternal weight on the glucose content of breast milk and its impact on infant weight gain and metabolism.

The association between maternal obesity and dyslipidemia has been extensively described [35–37], and it likely contributes to vascular diseases including preeclampsia and the development of macrosomia [38]. The present study also found increased of dyslipidemia markers in higher BMI groups in colostrum samples, given that in obese and overweight groups this secretion contained higher fat and calorie content compared to normal weight women. The effects of maternal BMI on the energy content of breast milk are controversial, with studies showing that fat content in the milk of obese women does not differ from that of other weight classes [39], whereas others report lower fat content in milk from overweight mothers [28].

The immaturity of the immune system of newborns makes it susceptible to infections by viruses and bacteria. Accordingly, the transfer of antibodies *via* placenta during uterine life and then *via* colostrum and breast milk after birth is important in reducing this deficiency [30]. In the present study, overweight and obese mothers exhibited higher IgA concentrations in serum and sIgA concentrations in colostrum than normal weight women. Earlier studies report that obesity increases serum IgA concentrations in both sexes [40]. The present study is the first to evaluate the concentrations of antibodies and complement proteins in colostrum of overweight pregnant women. The increase in sIgA concentrations in colostrum might be associated with conditions determined by the metabolic syndrome, including hyperglycemia, hypertriglyceridemia and abdominal obesity. The mechanisms by which obesity increases sIgA concentrations are not known, but they are

possibly associated with chronic low-grade inflammation, characterized by elevated concentrations of serum pro-inflammatory marker IL-6 [40]. IL-6 is one of the main cytokines in human milk, and its content has been shown to correlate with sIgA concentrations in colostrum in other studies [41, 42].

Unlike IgG, which is transferred transplacentally, the action of immunoprotective components of colostrum and milk is usually local, in the newborn's intestinal mucosa [3]. sIgA is able to inhibit bacterial adhesion and neutralize virus infection in the intestinal mucosa, preventing tissue damage and loss of energy [43] through a non-inflammatory process called immune exclusion [44]. The IgG antibodies activate the complement system and granulocytes and induce cytokine production, which results in inflammation. sIgA can also act as opsonin, signaling the presence of antigens to phagocytes by binding to the surface of bacteria and facilitating aggregation. The opsonizing activity of sIgA is of great biological significance, and given that colostrum is the secretion containing the highest concentration of this antibody class, it provides a complete micro-environment where components found in both its soluble portion and cells act together [3, 44].

The increased serum C3 concentrations in overweight and obese women and serum C4 in the obese group was not accompanied by an increase in these concentrations in colostrum. It was previously reported that obese individuals exhibit higher concentrations of circulating C3 [45, 46] and C4 [47]. The complement system consists of proteins that interact to provide many of the effector functions of humoral immunity and inflammation [45]. C3 and C4, the central components of the complement pathway of the immune system, are synthesized by stimulation of pro-inflammatory cytokines [46]. The C3 and C4 proteins are mainly produced in the liver, but they can also be synthesized and expressed in other tissues such as the adipose [47]. It has been suggested that diagnosis of chronic low-grade inflammation, which characterizes obesity, is responsible for activation of the complement system, which, in turn, would cause the associated metabolic complications [48].

Obese mothers exhibited higher concentrations of serum CRP, but not in colostrum. CRP secretion by the liver is stimulated by several inflammatory cytokines, which are released in response to trauma, infection and inflammation, and this protein rapidly reduces the resolution of these conditions [49]. Another study found an association between serum CRP concentrations and prepregnancy BMI [50]. High CRP concentrations in the amniotic fluid of obese mothers expose the fetus to high amounts of inflammatory mediators, which may contribute to fetal programming, account for various complications during pregnancy and impact health condition in adulthood [51].

It should be considered that these data were evaluated in one period of collection and only one milk maturation stage that may be considered a limitation of this study. It is necessary to continue investigations focusing on other factors that may be involved during breastfeeding of the mothers with BMI alterations.

Conclusions

The data obtained in the present study support the hypothesis that metabolic changes promoted by obesity can change the biochemical and immunological parameters of breast milk. Nevertheless, we did not observe any changes that could cast doubt on the protection that breastfeeding provides to newborns or that could reflect the inflammatory state observed in maternal serum, because the only immunological component that increased in serum the obese women was IgA, which is known to be a non-inflammatory antibody. However, the increased calorie and fat content and glucose concentrations detected in colostrum from obese women deserve further attention.

Competing interests
The authors declare that they have no competing interests.

Authors' contributions
MF carried out the assay, participated in the sequence alignment, and drafted the manuscript. ELF participated in the design of the study and coordination and helped to draft the manuscript. VF participated in the collect of samples, carried out the assays. TCM participated in the collect of samples, carried out the assays and help to draft the manuscript. ACHF carried out the assay, conceived of the study, carried out the assays and participated in its design and coordination and help to draft the manuscript. LCA participated in the design of the study and helped to draft the manuscript. All authors read and approved the final manuscript.

Acknowledgments
This work was supported by Fundação de Amparo a Pesquisa de São Paulo (FAPESP-N° 2012-17843-8; N° 2012-16662-0) and Conselho Nacional de Desenvolvimento Científico e Tecnológico (CNPq-N° 308702/2013-1; N° 475238/2013-3).

Author details
[1]Department of Maternal and Child Health, School of Public Health, University of São Paulo, São Paulo, SP, Brazil. [2]Institute of Biological and Health Science, Federal University of Mato Grosso, Barra do Garças, MT, Brazil. [3]Laboratory of Scientific Writing, Department of Morphology and Physiology, School of Medicine of ABC, Santo André, SP, Brazil.

References
1.   World Health Organization. Obesity: preventing and managing the global epidemic. Report of a WHO consultation, World Health Organization Technical Report Series. Geneva, Switzerland: World Health Organization; 2000.
2.   França EL, Nicomedes TR, Calderon IMP, Honório-França AC. Time-dependent alterations of soluble and cellular components in human milk. Biol Rhythm Res. 2010;41:333–47.
3.   França EL, Bitencourt RV, Fujimori M, Morais TC, Calderon IMP, et al. Human colostral phagocytes eliminate enterotoxigenic Eschechia coli opsonized by colostrum supernatant. J Microbiol Immunol Infec. 2011;44:1–7.
4.   Newburg DS. Innate immunity and human milk. J Nutr. 2005;135:1308–12.
5.   Morceli G, Honorio-França AC, Fagundes DLG, Calderon IMP, França EL. Antioxidant effect of melatonin on the functional activity of colostral phagocytes in diabetic women. PLoS One. 2013;8:e56915.
6.   Fagundes DLG, França EL, Hara CCP, Honorio-França AC. Immunomodulatory effects of poly (ethylene glycol) microspheres adsorbed with cortisol on activity of colostrum phagocytes. Int J Pharmacol. 2012;8:510–8.
7.   Islam SK, Ahmed L, Khan MN, Huque S, Begum A, Yunus AB. Immune components (IgA, IgM, IgG immune cells) of colostrum of Bangladeshi mothers. Pediatr Int. 2006;48:543–8.
8.   Honorio-França AC, Hara CCP, Ormonde JVJ, Triches GN, França EL. Human colostrum melatonin exhibits a day-night variation and modulates the activity of colostral phagocytes. J Appl Biomed. 2013;11:153–62.
9.   Richani K, Soto E, Romero R, Espinoza J, Chaiworapongsa T, Nien JK, et al. Normal pregnancy is characterized by systemic activation of the complement system. J Matern Fetal Neonatal Med. 2005;17:239–45.
10. Fagundes DLG, França EL, Morceli G, Rudge MVC, Calderon IMP, Honório-França AC. The role of cytokines in the functional activity of phagocytes in blood and colostrum of diabetic mothers. Clin Develop Immunol. 2013;2013:1–8.
11. Massmann PF, França EL, Souza EG, Souza MS, Brune MFSS, Honorio-França AC. Maternal hypertension induces alterations in immunological factors of colostrum and human milk. Front Life Sci. 2013;7:155–63.
12. Kverka M, Burianova J, Lodinova-Zadnikova R, Kocourkova I, Cinova J, Tuckova L, et al. Cytokine profiling in human colostrum and milk by protein array. Clin Chem. 2007;53:955–62.
13. World Health Organization. Obesity and Overweight. Fact Sheet#311. 2013. (updated March 2013). [http://www.who.int/mediacentre/factsheets/fs311/en/].
14. Womack J, Tien PC, Feldman J, Shin JH, Fennie K, Anastos K, et al. Obesity and immune cell counts in women. Metabolism. 2007;56:998–1004.
15. Schmatz M, Madan J, Marino T, Davis J. Maternal obesity: the interplay between inflammation, mother and fetus. J Perinatol. 2010;30:441–6.
16. Kopelman P. Health risks associated with overweight and obesity. Obes Rev. 2007;8:13–7.
17. Andreasen KR, Andersen ML, Schantz AL. Obesity and pregnancy. Acta Obstet Gynecol Scand. 2004;83:1022–9.
18. Karlsson EA, Beck MA. The burden of obesity on infectious disease. Exp Biol Med (Maywood). 2010;235:1412–24.
19. Falagas ME, Kompoti M. Obesity and infection. Lancet Infect Dis. 2006;6:438–46.
20. Guelinckx I, Devlieger R, Beckers K, Vansant A. Maternal obesity: pregnancy complication, gestational weight gain and nutrition. Obes Rev. 2008;9:140–50.
21. Poston L, Harthoorn LF, Van der Beek EM. Obesity in pregnancy: implications for the mother and lifelong health of the child. A consensus statement. Pediatr Res. 2011;69:175–8.
22. Thornton CA, Jones RH, Doekhie A, Bryant AH, Beynon AL, Davies JS. Inflammation, obesity, and neuromodulation in pregnancy and fetal development. Adv Neuroimmune Biol. 2011;1:193–203.
23. Challier JC, Basu S, Bintein T, Minium J, Hotmire K, Catalano PM, et al. Obesity in pregnancy stimulates macrophage accumulation and inflammation in the placenta. Placenta. 2008;29:274–81.

24. World Health Organization. Physical status: the use and interpretation of athropometry, World Health Organization Technical Report Series 854. Geneva, Switzerland: World Health Organization; 1995.

25. Morceli G, França EL, Magalhães VB, Damasceno DC, Calderon IMP, Honorio França AC. Diabetes induced immunological and biochemical changes in human colostrum. Acta Paediatr. 2011;100:550–6.

26. Young DS. Effects of drugs on clinical laboratory tests 2. 5th ed. Washington DC: AACC Press; 2000.

27. Hassiotou F, Hepworth AR, Williams TM, Twigger AJ, Perrella S, Lai CT, et al. Breastmilk cell and fat contents respond similarly to removal of breastmilk by the infant. PLoS One. 2013;8:e78232.

28. Ali MA, Strandvik B, Palme-Kilander C, Yngve A. Lower polyamine levels in breast milk of obese mothers compared to mothers with normal body weight. J Hum Nutr Diet. 2013;26:164–70.

29. Bachour P, Yafawi R, Jaber F, Choueiri E, Abdel-Razzak Z. Effects of smoking, mother's age, body mass index, and parity number on lipid, protein, and secretory immunoglobulin A concentrations of human milk. Breastfeed Med. 2012;7:179–88.

30. França EL, Silva VA, Volpato RM, Silva PA, Brune MF, Honorio-França AC. Maternal anemia induces changes in immunological and nutritional components of breast milk. J Matern Fetal Neonatal Med. 2013;26:1223–7.

31. França EL, Calderon IMP, Vieira EL, Morceli G, Honorio-França AC. Transfer of maternal immunity to newborns of diabetic mothers. Clin Develop Immunol. 2012;2012:928187.

32. França EL, Morceli G, Fagundes DLG, Rudge MVC, Calderon IMP, Honorio França AC. Secretory IgA Fcα receptor interaction modulating phagocytosis and microbicidal activity by phagocytes in human colostrum of diabetics. APMIS. 2011;119:710–9.

33. Ahuja S, Boylan M, Hart LS, Román-Shriver C, Spallholz JE, Pence BC, et al. Glucose and insulin levels are increased in obese and overweight mothers' breast-milk. J Nutr Food Sci. 2011;2:201–6.

34. Plagemann A, Harder T, Franke K, Kohlhoff R. Long-term impact of neonatal breast-feeding on body weight and glucose tolerance in children of diabetic mothers. Diabetes Care. 2002;25:16–22.

35. Meyer BJ, Stewart FM, Brown EA, Cooney J, Nilsson S, Olivecrona G, et al. Maternal obesity is associated with the formation of small dense LDL and hypoadiponectinemia in the third trimester. J Clin Endocrinol Metab. 2013;98:643–52.

36. Sanchez-Vera I, Bonet B, Viana M, Quintanar A, Martin MD, Blanco P, et al. Changes in plasma lipids and increased low-density lipoprotein susceptibility to oxidation in pregnancies complicated by gestational diabetes: consequences of obesity. Metab Clin Exp. 2007;56:1527–33.

37. Ramsay JE, Ferrell WR, Crawford L, Wallace AM, Greer IA, Sattar N. Maternal obesity is associated with dysregulation of metabolic, vascular, and inflammatory pathways. J Clin Endocrinol Metab. 2002;87:4231–7.

38. Knopp RH, Magee MS, Walden CE, Bonet B, Benedetti TJ. Prediction of infant birth weight by GDM screening tests. Importance of plasma triglyceride. Diabetes Care. 1992;15:1605–13.

39. Ray J, Diamond P, Singh G, Bell C. Brief overview of maternal triglycerides as a risk factor for pre-eclampsia. BJOG. 2006;113:379–86.

40. Marín MC, Sanjurjo A, Rodrigo MA, de Alaniz MJ. Long-chain polyunsaturated fatty acids in breast milk in La Plata, Argentina: relationship with maternal nutritional status. Prostaglandins Leukot Essent Fatty Acids. 2005;73:355–60.

41. Gonzalez-Quintela A, Alende R, Gude F, Campos J, Rey J, Meijide LM, et al. Serum levels of mmunoglobulins (IgG, IgA, IgM) in a general adult population and their relationship with alcohol consumption, smoking and common metabolic abnormalities. Clin Exp Immunol. 2008;151:42–50.

42. Fujihashi K, McGhee JR, Lue C, Beagley KW, Taga T, Hirano T, et al. Human appendix B cells naturally express receptors for and respond to interleukin 6 with selective IgA1 and IgA2 synthesis. J Clin Invest. 1991;88:248–52.

43. Honorio-França AC, Launay P, Carneiro-Sampaio MMS, Monteiro RC. Colostral neutrophils express IgA Fc receptors (CD89) lacking γ chain association that mediate non-inflammatory properties of secretory IgA. J Leuk Biol. 2001;69:289–96.

44. Honorio-França AC, Carvalho MP, Isaac L, Trabulsi LR, Carneiro-Sampaio MM. Colostral mononuclear phagocytes are able to kill enteropathogenic Escherichia coli opsonized with colostral IgA. Scand J Immunol. 1997;46:59–66.

45. Hernández-Mijares A, Jarabo-Bueno MM, López-Ruiz A, Solá-Izquierdo E, Morillas-Ariño C, Martínez-Triguero ML. Levels of C3 in patients with severe, morbid and extreme obesity: its relationship to insulin resistance and different cardiovascular risk factors. Int J Obes (Lond). 2007;31:927–32.

46. Ritchie RF, Palomaki GE, Neveux LM, Navolotskaia O, Ledue TB, Craig WY. Reference distributions for complement proteins C3 and C4: a practical, simple and clinically relevant approach in a large cohort. J Clin Lab Anal. 2004;18:1–8.

47. Gabrielsson BG, Johansson JM, Lönn M, Jernås M, Olbers T, Peltonen M, et al. High expression of complement components in omental adipose tissue in obese men. Obes Res. 2003;11:699–708.

48. Andrews E, Feldhoff P, Feldhoff R, Lassiter H. Comparative effects of cytokines and cytokine combinations on complement component C3 secretion by HepG2 cells. Cytokine. 2003;23:164–9.

49. Das UN. Is obesity an inflammatory condition? Nutrition. 2001;17:953–66.

50. Stewart FM, Freeman DJ, Ramsay JE, Greer IA, Caslake M, Ferrell WR. Longitudinal assessment of maternal endothelial function and markers of inflammation and placental function throughout pregnancy in lean and obese mothers. J Clin Endocrinol Metab. 2007;92:969–75.

51. Bugatto F, Fernández-Deudero A, Bailén A, Fernández-Macías R, Hervías-Vivancos B, Bartha JL. Second-trimester amniotic fluid proinflammatory cytokine levels in normal and overweight women. Obstet Gynecol. 2010;115:127–33.

Change in level of physical activity during pregnancy in obese women: findings from the UPBEAT pilot trial

Louise Hayes[1*], Catherine Mcparlin[1,3], Tarja I Kinnunen[4], Lucilla Poston[5], Stephen C Robson[2], Ruth Bell[1] and On behalf of the UPBEAT Consortium

Abstract

Background: Maternal obesity is associated with an increased risk of pregnancy complications, including gestational diabetes. Physical activity (PA) might improve glucose metabolism and reduce the incidence of gestational diabetes. The purpose of this study was to explore patterns of PA and factors associated with change in PA in obese pregnant women.

Methods: PA was assessed objectively by accelerometer at 16 – 18 weeks' (T0), 27 – 28 weeks' (T1) and 35 – 36 weeks' gestation (T2) in 183 obese pregnant women recruited to a pilot randomised trial of a combined diet and PA intervention (the UPBEAT study).

Results: Valid PA data were available for 140 (77%), 76 (42%) and 54 (30%) women at T0, T1 and T2 respectively. Moderate and vigorous physical activity as a proportion of accelerometer wear time declined with gestation from a median of 4.8% at T0 to 3% at T2 ($p < 0.05$). Total activity as a proportion of accelerometer wear time did not change. Being more active in early pregnancy was associated with a higher level of PA later in pregnancy. The intervention had no effect on PA.

Conclusions: PA in early pregnancy was the factor most strongly associated with PA at later gestations. Women should be encouraged to participate in PA before becoming pregnant and to maintain their activity levels during pregnancy. There is a need for effective interventions, tailored to the needs of individuals and delivered early in pregnancy to support obese women to be sufficiently active during pregnancy.

Keywords: Maternal obesity, Accelerometer, MVPA, Socio-demographic factors

Background

Gestational diabetes (GDM; defined as diabetes or impaired glucose tolerance that is first recognised during pregnancy [1]) is associated with maternal obesity [2]. Physical activity (PA) during pregnancy might reduce GDM risk. A meta-analysis reported a 24% reduction in GDM incidence among women (unselected for BMI status) who were active in early pregnancy compared to those who were inactive [3]. Current guidance for pregnant women recommends 30 minutes of daily moderate intensity PA [4,5].

Data on objectively measured PA during pregnancy are sparse but indicate that PA declines with gestation [6-8]. Data on obese pregnant women are even more limited but suggest a similar, or greater, decline in PA [9,10]. A recent systematic review concluded that more detailed description of PA in this population was needed [11].

Effective interventions that impact on GDM incidence by supporting obese pregnant women to be active are lacking [12,13]. A better understanding of factors influencing PA during pregnancy would help to inform the development of such interventions.

* Correspondence: louise.hayes@ncl.ac.uk
[1]Institute of Health & Society, Newcastle University, Baddiley-Clark Building, Richardson Road, Newcastle upon Tyne NE2 4AX, UK
Full list of author information is available at the end of the article

We aimed to describe objectively measured PA during pregnancy in obese women enrolled in the UK Pregnancies Better Eating and Activity (UPBEAT) pilot trial [14] and to explore factors associated with PA in these women.

Methods

The UPBEAT trial

UPBEAT aims to improve glycaemic control in obese women through a combined behaviour change intervention targeting PA and diet. (Current Controlled Trials ISRCTN89971375; registered 28/11/2008). A pilot study to determine the effect of the intervention on diet and PA behaviours was undertaken in one hundred and eighty-three obese (BMI $\geq$30 kg/m^2) women, with a singleton pregnancy of 15 to 18 weeks' gestation [14]. Women were recruited from four ante-natal clinics within the UK between March 2009 and May 2011, and were randomised to receive the intervention or standard care. The methods have been reported previously [14]. There was no statistically significant difference between the intervention and control groups in PA measured by accelerometry at baseline or follow-up in the UPBEAT pilot trial. Median (interquartile range) minutes per day active at baseline was 217.4 (171.3, 268.3) in women in the intervention group and 213.7 (167.7, 263.7) in the control group (p = 0.638). At first follow-up the figures were 188.1 (151.6, 244.2) and 199.2 (147.0, 237.9) respectively (p = 0.316) and at second follow-up 202.7 (178.6, 228.6) and 189.7 (130.3, 236.6) respectively (p = 0.455). As PA at baseline and follow-up was similar in women in the intervention and control groups, data from the intervention and control arms of the trial were combined for this study. This was a post-hoc decision, made after examination of the data.

PA measurement

PA was measured using an Actigraph™ accelerometer at $16^{+0} - 18^{+6}$ weeks' gestation (T0), $27^{+0} - 28^{+6}$ weeks' gestation (T1) and $35^{+0} - 36^{+6}$ weeks' gestation (T2). The Actigraph is considered appropriate for use in pregnancy and has previously been used to measure PA in overweight and obese pregnant women [15,16]. Data were processed using Actilife software [17]. Freedson's cut points were used to categorise time as sedentary (SED; <100 counts per minute (cpm)), light activity (LPA; 100–1951 cpm), and moderate or vigorous intensity activity (MVPA; >1951 cpm) [18]. All activity (ACTIVE; $\geq$100 cpm) was also calculated. Data from participants recording $\geq$3 days of valid ($\geq$500 minutes per day) accelerometry were included in the analysis. PA data for each individual were summarised as median minutes per day in each intensity category. Change in time spent in different PA intensities was calculated as the difference in minutes per day recorded in each intensity

(T1 −T0 and T2 −T0). As accelerometer wear time (valid minutes of data recorded) decreased from baseline to follow-up, PA of different intensities as a proportion of total wear time was also calculated (mins per day in each activity intensity/mins per day accelerometer worn). Previous work reports that total activity, rather than sub-components of activity, is most strongly associated with glucose homeostasis [19]. We therefore sought to identify factors associated with proportion of accelerometer wear time $\geq$100 cpm recorded (%ACTIVE). Women were categorised as recording above or below median %ACTIVE at each time point. They were further categorised as reducing %ACTIVE by greater than or less than the median at T1 (−1.5%) and T2 (−0.5%).

Statistical analysis

Data analysis was performed using SPSS version 21.0. Variables were checked for normal distribution using the Shapiro-Wilk test. Descriptive statistics are presented as mean (SD), median (inter-quartile range) or proportions, as appropriate. Wilcoxon matched-pairs signed rank tests were used to assess change in PA. Logistic regression was used to explore associations of maternal characteristics with absolute duration of and change in PA.

The following variables were included in the analyses: BMI (kg/m^2) at T0; age (years) at T0; parity (nulliparous or parous); smoking status (self-reported never or ex/current smoker at T0); ethnicity (White or non-White); marital status (married/cohabiting or single/divorced/separated); highest educational attainment (degree or higher or no degree); employment status (in paid employment or not in paid employment); living accommodation (owner occupier/private rented or council rented); Index of Multiple Deprivation (IMD; quintile 5 [most deprived] compared to quintile 1–4). All data were collected at baseline by the research midwife and entered immediately into the study database.

Ethics

Research Ethics Committee approval was obtained in all participating centres (London, Newcastle and Glasgow), UK Integrated Research Application System; reference 09/H0802/5 (South East London Research Ethics Committee). Written informed consent for participation in the study was obtained from all participants.

Results

One hundred and forty of 183 (77%) women recruited to the study provided sufficient PA data to be included at T0. Median BMI was 33.8 (IQR 31.9, 37.6) and median age was 32 years (IQR 26, 35 years) (Table 1).

At T1, 76 (42%) women and at T2, 54 (30%) women provided valid PA data. Women who provided valid accelerometry data at all 3 data collection points were

Table 1 Baseline characteristics of participants with valid accelerometry data at T0, T1 and T2

	T0		T1		T2	
	16^{+0} – 18^{+6} weeks' gestation		27^{+0} – 28^{+6} weeks' gestation		35^{+0} – 36^{+6} weeks' gestation	
≥3 days valid data (% consented)	140	(76.5)	76	(41.5)	54	(29.5)
BMI at T0 (Kg/m^2)[1]	33.8	(31.9, 37.6)	34.1	(32.4, 37.1)	35.6	(33.4, 38.4)**
Age (years) [1]	32	(26, 35)	32	(28, 35)	33	(28, 36)**
Parity						
Nulliparous	62	(45.9)	26	(34.7)*	17	(31.5)**
Parous	73	(54.1)	49	(65.3)	37	(68.5)
Smoking status						
Current or ex-smoker	46	(34.1)	30	(40.0)	20	(37.0)
Never smoked	89	(65.9)	45	(60.0)	34	(63.0)
Ethnicity						
White	84	(62.2)	48	(64.0)	34	(63.0)
Black, Asian or other	51	(37.8)	27	(36.0)	20	(37.0)
Marital status						
Married/cohabiting	69	(51.1)	38	(50.7)	28	(51.9)
Single/divorced/separate	66	(48.9)	37	(49.3)	26	(48.1)
Educational achievement						
Degree or higher	62	(45.9)	35	(46.7)	26	(48.1)
No degree	73	(54.1)	40	(53.3)	28	(51.9)
Employment status						
Paid or self employment	92	(68.7)	50	(66.7)	40	(74.1)
Not in paid employment	42	(31.3)	25	(33.3)	14	(25.9)
Living accommodation						
Owned or private rented	76	(54.3)	48	(63.2)*	36	(66.7)**
Rented (council)	64	(45.7)	28	(36.8)	18	(33.3)
IMD quintile						
1 (least deprived)	4	(3.4)	4	(6.2)	3	(6.5)
2	4	(3.4)	2	(3.1)	1	(2.2)
3	14	(12.1)	7	(10.8)	4	(8.7)
4	44	(37.9)	26	(40.0)	21	(45.7)
5 (most deprived)	50	(43.1)	26	(40.0)	17	(37.0)
Weight gain[2]						
Above IOM guideline					23	(45.1)
Within or below IOM guideline					28	(54.9)

Figures are n(%); [1]Median (inter-quartile range); [2]The American Institute of Medicine (IOM) recommends that obese women should gain between 5–9 kg during pregnancy.
*p < 0.05 for difference between baseline and 28 weeks.
**p < 0.05 for difference between baseline and 35 weeks.

similar to women who did not in degree of obesity (p = 0.092), ethnicity (p = 0.712), and IMD score (p = 0.604), but were older (33 years vs 32 years; p = 0.020), more likely to have at least one child (p = 0.001) and less likely to live in council rented accommodation (p = 0.004).

The number of minutes spent in SED, LPA, MVPA and ACTIVE was lower at T1 than at T0 (Table 2). At T2 time spent in SED, MVPA and ACTIVE was lower than at T0. MVPA also declined between T1 and T2. A decrease in total MVPA from a median (inter-quartile range) at T0 of 39 mins/day (25, 52) to 34.5 (24, 44) at T1 and 23 (18, 38) at T2 was recorded. MVPA as a proportion of wear time (%MVPA), but not %LPA or %ACTIVE, also decreased with gestation (Table 2).

Having at least one child (OR 2.73; 95% CI 1.36, 5.48) and not having a degree (OR 4.03; 95% CI 1.96, 8.28) were associated with greater than median %ACTIVE at T0 (Table 3). At T1 non-white ethnicity was associated

Table 2 Change between T0, T1 and T2 in sedentary time, LPA, MVPA and total time active

	T0 (n = 140)	T1 (n = 76)	Change (T1-T0)	T2 (n = 54)	Change (T2-T0)
Absolute values (min/day)					
SED	576.5	555.1	−21.5*	571.8	−4.7*
	(510.6, 642.8)	(505.6, 635.3)		(507.5, 615.9)	
LPA	174.8	154.8	−20.0*	169.7	−5.1
	(140.3, 222.2)	(124.9, 191.7)		(142.7, 199.2)	
MVPA	39.0	34.5	−4.5*	23.3	−15.7*†
	(24.7, 51.9)	(23.9, 43.5)		(18.0, 38.0)	
ACTIVE	215.6	194.8	−20.8*	198.6	−17.0*
	(168.2, 264.9)	(146.2, 228.3)		(163.4, 228.6)	
Proportion of time accelerometer worn (% worn time)					
%SED	73.2	75.3	1.3	73.8	0.5
	(68.5, 78.4)	(70.5, 80.5)	(−2.5, 5.8)	(70.6, 79.9)	(−2.2, 4.1)
%LPA	21.5	20.1	−0.5	21.9	0.9
	(17.6, 25.8)	(16.3, 25.5)	(−4.1, 1.9)	(17.8, 25.4)	(−2.7, 2.8)
%MVPA	4.8	4.3	−0.4	3.0	−1.1*†
	(3.1, 6.3)	(2.9, 5.2)	(−1.3, 0.6)	(2.3, 4.6)	(−2.5, −0.3)
%ACTIVE	26.8	24.7	−1.5	26.3	−0.5
	(21.6, 31.5)	(19.6, 29.5)	(−5.8, 2.7)	(20.1, 29.4)	(−4.1, 2.2)
Mean counts per minute (SD)	299	278	-	248*	-
	(114)	(119)		(93)	

Figures are median (IQR) or mean (SD); Wilcoxon Signed Ranks Test or Paired Samples t-test used to test for differences.
Definition of PA intensity: <100 cpm = Sedentary (SED); 100-1951 cpm = Light PA (LPA); >1951 cpm = Moderate + vigorous PA (MVPA); ≥100 cpm = total activity (ACTIVE).
*$p < 0.05$ for change in median or mean between T0 and T1 or T0 and T2.
†$p < 0.05$ for change in median or mean between T1 and T2.
T0 = 16^{+0} – 18^{+6} weeks' gestation; T1 = 27^{+0} – 28^{+6} weeks' gestation; T2 = 35^{+0} – 36^{+6} weeks' gestation.

with greater than median %ACTIVE (OR 3.96; 95% CI 1.44, 10.89). A recording greater than median %ACTIVE at T0 was strongly associated with %ACTIVE at T1 (OR 5.85; 2.16, 15.86) and T2 (OR 5.95; 1.80, 19.70). A recording greater than median %ACTIVE at T1 was strongly associated with %ACTIVE at T2 (OR 4.61; 1.39, 15.24).

A recording greater than median %ACTIVE at T0 was also strongly associated with a greater than median reduction in %ACTIVE (T1: OR 4.0; 1.53, 10.46; T2: OR 4.16; 1.31, 13.17) (Table 4). There was a strong negative correlation between %ACTIVE at T0 and change in %ACTIVE at T1 (−0.52, $p < 0.001$) and T2 (−0.56, $p < 0.001$).

Discussion

Objectively measured MVPA, but not light or total activity, decreased with gestation in this cohort of obese pregnant women. Our finding is consistent with previous studies of objectively measured PA in non-obese pregnant women [6], and with previous cross-sectional pedometer studies showing lower activity at later gestation in obese pregnant women [10]. This might be attributable to difficulties in maintaining PA as physical discomfort increases as pregnancy progresses [14].

Results from a number of recent trials of lifestyle interventions in overweight and obese pregnant women have demonstrated positive effects. For example, in the TOP (Treatment of Obese Pregnant women) study of 425 obese pregnant women in Denmark, gestational weight gain was lower in women randomised to receive a physical activity intervention, either with or without a dietary component, than in those receiving standard care [20]. In the LIMIT RCT of a combined diet and physical activity lifestyle advice intervention in 2212 overweight and obese pregnant Australian women, fewer macrocosmic infants were born to women randomised to receive lifestyle advice than to those receiving standard care [21]. These findings reinforce the importance of identifying ways of supporting obese pregnant women to make healthy lifestyle choices. However, the intervention in the UPBEAT pilot trial did not have an impact on objectively measured PA. Other trials have reported similar findings. For example, the Fitfor2 study reported no effect of a supervised PA intervention in overweight pregnant women on objectively measured PA [16]. The UPBEAT intervention focused on walking to increase PA. It is possible that in the pilot trial the need to walk

Table 3 Unadjusted odds ratio of recording more than median time ACTIVE at T0, T1 and T2 as proportion of accelerometer wear time, by baseline characteristics

	T0		T1		T2	
	OR	95% CI	OR	95% CI	OR	95% CI
Intervention status						
Intervention	Ref		Ref		Ref	
Control	0.89	0.46, 1.73	0.81	0.33, 1.99	0.86	0.30, 2.51
Body Mass Index (Kg/m^2)						
30-34.9	Ref		Ref		Ref	
35+	1.81	0.89, 3.66	0.85	0.34, 2.14	1.25	0.42, 3.70
Age (years)						
<35	Ref		Ref		Ref	
≥35	0.78	0.37, 1.67	1.40	0.52, 3.77	0.53	0.17, 1.62
Parity						
Nulliparous	Ref		Ref		Ref	
Parous	**2.73**	**1.36, 5.48**	1.04	0.40, 2.70	1.19	0. 38, 3.75
Smoking status						
Current or ex-smoker	1.46	0.71, 2.98	1.20	0.47, 3.01	0.53	0.17, 1.62
Never smoked	Ref		Ref		Ref	
Ethnicity						
White	Ref		Ref		Ref	
Black, Asian or other	1.09	0.54, 2.19	**3.96**	**1.44, 10.89**	0.53	0.17, 1.62
Marital status						
Married/cohabiting	Ref		Ref		Ref	
Single/divorced/separate	0.72	0.37, 1.42	1.17	0.47, 2.90	1.00	0.34, 2.91
Educational achievement						
Degree or higher	Ref		Ref		Ref	
No degree	**4.03**	**1.96, 8.28**	1.80	0.72, 4.51	1.82	0.62, 5.35
Employment status						
Paid or self employment	Ref		Ref		Ref	
Not in paid employment	1.46	0.70, 3.04	1.76	0.67, 4.67	2.20	0.63, 7.74
Living accommodation						
Owned or private rented	Ref		Ref		Ref	
Rented (council)	1.00	0.51, 1.95	1.00	0.39, 2.54	0.72	0.23, 2.23
IMD quintile						
1-4	Ref		Ref		Ref	
5 (most deprived)	1.53	0.73, 3.20	1.23	0.45, 3.32	1.05	0.32, 3.48
Baseline ACTIVE						
Below median	-		Ref		Ref	
Above median	-		5.85	2.16, 15.86	5.95	**1.80, 19.70**
28 week ACTIVE						
Below median	-		-		Ref	
Above median	-		-		**4.61**	**1.39, 15.24**

Statistically significant relationships (p < 0.05) are in **bold**.
'ACTIVE' defined as ≥100 cpm; Median %ACTIVE at T0 = 26.8%; at T1 = 24.7%; at T2 = 26.3%.
T0 = 16^{+0} – 18^{+6} weeks' gestation; T1 = 27^{+0} – 28^{+6} weeks' gestation; T2 = 35^{+0} – 36^{+6} weeks' gestation.

Table 4 Unadjusted odds ratio of reducing ACTIVE as proportion of accelerometer wear time by more than median at T1 and T2 by baseline characteristics

	OR	95% CI	OR	95% CI
Intervention status				
Intervention	Ref		Ref	
Control	0.44	0.18, 1.12	1.57	0.53, 5.60
Body Mass Index (Kg/m^2)				
30-34.9	Ref		Ref	
35+	1.25	0.49, 3.18	2.33	0.77, 7.09
Age (years)				
<35	Ref		Ref	
≥35	1.58	0.59, 4.27	1.38	0.54, 4.17
Parity				
Nulliparous	Ref		Ref	
Parous	1.17	0.45, 3.04	0.60	0.19, 1.90
Smoking status				
Current or ex-smoker	1.37	0.54, 3.48	1.38	0.45, 4.17
Never smoked	Ref		Ref	
Ethnicity				
White	Ref		Ref	
Black, Asian or other	1.48	0.57, 3.88	1.90	0.62, 5.83
Marital status				
Married/cohabiting	Ref		Ref	
Single/divorced/separate	0.47	0.18, 1.18	0.40	0.14, 1.21
Educational achievement				
Degree or higher	Ref		Ref	
No degree	1.94	0.77, 4.90	2.47	0.83, 7.39
Employment status				
Paid or self employment	Ref		Ref	
Not in paid employment	0.51	0.19, 1.38	1.00	0.30, 3.38
Living accommodation				
Owned or private rented	Ref		Ref	
Rented (council)	2.38	0.90, 6.27	1.96	0.62, 6.22
IMD quintile				
1-4	Ref		Ref	
5 (most deprived)	0.73	0.27, 2.00	1.39	0.42, 4.60
Baseline ACTIVE				
Below median	Ref		Ref	
Above median	**4.00**	**1.53, 10.46**	**4.16**	**1.31, 13.17**
28 week ACTIVE				
Below median	-		Ref	
Above median	-		2.84	0.91, 8.86

Statistically significant relationships (p < 0.05) are in **bold**.
(median reduction in %ACTIVE was 1.5% at T1 and 0.5% at T2).
T0 = 16^{+0} – 18^{+6} weeks' gestation; T1 = 27^{+0} – 28^{+6} weeks' gestation; T2 = 35^{+0} – 36^{+6} weeks' gestation.

at an appropriate (i.e. moderate) intensity was not emphasised sufficiently; women in the intervention group in the UPBEAT pilot trial self-reported an increase in light physical activity [14].

We examined total activity as it has been found to be more strongly associated with insulin sensitivity during pregnancy than sub-components of PA and may be the most appropriate target for interventions to improve glucose tolerance [19]. Baseline activity was the strongest predictor of PA throughout pregnancy. Despite a greater reduction in PA in women who were more active at baseline, this group of women still had a substantially increased likelihood of remaining active throughout pregnancy.

Although this is the first study to consider factors associated with change in objectively measured PA during pregnancy in a cohort of obese women, it has several limitations.

Only 20% of eligible women participated in the UPBEAT pilot trial, raising the possibility of selection bias and attrition was high with less than 40% of women providing data at all time points. However, as women who dropped out of the study did not differ in terms of demographic factors from those who remained in the study, it is unlikely that this affected the findings. The small sample size means type II errors are possible. Accelerometers underestimate upper body activities and cannot capture water-based activities [22]. However accelerometry remains a useful way of measuring PA during pregnancy and in particular intra-individual change [8].

We aimed to identify factors associated with low levels of PA that could help clinicians identify women most likely to benefit from intervention. PA at baseline was the factor most strongly associated with PA during pregnancy. This suggests that an objective assessment of PA in early pregnancy and intervention to support women with low PA to increase their PA and to encourage active women to maintain their PA is warranted. Pre-pregnancy PA has previously been identified as a predictor of PA during pregnancy and appears to be strongly associated with lower risk of GDM [3,23,24]. Population level interventions to encourage all women to be sufficiently physically active irrespective of pregnancy are clearly important.

Systematic review evidence demonstrates that goal setting, self-monitoring and feedback are important in achieving lifestyle behaviour change in pregnant and non-pregnant populations [25,26] and previous work suggests that obese pregnant women specifically require active involvement in setting individualised goals and intensive support and feedback to make behaviour changes [11,25]. Previous qualitative work in the UK found obese pregnant women feel they do not receive adequate advice and support from health care providers around appropriate PA during pregnancy and would welcome more guidance [27]. Similar findings have been reported from the US [28]. Pain during pregnancy can be severe enough to impact on usual daily activities [19]. These findings present several modifiable barriers to PA that could be addressed in the development of interventions to support women to be active during pregnancy. Interventions should include appropriate advice on the benefits of PA and support to set and monitor PA goals from health care professionals and advice on coping with pregnancy-related pain.

Conclusion

Identifying ways of supporting women to be sufficiently active during pregnancy remains a challenge. The clearest predictor of change in PA during pregnancy in this study was level of PA at baseline. Women who were most active at the beginning of their pregnancy maintained their activity level better than those who were less active. This indicates the importance of emphasising the health benefits associated with physical activity to obese women within pre-conception planning when the opportunity arises, and at booking appointments.

Competing interests

The authors declare that they have no competing interests.

Authors' contributions

LP, RB and TK conceived the study, participated in its design and coordination and helped to draft the manuscript. LH performed the analyses and drafted the manuscript. CM and SCR contributed to drafting the manuscript. All authors read and approved the final manuscript.

Acknowledgements

We thank the research midwives and health trainers and all the pregnant women who took part in this study. This manuscript presents independent research commissioned by the National Institute for Health Research (NIHR) (UK) under the Programme Grants for Applied Research programme RP-0407-10452. The views expressed in this paper are those of the authors and not necessarily those of the National Health Service, the NIHR or the Department of Health. The study was also supported by Guys and St. Thomas' Charity; Reg Charity 251983, UK; Chief Scientist Office, Scottish Government Health Directorates, Edinburgh, UK and Tommy's Charity; Reg Charity 1060508, UK.

Author details

[1]Institute of Health & Society, Newcastle University, Baddiley-Clark Building, Richardson Road, Newcastle upon Tyne NE2 4AX, UK. [2]Institute of Cellular Medicine, Newcastle University, Newcastle upon Tyne, UK. [3]Newcastle-upon-Tyne Hospitals NHS Foundation Trust, Newcastle upon Tyne, UK. [4]School of Health Sciences, University of Tampere, Tampere, Finland. [5]Division of Women's Health, Women's Health Academic Centre, King's College, London, UK.

References

1. American Diabetes Association. Diagnosis and Classification of Diabetes Mellitus. Diabetes Care. 2010;33 Suppl 1:S62–9.
2. Chu SY, Kim SY, Lau J, Schmid CH, Dietz PM, Callaghan WM, et al. Maternal obesity and risk of gestational diabetes mellitus. Diabetes Care. 2007;30(8):2070–6.
3. Tobias DK, Zhang C, van Dam RM, Bowers K, Hu FB. Physical activity before and during pregnancy and risk of gestational diabetes mellitus: a meta-analysis. Diabetes Care. 2011;34(1):223–9.
4. ACOG. Exercise during pregnancy and the postpartum period. Clin Obstet Gynecol. 2003;46(2):469–99.
5. Royal College of Obstetricians and Gynaecologists. Exercise in pregnancy. Statement No.4. London: Royal College of Obstetricians and Gynaecologists; 2006.
6. Downs DS, LeMasurier GC, DiNallo JM. Baby steps: pedometer-determined and self-reported leisure-time exercise behaviors of pregnant women. J Phys Act Health. 2009;6(1):63–72.
7. Evenson KR, Wen F. Prevalence and correlates of objectively measured physical activity and sedentary behavior among US pregnant women. Prev Med. 2011;53(1–2):39–43.
8. Rousham EK, Clarke PE, Gross H. Significant changes in physical activity among pregnant women in the UK as assessed by accelerometry and self-reported activity. Eur J Clin Nutr. 2006;60(3):393–400.
9. McParlin C, Robson SC, Tennant PWG, Besson H, Rankin J, Adamson AJ, et al. Objectively measured physical activity during pregnancy: a study in obese and overweight women. BMC Pregnancy Childbirth. 2010;10:76.
10. Renault K, Nørgaard K, Andreasen KR, Secher NJ, Nilas L. Physical activity during pregnancy in obese and normal-weight women as assessed by pedometer. Acta Obstet Gynecol Scand. 2010;89(7):956–61.
11. Sui Z, Dodd JM. Exercise in obese pregnant women: positive impacts and current perceptions. Int J Womens Health. 2013;5:389–98.
12. Dodd JM, Crowther CA, Robinson JS. Dietary and lifestyle interventions to limit weight gain during pregnancy for obese or overweight women: a systematic review. Acta Obstet Gynecol Scand. 2008;87(7):702–6.
13. Choi J, Fukuoka Y, Lee JH. The effects of physical activity and physical activity plus diet interventions on bodyweight in overweight or obese women who are pregnant or in postpartum: A systematic review and meta-analysis of randomized controlled trials. Preventive Medicine. 2013;56(6):351–64.
14. Poston L, Briley AL, Barr S, Bell R, Croker H, Coxon K, et al. Developing a complex intervention in obese pregnant women; assessment of behavioural change and process evaluation through a randomised controlled exploratory trial. BMC Pregnancy Childbirth. 2013;13(1):148.
15. Harrison CL, Thompson RG, Teede HJ, Lombard CB. Measuring physical activity during pregnancy. Int J Behav Nutr Phys Act. 2011;8:19.
16. Oostdam N, van Poppel MN, Wouters MG, Eekhoff EM, Bekedam DJ, Kuchenbecker WKH, et al. No effect of the FitFor2 exercise programme on blood glucose, insulin sensitivity, and birthweight in pregnant women who were overweight and at risk for gestational diabetes: results of a randomised controlled trial. Br J Obstet Gynaecol. 2012;119:1098–107.
17. ActiLife5.lnk [computer program]. Version 5.10.0;2010-2011. Available from http://www.actigraphcorp.com/support/software/
18. Freedson PS, Melanson E, Sirard J. Calibration of the computer science and applications, inc. accelerometer. Med Sci Sports Exerc. 1998;30:777–81.
19. Gradmark A, Pomeroy J, Renstrom F, Steiginga S, Persson M, Wright A, et al. Physical activity, sedentary behaviors, and estimated insulin sensitivity and secretion in pregnant and non-pregnant women. BMC Pregnancy Childbirth. 2011;11:44.
20. Renault KM, Norgaard K, Nilas L, Carlsen EM, Cortes D, Pryds O, et al. The Treatment of Obese Pregnant Women (TOP) study: a randomized controlled trial of the effect of physical activity intervention assessed by pedometer with or without dietary intervention in obese pregnant women. Am J Obstet Gynecol. 2014;210(2):134. e131-139.
21. Dodd JM, McPhee AJ, Turnbull D, Yelland LN, Deussen AR, Grivell RM, et al. The effects of antenatal dietary and lifestyle advice for women who are overweight or obese on neonatal health outcomes: the LIMIT randomised trial. BMC Med. 2014;12:163.
22. Troiano RP. Translating accelerometer counts into energy expenditure: advancing the quest. J Appl Physiol. 2006;100(4):1107–8.
23. Ning Y, Williams MA, Dempsey JC, Sorensen TK, Frederick IO, Luthy DA. Correlates of recreational physical activity in early pregnancy. J Matern Fetal Neonatal Med. 2003;13(6):385–93.
24. Pereira MA, Rifas-Shiman SL, Kleinman KP, Rich-Edwards JW, Peterson KE, Gillman MW. Predictors of change in physical activity during and after pregnancy: Project Viva. Am J Prev Med. 2007;32(4):312–9.
25. Brown MJ, Sinclair M, Liddle D, Hill AJ, Madden E, Stockdale J. A systematic review investigating healthy lifestyle interventions incorporating goal

setting strategies for preventing excess gestational weight gain. PLoS ONE [Electronic Resource]. 2012;7(7):e39503.

26. National Institute for Health and Clinical Excellence (NICE). Behaviour change at population, community and individual levels. London: Department of Health; 2007.

27. Brown A, Avery A. Healthy weight management during pregnancy: what advice and information is being provided. J Hum Nutr Diet. 2012;25(4):378–87.

28. Stengel MR, Kraschnewski JL, Hwang SW, Kjerulff KH, Chuang CH. "What my doctor didn't tell me": examining health care provider advice to overweight and obese pregnant women on gestational weight gain and physical activity. Womens Health Issues. 2012;22(6):e535–40.

Pre-pregnancy obesity and non-adherence to multivitamin use: findings from the National Pregnancy Risk Assessment Monitoring System (2009–2011)

Saba W. Masho[1,2,3*], Amani Bassyouni[1] and Susan Cha[1]

Abstract

Background: Although adequate folic acid or multivitamins can prevent up to 70 % of neural tube defects, the majority of U.S. non-pregnant women of childbearing age do not use multivitamins every day. Factors influencing consistent multivitamin use are not fully explored. This study aims to investigate the association between pre-pregnancy body mass index (BMI) and multivitamin use before pregnancy using a large, nationally representative sample of women with recent live births.

Methods: The national 2009–2011 Pregnancy Risk Assessment Monitoring System data were analyzed. The sample included women with recent singleton live births ($N = 104,211$). The outcome of interest was multivitamin use which was categorized as no multivitamin use, 1–3 times/week, 4–6 times/week, and daily use. Maternal BMI was examined as underweight (<18.50 kg/m^2), normal weight (18.50–24.99 kg/m^2), overweight (25.00–29.99 kg/m^2), and obese (≥ 30.00 kg/m^2). Multinomial logistic regression was conducted, and adjusted odds ratios and 95 % confidence intervals were calculated.

Results: Compared to women with normal weight, overweight and obese women had significantly increased odds of not taking multivitamins after adjusting for confounding factors. Further, the lack of multivitamin use increased in magnitude with the level of BMI (OR$_{overweight}$ = 1.2, 95 % CI = 1.1–1.3; OR$_{obese}$ = 1.4, 95 % CI = 1.2–1.5).

Conclusions: Obese and overweight women were less likely to follow the recommendation for preconception multivitamin use compared to normal weight women. All health care professionals must enhance preconception care with particular attention to overweight and obese women. Preconception counseling may be an opportunity to discuss healthy eating and benefits of daily multivitamin intake before pregnancy.

Keywords: Obesity, Body mass index, Vitamins, Dietary supplements, Preconception care, PRAMS

Background

Multivitamin use has increased over the past decade and is the most commonly used dietary supplement in the United States [1]. According to the Centers for Disease Control and Prevention (CDC), approximately 34 % of women aged 20–39 used a dietary supplement containing folic acid and 30 % reported using supplemental vitamin D in 2003–2006 [2]. Additionally, nationally representative data that come from the Behavioral Risk Factor Surveillance System (BRFSS) indicate 78 % of pregnant women and 47 % of non-pregnant women of childbearing age (18–44) use multivitamins daily [3]. Since 1991, the U.S. Public Health Service has recommended that all women who plan on becoming pregnant consume 400 μg of folic acid daily beginning one month before trying to get pregnant [4, 5]. However, a recent report from the CDC finds that more than 63 % of women do not

* Correspondence: saba.masho@vcuhealth.org
[1]Division of Epidemiology, Department of Family Medicine and Population Health, School of Medicine, Virginia Commonwealth University, 830 E. Main Street, 8th Floor, P.O. Box 980212, Richmond, VA 23298-0212, USA
[2]Department of Obstetrics and Gynecology, School of Medicine, Virginia Commonwealth University, Richmond, VA, USA
Full list of author information is available at the end of the article

take multivitamins during the month before pregnancy [6]. The lack of multivitamin use is a public health concern given that adequate folic acid or multivitamins can prevent 50to 70 % of pregnancies affected by serious birth defects, (i.e., spina bifida and anencephaly) [7]. For instance, one hospital-based case–control study reported the use of folic acid (0.4 mg daily for three months before and after conception, and continuing for at least one month) was associated with decreased neural tube defects (OR = 0.32, 95 % CI = 0.17–0.58), but the protective effects of folic acid supplementation was attenuated for overweight or obese women [8]. Similarly, a recent Cochrane review, women receiving folic acid with micronutrients were less likely to have infants with neural tube defects than women receiving other or same micronutrients without folic acid (RR = 0.31, 95 % CI = 0.16–0.60; RR = 0.29, 95 % CI = 0.12–0.70) [9].

Additionally, prenatal iron deficiency anemia during pregnancy has detrimental effects on infant mental development. A cohort study that followed women during the last trimester to 24 months after delivery reported a lower mental development index among children exposed to prenatal iron deficiency anemia at 12, 18, and 24 months of age; however, supplementation with sufficient iron was found to be protective [10]. Prenatal vitamin intake during pregnancy has been shown to significantly reduce the risk of birth defects, low birth weight, small for gestational age, and spontaneous preterm birth [11–14].

Despite the benefits of multivitamins or folic acid use before pregnancy, non-adherence to recommendations has been observed in some populations. A large proportion of women who are younger (under 20 years of age), of racial/ethnic minority group, or without history of neural tube defects do not take folic acid supplements before pregnancy [15]. Other risk factors for inconsistent or no use of multivitamin during pregnancy include low income and below high school educational attainment [3, 16]. One study conducted among African-American and Hispanic women identified adverse side effects, large size of pills, and bad taste and smell as possible barriers to multivitamin use [17]. Lack of knowledge regarding multivitamin use, dose, duration, timing and efficacy can also lead to non-adherence to multivitamin use during pregnancy [18]. On the other hand, Kimmons et al. reported that obese women were less likely to use multivitamins than normal weight women [19].

To the authors' knowledge, only a few studies have assessed the relationship between obesity and multivitamin use [20–22]. For example, a nested retrospective cohort study conducted by Farah et al. found that obese and overweight women reported less folic acid use before pregnancy compared to women of normal weight

[20]. In yet another study, Case et al. used data from the Texas Behavioral Risk Factor Surveillance System (1999–2003) and found that obese but not overweight women were less likely to take folic acid every day compared to normal weight/underweight women [21]. Kimmons et al. examined the association between body mass index (BMI) and serum micronutrient levels among U.S. adults and found that premenopausal women who were overweight and obese were more likely to have low levels of micronutrients (e.g., folate) than normal weight premenopausal women [22]. Decreased folic acid intake may be due to unplanned pregnancies and failed contraceptive methods prevalent in obese women [23]. Although findings in these studies provide critical evidence, these studies have notable limitations. The study by Farah et al. had a small sample size ($n = 288$) and included only Caucasian women, making it less generalizable to minorities who may be at risk for poor pregnancy outcomes [20]. Similarly, Case et al. only considered women from Texas and excluded those who were younger than 18 years old [21]. In the study by Kimmons et al., micronutrient intake was not taken into consideration, and any adult women (≥19 years) were categorized as premenopausal if they reported menstruation in the previous 12 months, possibly including older women who were no longer of reproductive age (15–44) [22]. The observed shortcomings in the study designs, problems related to small sample sizes and homogenous study populations, warrant further investigation of the relationship between obesity and multivitamin use.

This study aims to investigate the association between pre-pregnancy BMI and multivitamins use before pregnancy using a large, nationally representative sample of women with recent live births.

Methods
The 2009–2011 Pregnancy Risk Assessment Monitoring System (PRAMS) [24] was analyzed to assess the relationship between pre-pregnancy BMI and multivitamin use before pregnancy. PRAMS is an ongoing national surveillance program through the CDC in collaboration with participating state health departments. Data on women with recently delivered live-born infants are drawn from state birth certificate files. PRAMS utilizes a complex multistage sampling design and oversamples women from minority groups and high risk populations to ensure adequate numbers for analyses (e.g., low weight births). Accordingly, oversampling is accounted for by analysis weights provided by CDC to obtain nationally representative estimates. Women are contacted by mail or telephone to participate, and information regarding their attitudes, behaviors, and experiences before and during pregnancy, and a few months after birth are

obtained from those who consent to participate. In order to ensure comparability of data, PRAMS establishes standardized surveillance methods and tools for data collection.

A total of 112,358 women (unweighted N) participated in PRAMS for 2009 to 2011. For this analysis women with singleton live births and valid responses to questions on pre-pregnancy BMI and multivitamin use a month prior to pregnancy were included. The study sample consisted of 104,211 women (unweighted number) representing 5,032,562 women (weighted number). Women who delivered multiple births (e.g., twins, triplets) were excluded from the analysis, as consistent with the literature [25, 26]. This study analyzed a de-identified publicly available data and was approved as exempt by the Institutional Review Board at Virginia Commonwealth University.

The exposure, maternal pre-pregnancy BMI was determined by self-report weight and height prior to pregnancy (kilograms/meters^2). Participants were asked, "Just before you got pregnant with your new baby, how much did you weigh?" and "How tall are you without shoes?" Using BMI classifications from the World Health Organization, pre-pregnancy BMI was categorized as underweight (<18.5 kg/m^2), normal weight (18.5–24.9 kg/m^2), overweight (25.0–29.9 (kg/m^2) and obese (≥ 30.0 kg/m^2) [27].

The outcome of interest was the frequency of multivitamin use one month prior to pregnancy. Women were asked, "During the month before you got pregnant with your new baby, how many times a week did you take a multivitamin, a prenatal vitamin, or a folic acid vitamin?" Consistent with the literature, responses were categorized into four levels: "I didn't take a multivitamins, prenatal vitamins or folic acid vitamins at all" (i.e., Not at all), "1 to 3 times a week", "4 to 6 times a week", or "every day of the week" [28].

Covariates examined included maternal socio-demographic factors, access to resources and care, behavioral and lifestyle factors, reproductive health factors and medical complications [15, 29–31]. Socio-demographic factors included maternal age (≤ 19; 20–24; 25–29; 30–35; >35), race/ethnicity (White non-Hispanic; Black non-Hispanic; Hispanic; other non-Hispanic), education ($<$high school; high school; $>$high school), marital status (married; not married), and household income level ($<20,000$; 20,000–34,999; 35,000–49,999; $\geq 50,000$). Factors related to access to care and services included health insurance 12 months before pregnancy (private; Medicaid; multiple; other; none). Maternal health behaviors prior to pregnancy consisted of smoking (yes; no), drinking alcohol (yes; no), dieting, i.e., changing eating habits any time during the 12 months prior to pregnancy (yes; no), and exercise habits, i.e., exercising three or more days of the week

any time during the last 12 months before pregnancy (yes; no). Maternal health conditions included preconception morbidities such as diabetes (yes; no) and hypertension (yes; no). Previous live pregnancy, pregnancy intention and intimate partner violence were also evaluated as confounders.

All analyses were conducted using SAS statistical software version 9.4 to account for the complex survey design. Descriptive statistics including unweighted frequencies and weighted percentages were generated to assess the distribution of maternal characteristics and multivitamin use. Multinomial logistic regression models for the outcome of interest were used to obtain crude and adjusted odds ratios (COR and AOR, respectively) and 95 % confidence intervals (CI). Adjusted estimates controlled for domains of covariates such as maternal socio-demographic characteristics, medical-reproductive factors, and socio-behavioral characteristics.

Results

The majority of the study population was between the ages of 20–29 years (53 %), Non-Hispanic White (60 %), married (61 %), reported high school or more education (58 %), earned less than $50,000 (64 %), and privately insured (56 %) (Table 1). Approximately 4.4 % of women were underweight, 50.4 % were normal weight, 24.1 % were overweight, and 21.2 % obese. More than half of women (55.4 %) did not take multivitamins at any time, 8.4 % used multivitamins 1–3 times per week, 6.1 % used multivitamins 4–6 times per week, and 30.2 % used multivitamins every day. Multivitamin intake was strongly associated with socio-demographic characteristics (e.g., marital status, income, race/ethnicity), medical-reproductive (e.g., parity, pre-pregnancy diabetes), and social-behavioral factors (e.g., smoking prior to pregnancy, intimate partner violence) (Table 2). Pre-pregnancy BMI was significantly associated with age, race, marital status, education, income, insurance, parity, pre-pregnancy diabetes, pre-pregnancy hypertension, pregnancy intention, smoking prior to pregnancy, alcohol use, exercise, dieting, and intimate partner violence (Table 3).

The unadjusted analyses showed a statistically significant association between pre-pregnancy BMI and multivitamin use (Table 4). Underweight and obese women were 1.6 times as likely to report no multivitamin use compared to women of normal weight (COR = 1.6, 95 % CI = 1.4–1.8; COR = 1.6, 95 % CI = 1.5–1.7, respectively). In addition, overweight women had 1.3 times the odds of reporting no intake compared to women with normal BMI (COR = 1.3, 95 % CI = 1.2–1.4). When controlling for socio-demographic characteristics such as maternal age, race, marital status, education, income, and health insurance, the odds of non-adherence to multivitamin

Table 1 Distribution of the study population characteristics

	Total Weighted N = 5 032 562 %
Age	
≤ 19	9.3
20–24	22.9
25–29	29.7
30–35	24.7
> 35	13.9
Race/Ethnicity	
White, non-Hispanic	60.4
Black, non-Hispanic	13.7
Hispanic	17.8
Other, non-Hispanic	8.2
Married	61.0
Education	
< High school	15.8
High school	26.3
> High school	57.9
Income	
< $20,000	36.2
$20,000–34,999	17.0
$35,000–49,999	10.3
v ≥ $50,000	36.5
Pre-pregnancy Insurance	
Private	55.9
Medicaid	15.6
Other	1.9
Multiple	3.4
No insurance	23.2
Previous live birth	
0	42.0
v1 - 2	47.5
≥ 3	10.6
Pre-pregnancy diabetes	2.2
Pre-pregnancy hypertension	8.9
Unintended pregnancy	42.5
Pre-pregnancy smoking	24.6
Average number of alcohol drink/week	
None	17.0
Up to 3	67.7
4 or more	15.3
Pre-pregnancy dieting	28.5
Pre-pregnancy exercising	42.2
Intimate partner violence	3.0

Weighted N = adjusted for the complex sampling design and represents the total population that the sampled was derived from

use stayed significant for overweight and obese women (AOR = 1.2, 95 % CI = 1.1–1.3; AOR = 1.4, 95 % CI = 1.3–1.5, respectively). However, estimates were no longer significant for the underweight group (AOR = 1.2, 95 % CI = 1.0–1.4). After additionally adjusting for medical-reproductive factors such as previous live birth, pregnancy intention, pre-pregnancy diabetes, and pre-pregnancy hypertension, the estimates remained consistent for overweight (AOR = 1.2, 95 % CI = 1.2–1.3) and obese women (AOR = 1.5, 95 % CI = 1.03–1.6). In fact, overweight and obese women were significantly more likely to report no multivitamin use compared to normal weight women (AOR = 1.2, 95 % CI = 1.1–1.3; AOR = 1.4, 95 % CI = 1.2–1.5, respectively) even after controlling for all covariates including socio-demographic characteristics, medical-reproductive factors, and socio-behavioral characteristics (i.e., smoking, alcohol consumption, diet, exercise, and intimate partner violence).

The odds of inadequate multivitamin supplementation, specifically 1–3 times per week, were higher for obese women compared to normal weight women (COR = 1.3, 95 % CI = 1.1–1.4). Similar estimates were obtained after adjusting for socio-demographic and medical-reproductive factors (AOR = 1.2, 95 % CI = 1.1–1.3). However, there were no longer significant differences between obese and normal weight women in fully adjusted models (AOR = 1.1, 95 % CI = 0.9–1.3). The odds of multivitamin use (4–6 times per week) remained non-significant for all different weight groups, even after controlling for all aforementioned factors.

Discussion

We found that obese and overweight women were less likely to follow the recommended use of preconception multivitamins compared to normal weight women. These findings are consistent with previous studies [20, 21]. Unlike previous studies, this analysis employed data from a national survey that provided a large sample size and representative study population. For instance, contrary to findings from Farah et al. which were based on a small sample of Caucasian women, the current study provided estimates that are more generalizable to the U.S. population [20].

Adequate multivitamin use one month prior to pregnancy has well-known positive benefits for both mothers and developing infants. However, the CDC reported that 63 % of women do not take the recommended amount of multivitamin one month prior to pregnancy [6]. This is consistent with our study finding that more than half of the women did not take multivitamin during the preconception period. While there are several possible reasons for lack of multivitamin use (e.g., simply forgetting), a growing body of literature has attributed this lack of adherence to unintended pregnancies [32–34].

Table 2 Prevalence of multivitamin intake by maternal characteristics

	No intake $n = 2\ 946\ 523$	1–3 times/week $n = 444\ 399$	4–6 times/week $n = 323\ 867$	Every day $n = 1\ 607\ 653$	P-value
		Weighted row %			
Body mass index					<.0001
Underweight	61.6	8.5	4.6	25.3	
Normal Weight	51.09	8.50	6.92	33.49	
Overweight	56.47	8.33	6.07	29.13	
Obese	60.9	8.3	5.0	25.8	
Socio-demographic					
Age					<.0001
≤ 19	77.6	5.6	1.9	14.9	
20–24	71.8	7.3	3.8	17.1	
25—29	54.3	8.7	6.2	30.8	
30–35	42.3	9.2	8.0	40.5	
> 35	38.5	9.8	8.9	42.8	
Race/Ethnicity					<.0001
White, non-Hispanic	49.2	8.6	7.5	34.7	
Black, non-Hispanic	66.6	9.1	3.5	20.8	
Hispanic	66.0	7.2	3.9	22.9	
Other, non-Hispanic	54.1	8.2	6.1	31.6	
Married					<.0001
Yes	43.5	9.2	8.2	39.1	
Other	73.2	7.1	2.9	16.8	
Education					<.0001
< High school	71.0	6.7	2.9	19.4	
High school	68.6	7.1	3.6	20.7	
> High school	44.2	9.5	8.2	38.1	
Income					<.0001
< $20,000	72.2	7.5	3.1	17.2	
$20,000–34,999	62.7	8.6	5.2	23.5	
$35,000–49,999	53.1	9.6	7.6	29.7	
≥ $50,000	33.0	9.0	9.8	48.2	
Pre-pregnancy Insurance					<.0001
Private	42.8	9.0	8.2	40.0	
Medicaid	66.8	8.1	3.6	21.5	
Other	61.3	8.7	4.5	25.5	
Multiple	57.4	8.1	3.9	30.6	
No insurance	73.5	7.2	3.6	15.7	
Medical-reproductive					
Previous live birth					<.0001
0	54.8	7.1	5.4	32.7	
1–2	54.6	9.0	6.6	29.8	
≥ 3	60.94	10.1	6.5	22.54	

Table 2 Prevalence of multivitamin intake by maternal characteristics *(Continued)*

Pre-pregnancy diabetes					<.0001
No	55.5	8.3	6.1	30.1	
Yes	50.9	8.6	4.7	35.8	
Pre-pregnancy hypertension					<.0001
No	56.1	8.3	6.2	29.4	
Yes	47.3	8.7	4.9	39.1	
Pregnancy intention					<.0001
Unintended	71.9	8.1	4.00	16.0	
Intended	43.0	8.5	7.6	40.9	
Socio-behavioral					
Pre-pregnancy smoking					<.0001
No	49.9	8.8	6.8	34.5	
Yes	72.5	6.9	3.9	16.7	
Average # of alcohol drink/week					<.0001
None	55.1	6.9	5.2	32.8	
Up to 3	52.5	8.6	7.2	31.7	
v4 or more	58.5	8.1	7.0	26.4	
Pre-pregnancy dieting					<.0001
No	57.2	7.8	5.7	29.3	
Yes	50.6	9.8	7.1	32.5	
Pre-pregnancy exercising					<.0001
No	63.1	7.8	4.8	24.3	
Yes	44.5	9.0	7.9	38.6	
Intimate partner violence					<.0001
No	54.6	8.4	6.2	30.8	
Yes	72.9	7.4	3.1	16.6	

Weighted *N* = adjusted for the complex sampling design and represents the total population that the sampled was derived from

Previous studies reported that obese women have higher rates of unintended pregnancies compared to their normal weight counterpart. Huber et al. analyzed PRAMS database and reported that obese women are at higher risk of unintended pregnancy compared to normal weight women (AOR = 1.75, 95 % CI = 1.21–2.52) [33]. Similarly, Garbers et al. found that obese women had more than twice the odds of unintended pregnancy (AOR = 2.81, 95 % CI = 1.41–5.60) [35]. Nevertheless, findings from the current study demonstrated that obese women had a higher odds of not using multivitamins even after adjusting for pregnancy intention.

Another possible explanation for the association between obesity and lack of multivitamin use may be that overweight and obese women are less likely to take dietary supplements. This was demonstrated by Radimer et al. who reported that obese adults were less likely to engage in healthy behaviors including multivitamin use [36]. Furthermore, it is also possible that overweight and obese women may not receive the appropriate counseling for preconception multivitamin use. The CDC reports that obese/overweight women are more likely to receive suboptimal preconception care in contrast to normal weight women [6]. Health care providers may play an important role in multivitamin use prior to pregnancy. However, only one of six obstetrician/gynecologists or family physicians provides preconception care to prenatal care patients [37].

The strengths of this study consist of having a large nationally-representative data that utilizes standardized methods of data collection. These methods allow for optimal comparison among participating states. The PRAMS data also allowed this study to account for important socio-demographic, medical, and high-risk behavioral factors. Despite these strengths, the study has some limitations. The cross-sectional design makes it difficult to determine causality between exposure and outcome. However, this study included women who had a live birth and the question about preconception multivitamin use clearly referred to one month prior to

Table 3 Maternal characteristics by Body Mass Index

	Underweight $n = 219\ 560$	Normal Weight $n = 2\ 534\ 187$	Overweight $n = 1\ 212\ 554$	Obese $n = 1\ 066\ 261$	P-value
		Weighted row %			
Socio-demographic					
Age					<.0001
≤ 19	17.4	10.9	7.4	5.8	
20–24	30.9	22.2	23.1	22.7	
25–29	26.7	28.5	29.8	31.0	
30–35	16.8	25.0	24.7	25.4	
> 35	8.3	13.4	15.0	15.1	
Race/Ethnicity					<.0001
White, non-Hispanic	60.4	63.7	56.0	56.2	
Black, non-Hispanic	11.7	10.8	15.6	18.7	
Hispanic	14.8	16.0	20.4	19.8	
Other, non-Hispanic	13.1	9.4	7.1	5.4	
Married					<.0001
Yes	52.2	63.5	60.5	57.4	
Other	47.8	36.5	39.5	42.6	
Education					<.0001
< High school	22.2	15.1	16.1	16.0	
High school	29.4	23.6	27.2	31.2	
> High school	48.4	61.4	56.6	52.9	
Income					<.0001
< $20,000	48.9	32.9	36.7	40.8	
$20,000–34,999	15.0	15.4	17.7	20.4	
$35,000–49,999	9.1	9.8	10.6	11.3	
≥ $50,000	27.0	41.9	35.1	27.5	
Pre-pregnancy Insurance					<.0001
Private	45.3	60.0	54.8	49.3	
Medicaid	20.9	13.9	15.2	19.1	
Other	2.11	1.9	1.9	2.1	
Multiple	3.6	3.2	3.3	3.9	
No insurance	28.0	21.0	24.8	25.6	
Medical-reproductive					
Previous live birth					<.0001
0	51.6	45.8	38.7	34.7	
1–2	40.8	45.7	49.0	51.4	
≥ 3	7.6	8.6	12.3	13.9	
Pre-pregnancy diabetes	1.6	1.4	2.2	3.9	<.0001
Pre-pregnancy hypertension	7.1	7.1	9.0	13.3	<.0001
Unintended Pregnancy	50.0	40.6	42.0	45.9	<.0001
Socio-behavioral					
Pre-pregnancy smoking	30.7	22.5	24.5	28.3	<.0001

Table 3 Maternal characteristics by Body Mass Index *(Continued)*

Average # of alcohol drink/week					<.0001
None	17.7	15.6	17.2	19.8	
Up to 3	68.9	67.5	67.3	68.3	
4 or more	11.4	15.0	13.4	10.3	
Pre-pregnancy dieting	8.1	21.0	36.5	41.4	<.0001
Pre-pregnancy exercising	31.0	45.8	42.8	35.3	<.0001
Intimate partner violence	4.4	2.8	3.2	3.2	0.0085

Weighted *N* = adjusted for the complex sampling design and represents the total population that the sampled was derived from

pregnancy. Another limitation of the study is that BMI and multivitamin use were both self-reported. It is possible that overweight and obese women may be under-reporting their weight because of social desirability bias which may bias the estimate toward the null. Additionally, PRAMS questionnaire is administered several months after delivery, making women's answers subject to recall bias. However, limiting the recall period to no longer than one year might minimize recall bias. In fact, PRAMS typically contacts women two to four months

Table 4 Adjusted logistic regression models for non-adherence to multivitamin use among BMI Groups

	Underweight	Overweight	Obese
COR[a]			
No intake	**1.6 (1.4–1.8)**	**1.3 (1.2–1.4)**	**1.6 (1.5–1.7)**
1–3 times/week	1.3 (1.0–1.6)	1.1 (1.0–1.2)	**1.3 (1.1–1.4)**
4–6 times/week	0.9 (0.7–1.1)	1.0 (0.9–1.1)	0.9 (0.8–1.1)
AOR[b]			
No intake	1.2 (1.0–1.4)	**1.2 (1.1–1.3)**	**1.4 (1.3–1.5)**
1–3 times/week	1.2 (1.0–1.5)	1.1 (1.0–1.2)	1.2 (1.0–1.3)
4–6 times/week	1.0 (0.8–1.2)	1.0 (0.9–1.1)	1.0 (0.9–1.1)
AOR[c]			
No intake	1.2 (1.0–1.4)	**1.2 (1.2–1.3)**	**1.5 (1.3–1.6)**
1–3 times/week	1.2 (1.0–1.5)	1.1 (1.0–1.2)	**1.2 (1.1–1.3)**
4–6 times/week	1.0 (0.8–1.3)	1.0 (0.9–1.1)	1.0 (0.9–1.2)
AOR[d]			
No intake	1.1 (0.9–1.4)	**1.2 (1.1–1.3)**	**1.4 (1.2–1.5)**
1–3 times/week	1.4 (1.0–1.8)	1.1 (0.9–1.2)	1.1 (0.9–1.3)
4–6 times/week	1.1 (0.8–1.5)	1.0 (0.9–1.2)	1.0 (0.9–1.2)

Daily intake is referent outcome group; bolded estimates indicate statistical significance
[a]Crude odds ratio of multivitamin intake
[b]Adjusted for socio-demographic characteristics (age, marital status, race/ethnicity, education, income, and health insurance)
[c]Adjusted for socio-demographic characteristics and medical-reproductive factors (previous live birth, pregnancy intention, pre-pregnancy diabetes, and pre-pregnancy hypertension)
[d]Adjusted for socio-demographic characteristics, medical-reproductive factors, and socio-behavioral characteristics (pre-pregnancy smoking, average # of alcohol drink per week, pre-pregnancy dieting, pre-pregnancy exercising, and intimate partner violence)

after delivery [38, 39]. Lastly, the effect of preconception counseling on multivitamin use may have affected the results but were unavailable in the data. Health education and counseling on positive health behaviors during perinatal care visits may be of interest for future research.

Conclusions

In summary, overweight and obese women are less likely to follow the universal recommendation for multivitamin use one month before pregnancy. This behavior might increase the risk for serious but preventable outcomes in infants, such as neural tube defects, anencephaly, multiple birth defects, small for gestation, and low birth weight. More research and well-designed studies are needed to investigate in detail the reasons for inadequate multivitamin use in obese/overweight women during the preconception period. Knowing the motivations underlying this problem would help health policy makers implement a proper intervention. However, health care providers and policy makers need to raise awareness of this significant health problem. Furthermore, all health care professional should enhance preconception care during well–woman visits or other routine visits, and particular attention should be given to obese women. Preconception counseling presents an opportunity to discuss healthy eating and healthy weight, as well as the benefit of daily multivitamin intake before pregnancy.

Abbreviations
AOR, adjusted odds ratio; BMI, body mass index; BRFSS, behavioral risk factor surveillance system; CDC, centers for disease control and prevention; CI, confidence interval; COR, crude odds ratio; OR, odds ratio; PRAMS, pregnancy risk assessment monitoring system

Acknowledgements
We would like to thank the PRAMS Working Group: Alabama—Izza Afgan, MPH; Alaska—Kathy Perham-Hester, MS, MPH; Arkansas— Mary McGehee, PhD; Colorado—Alyson Shupe, PhD; Connecticut — Jennifer Morin, MPH; Delaware— George Yocher, MS; Florida— Avalon Adams-Thames, MPH, CHES; Georgia— Chinelo Ogbuanu, MD, MPH, PhD; Hawaii— Emily Roberson, MPH, PhD; Illinois—Theresa Sandidge, MA; Iowa —Sarah Mauch, MPH; Louisiana— Amy Zapata, MPH; Maine—Tom Patenaude, MPH; Maryland— Diana Cheng, MD; Massachusetts— Emily Lu, MPH; Michigan—Cristin Larder, MS; Minnesota—Judy Punyko, PhD, MPH; Mississippi— Brenda Hughes, MPPA; Missouri—Venkata Garikapaty, MSc, MS, PhD, MPH; Montana—JoAnn Dotson;

Nebraska—Brenda Coufal; New Hampshire—David J. Laflamme, PhD, MPH; New Jersey—Lakota Kruse, MD; New Mexico—Eirian Coronado, MPH; New York State—Anne Radigan-Garcia; New York City—Candace Mulready-Ward, MPH; North Carolina— Kathleen Jones-Vessey, MS; North Dakota—Sandra Anseth; Ohio—Connie Geidenberger PhD; Oklahoma—Alicia Lincoln, MSW, MSPH; Oregon—Kenneth Rosenberg, MD, MPH; Pennsylvania—Tony Norwood; Rhode Island—Sam Viner-Brown, PhD; South Carolina—Mike Smith, MSPH; Texas—Rochelle Kingsley, MPH; Tennessee—David Law, PhD; Utah—Lynsey Gammon, MPH; Vermont—Peggy Brozicevic; Virginia—Marilyn Wenner; Washington—Linda Lohdefinck; West Virginia—Melissa Baker, MA; Wisconsin—Katherine Kvale, PhD; Wyoming—Amy Spieker, MPH; CDC PRAMS Team, Applied Sciences Branch, Division of Reproductive Health.

Funding
None.

Authors' contributions
SM conceptualized the study and framed the study design, guided the analysis and interpretation of the results, and drafted sections of the article. SC and AB contributed to the acquisition, analysis and interpretation of the data, drafted sections of the article, and all authors reviewed and approved the final version of the article.

Competing interests
The authors declare that they have no competing interests.

Consent for publication
Not applicable.

Author details
[1]Division of Epidemiology, Department of Family Medicine and Population Health, School of Medicine, Virginia Commonwealth University, 830 E. Main Street, 8th Floor, P.O. Box 980212, Richmond, VA 23298-0212, USA. [2]Department of Obstetrics and Gynecology, School of Medicine, Virginia Commonwealth University, Richmond, VA, USA. [3]Virginia Commonwealth University Institute for Women's Health, Richmond, VA, USA.

References
1. Rock CL. Multivitamin-multimineral supplements: who uses them? Am J Clin Nutr. 2007;85(1):277S–9.
2. Gahche J, Bailey R, Burt V, et al. Dietary supplement use among U.S. adults has increased since NHANES III (1988–1994). NCHS Data Brief. 2011;61:1–8.
3. Sullivan KM, Ford ES, Azrak MF, Mokdad AH. Multivitamin use in pregnant and nonpregnant women: results from the behavioral risk factor surveillance system. Public Health Rep. 2009;124(3):384–90.
4. Centers for Disease Control and Prevention. Recommendations for the use of folic acid to reduce the number of cases of spina bifida and other neural tube defects. MMWR Morb Mortal Wkly Rep. 1992;41:1–7.
5. Centers for Disease Control and Prevention. Use of supplements containing folic acid among women of childbearing age–United States. MMWR Morb Mortal Wkly Rep. 2008;57:5–8.
6. Centers for Disease Control and Prevention. Preconception health indicators among women–Texas, 2002–2010. MMWR Morb Mortal Wkly Rep. 2012;61:550–5.
7. Crider K, Bailey L, Berry R. Folic acid food fortification- its history, effect, concerns, and future directions. Nutrients. 2011;3:370–84.
8. Wang M, Wang Z, Gao L, Gong R, Sun X, Zhao Z. Maternal body mass index and the association between folic acid supplements and neural tube defects. Acta Paediatr. 2013;102(9):908–13.

9. De-Regil LM, Peña-Rosas JP, Fernández-Gaxiola AC, Rayco-Solon P. Effects and safety of periconceptional oral folate supplementation for preventing birth defects. Cochrane Database Syst Rev. 2015;12: CD007950.
10. Chang S, Zeng L, Brouwer ID, Kok FJ, Yan H. Effect of iron deficiency anemia in pregnancy on child mental development in rural China. Pediatrics. 2013;131(3):e755–4763.
11. Correa A, Botto L, Liu Y, Mulinare J, Erickson JD. Do multivitamin supplements attenuate the risk for diabetes-associated birth defects? Pediatrics. 2003;111(5):1146–51.
12. Catov JM, Bodnar LM, Olsen J, Olsen S, Nohr EA. Periconceptional multivitamin use and risk of preterm or small-for- gestational- age births in the Danish National Birth Cohort. Am J Clin Nutr. 2011;94(3):906–12.
13. Li Z, Ye R, Zhang L, Li H, Lui J, Ren A. Periconceptional folic acid supplementation and the risk of preterm births in China: a large prospective cohort study. Int J Epidemiol. 2014;43(4):1132–9.
14. Ramakrishnan U, Grant FK, Imdad A, Bhutta ZA, Martorell R. Effect of multiple micronutrient versus iron-folate supplementation during pregnancy on intrauterine growth. Nestle Nutr Inst Workshop Ser. 2013;74:53–62.
15. Bestwick JP, Huttly WJ, Morris JK, Wald NJ. Prevention of neural tube defects: a cross-sectional study of the uptake of folic acid supplementation in nearly half a million women. PLoS One. 2014;9(2):e89354.
16. Short VL, Oza-Frank R, Conrey EJ. Preconception health indicators: a comparison between non-Appalachian and Appalachian women. Matern Child Health J. 2012;16(2):238–49.
17. Tessema J, Jefferds ME, Cogswell M, Carlton E. Motivators and barriers to prenatal supplement use among minority women in the United States. J Am Diet Assoc. 2009;109(1):102–8.
18. Mazza D, Chapman A. Improving the uptake of preconception care and periconceptional folate supplementation: what do women think? BMC Public Health. 2010;10(786):1–6.
19. Kimmons JE, Blanck HM, Tohill BC, Zhang J, Khan LK. Multivitamin use in relation to self-reported body mass index and weight loss attempts. Med Gen Med. 2006;8(3):3.
20. Farah N, Kennedy C, Turner C, O'Dwyer V, Kennelly MM, Turner MJ. Maternal obesity and pre-pregnancy folic acid supplementation. Obesity Facts. 2013;6(2):211–5.
21. Case AP, Ramadhani TA, Canfield MA, Beverly L, Wood R. Folic acid supplementation among diabetic, overweight, or obese women of childbearing age. J Obstet Gynecol Neonatal Nurs. 2007;36(4):335–41.
22. Kimmons JE, Blanck HM, Tohill BC, Zhang J, Khan LK. Associations between body mass index and the prevalence of low micronutrient levels among U.S. adults. Med Gen Med. 2006;8(4):59–69.
23. Huber LRB, Toth JL. Obesity and oral contraceptive failure: findings from the 2002 national survey of family growth. Am J Epidemiol. 2007;166(11):1306–11.
24. Pregnancy Risk Assessment Monitoring System. Centers for Disease Control and Prevention, Atlanta, GA. 2012. http://www.cdc.gov/prams/researchers. htm. Accessed 20 Jul 2015.
25. Guelinckx I, Devlieger R, Bogaerts A, Pauwels S, Vansant G. The effect of pre-pregnancy BMI on intention, initiation and duration of breast-feeding. Public Health Nutr. 2012;15(5):840–8.
26. Kitsantas P, Pawloski LR. Maternal obesity, health status during pregnancy, and breastfeeding initiation and duration. J Matern Fetal Neonatal Med. 2010;23(2):135–41.
27. World Health Organization. BMI Classification. http://apps.who.int/bmi/index. jsp?introPage=intro_3.html. Updated January 1, 2016. Accessed 21 Jan 2016.
28. Song Y, Xu Q, Park Y, Hollenbeck A, Schatzkin A, Chen H. Multivitamins, individual vitamin and mineral supplements, and risk of diabetes among older U.S. adults. Diabetes Care. 2011;34(1):108–14.
29. Jasti S, Siega-Riz A, Cogswell ME, Hartzema AG, Bentley ME. Pill count adherence to prenatal multivitamin/mineral supplement use among low-income women. J Nutr. 2005;135(5):1093–101.
30. Weiss LA, Chambers CD. Associations between multivitamin supplement use and alcohol consumption before pregnancy: pregnancy risk assessment monitoring system, 2004 to 2008. Alcohol Clin Exp Res. 2013;37(9):1595–600.
31. Scholl TO, Hediger ML, Bendich A, Schall JI, Smith WK, Krueger PM. Use of multivitamin/mineral prenatal supplements: Influence on the outcome of pregnancy. Am J Epidemiol. 1997;146(2):134–41.

32. Backhausen MG, Ekstrand M, Tydén T, et al. Pregnancy planning and lifestyle prior to conception and during early pregnancy among Danish women. Eur J Contracept Reprod Health Care. 2014;19(1):57–65.

33. Rosenberg KD, Gelow JM, Sandoval AP. Pregnancy intendedness and the use of periconceptional folic acid. Pediatrics. 2003;111(5):1142–5.

34. Stephenson J, Patel D, Barrett G, et al. How do women prepare for pregnancy? preconception experiences of women attending antenatal services and views of health professionals. PLoS One. 2014;9(7):e103085.

35. Garbers S, Chiasson MA. Class III obesity and unwanted pregnancy among women with live births in New York City, 2004–2007. Matern Child Health J. 2013;17(8):1459–67.

36. Radimer K, Bindewald B, Hughes J, Ervin B, Swanson C, Picciano MF. Dietary supplement use by US adults: data from the National Health and Nutrition Examination Survey, 1999–2000. Am J Epidemiol. 2004;160(4):339–49.

37. Johnson K, Posner SF, Biermann J, et al. Recommendations to improve preconception health and health care–United States: a report of the CDC/ATSDR preconception care work group and the select panel on preconception care. MMWR Morb Mortal Wkly Rep. 2006;55(RR06):1–23.

38. De Nicola F, Giné X. How accurate is recall data: evidence from coastal India. J Dev Econ. 2011;106:52–65.

39. Centers for Disease Control and Prevention. Methodology - PRAMS. http://www.cdc.gov/prams/methodology.htm. (accessed November 2014). Updated November 8, 2012. Accessed 21 Jan 2016.

Permissions

List of Contributors

Susie Dzakpasu and Sharon Bartholomew
Maternal and Infant Health Section, Health Surveillance and Epidemiology Division, Public Health Agency of Canada, 785 Carling Avenue, 6804A 4th Floor, Ottawa, Ontario K1A 0 K9, Canada

John Fahey
Reproductive Care Program of Nova Scotia, Halifax, Nova Scotia, Canada

Russell S Kirby
Department of Community and Family Health, College of Public Health, University of South Florida, Tampa, FL, U.S.A

Suzanne C Tough
Departments of Paediatrics and Community Health Sciences, Faculty of Medicine, University of Calgary, Calgary, Alberta, Canada

Beverley Chalmers
Department of Obstetrics and Gynaecology, Ottawa Hospital Research Institute, University of Ottawa, Ottawa, Ontario, Canada

Maureen I Heaman
College of Nursing, Faculty of Health Sciences, University of Manitoba, Winnipeg, Manitoba, Canada

Anne Biringer
Department of Family and Community Medicine, University of Toronto, Mount Sinai Hospital, Toronto, Ontario, Canada

Elizabeth K Darling
Midwifery Education Program, Laurentian University, Sudbury, Ontario, Canada

Lily S Lee
Perinatal Services British Columbia, Provincial Health Services Authority, Vancouver, British Columbia, Canada

Sarah D McDonald
Departments of Obstetrics & Gynecology, Radiology, and Clinical Epidemiology & Biostatistics, McMaster University, Hamilton, Canada

Miranda Davies-Tuck
The Ritchie Centre, Hudson Institute of Medical Research, Clayton, Vic 3168, Australia

Michelle Knight
Monash Health, Monash Medical Centre, Clayton, Australia

Lynne Stewart
Department of Obstetrics and Gynaecology, Monash University, Clayton, VIC, Australia

Joanne C. Mockler and Euan M. Wallace
The Ritchie Centre, Hudson Institute of Medical Research, Clayton, Vic 3168, Australia
Monash Health, Monash Medical Centre, Clayton, Australia
Department of Obstetrics and Gynaecology, Monash University, Clayton, VIC, Australia

Andrea R. Deussen
Discipline of Obstetrics & Gynaecology, and Robinson Research Institute, The University of Adelaide, Adelaide, South Australia, Australia

William Hague
Discipline of Obstetrics & Gynaecology, and Robinson Research Institute, The University of Adelaide, Adelaide, South Australia, Australia
Department of Perinatal Medicine, Women's and Children's Hospital, North Adelaide, South Australia, Australia

Jodie M. Dodd
Discipline of Obstetrics & Gynaecology, and Robinson Research Institute, The University of Adelaide, Adelaide, South Australia, Australia
Department of Perinatal Medicine, Women's and Children's Hospital, North Adelaide, South Australia, Australia
Discipline of Obstetrics & Gynaecology, and Robinson Institute, Women's & Children's Hospital, The University of Adelaide, 72 King William Road, North Adelaide, South Australia 5006, Australia

Rosalie M. Grivell
Discipline of Obstetrics & Gynaecology, and Robinson Research Institute, The University of Adelaide, Adelaide, South Australia, Australia
Department of Obstetrics & Gynaecology, Flinders Medical Centre and School of Medicine, Flinders University, Adelaide, Australia

Gustaaf Dekker
Discipline of Obstetrics & Gynaecology, and Robinson Research Institute, The University of Adelaide, Adelaide, South Australia, Australia
Lyell McEwin Hospital, Elizabeth Vale, South Australia, Australia

Jennie Louise
The University of Adelaide, School of Public Health, Adelaide, South Australia, Australia

Hara Nikolopoulos, Jessica MacIsaac and Rhonda C. Bell
Department of Agricultural, Food and Nutritional Sciences, University of Alberta, 4-126 Li Ka Shing Centre for Health Research Innovation, Edmonton, AB T6G 2E1, Canada

Maria Mayan
University of Alberta, Community University Partnership, Facility of Extension, 2nd Floor, 2-281 Enterprise Square, 10230 Jasper Avenue, Edmonton, AB T5J 4P6, Canada

Terri Miller
Healthy Living, Population, Public and Aboriginal Health, Reproductive Health, Healthy Children and Families, Alberta Health Services, 10101 Southport Road SW cubicle #1740, Calgary, AB T2W 3N2, Canada

Karen Louise Ellekjaer and Ellen Løkkegaard
Department of Obstetrics and Gynaecology, Nordsjællands Hospital, University of Copenhagen, Dyrehavevej 29, 3400 Hillerød, Denmark

Thomas Bergholt
Department of Obstetrics and Gynaecology, Rigshospitalet, University of Copenhagen, Blegdamsvej 9, 2100 Copenhagen, Denmark

Julie Boudet-Berquier and Benoit Salanave
Nutritional Surveillance and Epidemiology Team (ESEN), French Public Health Agency, Paris-13 University, Centre de Recherche en Epidémiologie et Statistiques, COMUE Sorbonne Paris Cité, SMBH Building, 1st floor, door 136, 74 rue Marcel Cachin, 93017 Bobigny Cedex, France

Jean-Claude Desenclos
French Public Health Agency (Agence nationale de Santé publique), Saint Maurice, France

Katia Castetbon
Centre de Recherche « Epidémiologie, Biostatistique et Recherche clinique », School of Public Health, Université libre de Bruxelles (ULB), Brussels, Belgium

Olha Lutsiv and Adam Hulman
Department of Obstetrics and Gynecology, McMaster University, 1280 Main Street West, Room 3N52B, Hamilton, ON L8S 4K1, Canada

Christy Woolcott and Linda Dodds
Departments of Obstetrics and Gynaecology, and Pediatrics, Dalhousie University, Halifax, NS, Canada

Joseph Beyene and Binod Neupane
Department of Clinical Epidemiology & Biostatistics, McMaster University, Hamilton, ON, Canada

Lucy Giglia
Department of Pediatrics, McMaster University, Hamilton, ON, Canada

B. Anthony Armson
Department of Obstetrics and Gynaecology, Dalhousie University, Halifax, NS, Canada

Sarah D. McDonald
Departments of Obstetrics and Gynecology, Radiology, and Clinical Epidemiology & Biostatistics, McMaster University, Hamilton, ON, Canada

Matteo C. Sattler
Institute of Sport Science, University of Graz, Mozartgasse 14, 8010, Graz, Austria

Judith G. M. Jelsma
Department of Public and Occupational Health, Amsterdam Public Health Research Institute, VU University Medical Centre, Amsterdam, the Netherlands

Mireille N. M. van Poppel
Institute of Sport Science, University of Graz, Mozartgasse 14, 8010, Graz, Austria
Department of Public and Occupational Health, Amsterdam Public Health Research Institute, VU University Medical Centre, Amsterdam, the Netherlands

Annick Bogaerts
Department of Development and Regeneration KULeuven, University of Leuven, Leuven, Belgium and Faculty of Medicine and Health Sciences, Centre for Research and Innovation in Care (CRIC), University of Antwerp, Belgium and Faculty of Health and Social Work, research unit Healthy Living, UC Leuven-Limburg, Leuven, Belgium

David Simmons
Institute of Metabolic Science, Addenbrookes Hospital, Cambridge, England and Macarthur Clinical School, Western Sydney University, Sydney, Australia

Gernot Desoye
Department of Obstetrics and Gynecology, Medizinische Universität Graz, Graz, Austria

Rosa Corcoy
Institut de Recerca de L'Hospital de la Santa Creu i Sant Pau, Barcelona, Spain
CIBER Bioengineering, Biomaterials and Nanotechnology, Instituto de Salud Carlos III, Zaragaza, Spain

Goele Jans
KU Leuven Department of Development and Regeneration: Pregnancy, Fetus and Neonate, Gynaecology and Obstetrics, University Hospitals, Leuven, Belgium

Sander Galjaard
KU Leuven Department of Development and Regeneration: Pregnancy, Fetus and Neonate, Gynaecology and Obstetrics, University Hospitals, Leuven, Belgium
Department of Obstetrics and Gynaecology Division of Obstetrics and Prenatal Medicine, Erasmus Medical Centre, Rotterdam, The Netherlands

David Hill
Recherche en Santé Lawson SA, Bronschhofen, Switzerland

Peter Damm and Elisabeth R. Mathiesen
Center for Pregnant Women with Diabetes, Departments of Endocrinology and Obstetrics, Rigshospitalet, University of Copenhagen, Copenhagen, Denmark

Ewa Wender-Ozegowska
Division of Reproduction, Poznan University of Medical Sciences, Poznan, Poland

Fidelma Dunne
National University of Ireland, Galway, Ireland

Dorte M. Jensen and Lise Lotte T. Andersen
Odense University Hospital, Odense, Denmark

Frank J. Snoek
Department of Medical Psychology, VU University Medical Centre, Amsterdam, the Netherlands
Department of Medical Psychology, Academic Medical Centre, Amsterdam, the Netherlands

Kirsti K. Garnæs
Department of Circulation and Medical Imaging, NTNU, Norwegian University of Science and Technology, Trondheim, Norway

Øyvind Salvesen
Department of Public Health and General Practice, NTNU, Norwegian University of Science and Technology, Trondheim, Norway

Siv Mørkved
Department of Public Health and General Practice, NTNU, Norwegian University of Science and Technology, Trondheim, Norway
Research Department, St. Olavs Hospital Trondheim University Hospital, Trondheim, Norway

Kjell Å. Salvesen
Institute of clinical and molecular medicine, Norwegian University of Science and Tecnology, Trondheim, Norway
Department of Obstetrics and Gynaecology, St. Olavs Hospital, Trondheim University Hospital, Trondheim, Norway

Trine Moholdt
Department of Circulation and Medical Imaging, NTNU, Norwegian University of Science and Technology, Trondheim, Norway
Department of Obstetrics and Gynaecology, St. Olavs Hospital, Trondheim University Hospital, Trondheim, Norway

C. Flannery and M. Byrne
Health Behaviour Change Research Group, School of Psychology, National University of Ireland, Galway, Ireland

S. McHugh, A. E. Anaba and P. M. Kearney
School of Public Health, University College Cork, Cork, Ireland

E. Clifford
Department of Nutrition & Dietetics, South Infirmary Victoria University Hospital, Cork, Ireland

M. O'Riordan
Department Obstetrics and Gynaecology, University College Cork, Cork, Ireland

L. C. Kenny
Department of Women's and Children's Health, Faculty of Health and Life Sciences, University of Liverpool, Liverpool, UK

F. M. McAuliffe
UCD Perinatal Research Centre, School of Medicine, University College Dublin, National Maternity Hospital, Dublin, Ireland

Michael L. Power
Research Department, American College of Obstetricians and Gynecologists, Washington, DC 20090-6920, USA
Smithsonian National Zoo and Conservation Biology Institute, Washington, DC, USA

Melisa L. Lott and A. Dhanya Mackeen
Geisinger, Department of Obstetrics and Gynecology, Division of Maternal-Fetal Medicine, Danville, PA, USA

Jessica DiBari
Health Resources and Services Administration, Maternal and Child Health Bureau, Office of Epidemiology and Research, Division of Research, Rockville, MD, USA

Jay Schulkin
Research Department, American College of Obstetricians and Gynecologists, Washington, DC 20090-6920, USA
Department of Obstetrics and Gynecology, University of Washington School of Medicine, Seattle, WA, USA

Tuija Hautakangas
Department of Obstetrics and Gynecology, Central Hospital of Central Finland, Keskussairaalantie 19, 40620 Jyväskylä, Finland

Outi Palomäki and Jukka Uotila
Department of Obstetrics and Gynecology, Tampere University Hospital, Tampere, Finland

Karoliina Eidstø
Kangasala Health Center, Kangasala, Finland

Heini Huhtala
School of Health Sciences, Tampere University, Tampere, Finland

Paul M. C. Lemmens, Francesco Sartor, Lieke G. E. Cox and Sebastiaan V. den Boer
Philips Research, High Tech Campus 34, 5656 AE Eindhoven, the Netherlands

Joyce H. D. M. Westerink
Philips Research, High Tech Campus 34, 5656 AE Eindhoven, the Netherlands
Eindhoven University of Technology, Het Eeuwsel, 5612 AZ Eindhoven, the Netherlands

Edyta Suliga
Department of Nutrition and Dietetics, Faculty of Medicine and Health Sciences, Jan Kochanowski University, Kielce, Poland

Wojciech Rokita and Olga Adamczyk-Gruszka
Department of Gynecological and Obstetric Prophylaxis, Faculty of Medicine and Health Sciences, Jan Kochanowski University, Kielce, Poland

Grażyna Pazera
Clinic of Neonatology at the Regional Polyclinic Hospital, Kielce, Poland

Elżbieta Cieśla
Department of Developmental Age Research, Faculty of Medicine and Health Sciences, Jan Kochanowski University, Kielce, Poland

Stanisław Głuszek
Department of Surgery and Surgical Nursing with the Scientific Research Laboratory, Faculty of Medicine and Health Sciences, Jan Kochanowski University, Kielce, Poland

Christine Sommer Kjersti Mørkrid and Kåre Inge Birkeland
Department of Endocrinology, Morbid Obesity and Preventive Medicine, Oslo University Hospital, Nydalen, N-0424 Oslo, Norway
Institute of Clinical Medicine, Faculty of Medicine, University of Oslo, Oslo, Norway

Line Sletner
Department of Child and Adolescents Medicine, Akershus University Hospital, Lørenskog, Norway

Anne Karen Jenum
Institute of Health and Society, Department of General Practice, Faculty of Medicine, University of Oslo, Oslo, Norway
Faculty of Health Sciences, Oslo and Akershus University College of Applied Sciences, Oslo, Norway

Anna Dencker, Sofie Dencker and Marie Berg
Centre for Person-Centred Care (GPCC), University of Gothenburg, Gothenburg, Sweden
Institute of Health and Care Sciences, Sahlgrenska Academy, University of Gothenburg, Gothenburg, Sweden

Åsa Premberg
Centre for Person-Centred Care (GPCC), University of Gothenburg, Gothenburg, Sweden
Institute of Health and Care Sciences, Sahlgrenska Academy, University of Gothenburg, Gothenburg, Sweden
Primary Health Care, Närhälsan, Gothenburg, Sweden

Ellinor K. Olander and Christine McCourt
Centre for Maternal and Child Health Research, City University London, London, UK

Karin Haby
Antenatal Health Care, Primary Health Care, Research and Development Unit, Närhälsan, Gothenburg, Sweden

Anna Glantz
Primary Health Care, Närhälsan, Gothenburg, Sweden

Marilyn Lacroix, Marie-Claude Battista, Julie Patenaude and Laetitia Guillemette
Department of Medicine, Université de Sherbrooke, 3001 12th Avenue North, Sherbrooke, Québec, Canada

Myriam Doyon, Julie Moreau and Julie Ménard
Centre de recherche du Centre Hospitalier Universitaire de Sherbrooke, 3001 12th Avenue North, wing 9, door 6, Sherbrooke, Québec, Canada

Jean-Luc Ardilouze and Patrice Perron
Department of Medicine, Université de Sherbrooke, 3001 12th Avenue North, Sherbrooke, Québec, Canada
Centre de recherche du Centre Hospitalier Universitaire de Sherbrooke, 3001 12th Avenue North, wing 9, door 6, Sherbrooke, Québec, Canada

Marie-France Hivert
Department of Medicine, Université de Sherbrooke, 3001 12th Avenue North, Sherbrooke, Québec, Canada
Centre de recherche du Centre Hospitalier Universitaire de Sherbrooke, 3001 12th Avenue North, wing 9, door 6, Sherbrooke, Québec, Canada
Diabetes Center, Massachusetts General Hospital, 50 Staniford Street, Boston, MA, USA
Department of Population Medicine, Harvard Medical School, Harvard Pilgrim Health Care Institute, 401 Park Drive, suite 401, Boston, MA, USA

Geraldine A Vaughan, Caroline SE Homer, Alex Wang, Zhuoyang Li, Nasrin Javid and Elizabeth Denney-Wilson
Faculty of Health, University of Technology Sydney, Broadway NSW, 2007 Sydney, Australia

Elizabeth A. Sullivan
Faculty of Health, University of Technology Sydney, Broadway NSW, 2007 Sydney, Australia
School of Women's and Children's Health, The University of New South Wales, Sydney, Australia

Jan E. Dickinson
School of Women's and Infants' Health, The University of Western Australia, Perth, Australia

Michael J. Peek
Department of Obstetrics and Gynaecology Medical School College of Medicine, Biology and Environment, The Australian National University, Canberra, Australia
Obstetrics and Gynaecology, Centenary Hospital for Women and Children, Canberra, Australia

David Ellwood
School of Medicine, Griffith University, Queensland, Australia
Gold Coast University Hospital, Queensland, Australia

Marian Knight
National Perinatal Epidemiology Unit, University of Oxford, Oxford, United Kingdom

Claire McLintock
Obstetrics and Gynaecology, National Women's Health, Auckland City Hospital, Auckland, New Zealand

Wendy Pollock
Judith Lumley Centre, La Trobe University, Melbourne, Australia
Department of Nursing, Melbourne School of Health Sciences, The University of Melbourne, Melbourne, Australia

Lisa Jackson Pulver
Muru Marri Indigenous Health Unit, School of Public Health and Community Medicine, The University of New South Wales, Sydney, Australia

Leonie Callaway
Royal Brisbane and Women's Hospital, Brisbane, Australia
School of Medicine, The University of Queensland, Brisbane, Australia

Mahmi Fujimori and Luiz C. de Abreu
Department of Maternal and Child Health, School of Public Health, University of São Paulo, São Paulo, SP, Brazil

Eduardo L. França and Adenilda C. Honorio-França
Institute of Biological and Health Science, Federal University of Mato Grosso, Barra do Garças, MT, Brazil

Tassiane C. Morais
Department of Maternal and Child Health, School of Public Health, University of São Paulo, São Paulo, SP, Brazil
Institute of Biological and Health Science, Federal University of Mato Grosso, Barra do Garças, MT, Brazil

Vanessa Fiorin
Laboratory of Scientific Writing, Department of Morphology and Physiology, School of Medicine of ABC, Santo André, SP, Brazil

Louise Hayes and Ruth Bell
Institute of Health & Society, Newcastle University, Baddiley-Clark Building, Richardson Road, Newcastle upon Tyne NE2 4AX, UK

Stephen C Robson
Institute of Cellular Medicine, Newcastle University, Newcastle upon Tyne, UK

Catherine Mcparlin
Institute of Health & Society, Newcastle University, Baddiley-Clark Building, Richardson Road, Newcastle upon Tyne NE2 4AX, UK
Newcastle-upon-Tyne Hospitals NHS Foundation Trust, Newcastle upon Tyne, UK

Tarja I Kinnunen
School of Health Sciences, University of Tampere, Tampere, Finland

Lucilla Poston
Division of Women's Health, Women's Health Academic Centre, King's College, London, UK

Amani Bassyouni and Susan Cha
Division of Epidemiology, Department of Family Medicine and Population Health, School of Medicine, Virginia Commonwealth University, 830 E. Main Street, 8th Floor, Richmond, VA 23298-0212, USA

Saba W. Masho
Division of Epidemiology, Department of Family Medicine and Population Health, School of Medicine, Virginia Commonwealth University, 830 E. Main Street, 8th Floor, Richmond, VA 23298-0212, USA
Department of Obstetrics and Gynecology, School of Medicine, Virginia Commonwealth University, Richmond, VA, USA
Virginia Commonwealth University Institute for Women's Health, Richmond, VA, USA

Index

A

Activity Monitor, 124-125, 129-131

Adverse Pregnancy Outcomes, 10-11, 13, 18, 20, 47, 58-59, 68, 78, 143, 153, 164-165

Antenatal Care, 28, 36, 47, 92, 98, 146, 160, 173

Antenatal Health Care, 154-155, 163

B

Behaviour Change Wheel, 94, 104, 106

Birth Weight, 11, 14, 18, 22, 24, 29, 38-42, 44, 47, 49-51, 53-57, 60-64, 66-70, 73, 79, 95, 105, 113-115, 120, 132, 134-135, 143-153, 162, 167, 178, 189, 199, 205

Body Composition, 27, 83-85, 91, 132, 145, 153

Body Mass Index (bmi), 1, 13-14, 22, 29, 37, 41, 61, 73, 84, 97, 107-108, 116, 135, 145, 154-155, 164-165, 173, 183-184, 198-199

C

cesarean section, 19, 116-117, 121-122, 143

Childbearing Age, 114, 198, 206

Colostrum, 182-189

Com-b Model, 94, 96, 98-100, 103-104, 106

Complement Protein, 182, 184, 186

D

Depression, 3-5, 24, 27, 72-74, 78-82, 100, 108-109

Diabetes, 10, 12-16, 18, 20, 22-24, 26-29, 37, 39-40, 47-48, 50, 54-56, 58-62, 65-67, 72-78, 80-81, 83-88, 90-95, 97-98, 105-106, 108-114, 117-125, 131-135, 142-144, 146-147, 149, 151-153, 165, 170-171, 173-183, 185-186, 189-196, 200-201, 203-206

Dietary Patterns, 134-137, 139, 142-143

Dystocia, 13, 15-20, 24, 37, 57-58, 116-122, 146, 152, 175

E

Early Pregnancy Bmi, 37-38, 113, 145-151

Excessive Weight Gain, 12, 20, 29, 35, 58, 61, 69, 71, 97, 115, 124, 130, 134-135, 142-144, 153, 160, 171

F

Fetal Health, 28-29, 33

G

Gestational Diabetes Mellitus (gdm), 13, 48, 81, 84, 94-95, 125, 165

Gestational Hypertension, 13, 15-16, 18, 62, 65, 109, 125, 174, 179

Gestational Weight Gain (gwg), 1, 28-29, 48, 61, 95, 107-108, 134, 164-165

H

Healthcare Providers, 28-29, 35, 78

Healthy Lifestyle Changes, 154, 157

High Bmi, 4, 6, 83, 116, 120, 155, 157, 160

I

Induction of Labor, 116, 118-122

Insulin Sensitivity, 21, 84, 165-166, 168-169, 171, 195-196

L

Large-for-gestational Age, 1

Late Pregnancy Gwg, 164, 166, 168-169

Leptin, 27, 164-171

Lifestyle Intervention, 26, 72-73, 81, 88, 92-93, 96, 104-105, 154-156, 159, 161

M

Maternal Body Weight, 28-29, 33

Maternal Fasting Glucose, 145, 148, 150-151

Maternal Glucose, 145-149, 151-152

Maternal Health, 20, 29, 35, 94, 108, 181, 200

Maternal Lipids, 145-146

Maternal Obesity, 11, 13-14, 17-20, 22, 27, 36-37, 43, 46-51, 53, 55-59, 73-74, 81, 92-93, 95, 105-106, 121-123, 143, 155, 162-163, 171, 177, 180-182, 187-188, 190, 206

Maternal Risks, 83

Maternal Socio-economic Disadvantage, 172

Maternal Super-obesity, 172-173

Maternal Weight, 1, 6, 10, 12, 24, 27, 33, 36, 61, 63, 70, 92, 105, 107, 114, 143, 153, 157, 162, 165-168, 170-171, 179, 183, 187

Mental Health, 33, 62, 65, 72-81, 105

Mid-gestational Weight Gain, 145-152

Midwife, 14, 30, 33, 49, 94, 96, 98, 101, 135, 154-155, 157-158, 160-162, 176, 191

Minimising Weight Gain, 154, 156

N

Neonatal Adiposity, 145, 151, 153

Neural Tube Defects, 198-199, 205-206

Newborn, 11, 27, 48-49, 56-57, 117, 119, 122, 142, 145-146, 151-153, 187

O

Obese Mothers, 20, 48, 182, 185-189

Obesity, 2, 4, 8-22, 27, 29, 35-37, 43-44, 46-59, 61, 70, 72-74, 78-84, 88, 92-95, 105-108, 115-117, 119-132, 135, 142-145, 152-156, 160-165, 171-173, 177-183, 187-192, 198-199, 203, 206-207

Obstetric Complications, 92, 155, 172-175, 177

Obstetrics, 11, 20-21, 23, 26-27, 37-38, 46, 59-60, 70, 80, 82-83, 92, 96, 105, 107, 115-116, 122, 135, 180-181, 198, 206

Offspring's Birth Weight, 145-146, 148, 152

P
Perinatal Care, 47-48, 205

Perinatal Outcomes, 11, 13-15, 17-20, 70-71, 105, 172-174, 177-180

Physical Activity, 23-24, 27, 29, 31-32, 34, 36, 57-58, 73, 75, 77, 80-87, 90-91, 93-106, 124-126, 128, 130-132, 135, 141, 143, 152-159, 161-162, 165-168, 170-171, 179, 190, 196-197

Placental Weight, 166-169

Poor Mental Health, 72-73, 78-79

Population Attributable Fraction, 1, 9

Postpartum Weight Retention, 29, 35, 48, 59, 83-84, 86, 89, 92-93, 142-144, 171, 181

Pre-pregnancy Overweight, 84, 95, 169

Preconception Care, 198, 203, 205-207

Preeclampsia, 13, 19-20, 37-38, 48, 54, 56, 59, 103, 109, 132, 165, 177, 187

Pregnancy Risk Assessment Monitoring System, 95, 143, 198-199, 205-206

Prenatal Care, 28, 34-35, 70, 115, 203

Prepregnancy Bmi, 3, 5-7, 11, 31, 36, 52-56, 58, 61, 84, 107, 111, 144, 148-149, 152-153, 166, 187

Prepregnancy Obesity, 46-47, 49, 51, 57-58, 81, 165

Prepregnancy Weight, 2, 47-50, 53, 57-58, 115, 146

Preterm Birth, 1, 4, 6, 8-9, 11-12, 15-16, 18-19, 24, 29, 48, 56, 61, 66-67, 69-71, 73, 78, 105, 115, 173, 176, 178, 199

Primipara, 37, 116, 185

S
Singleton Pregnancies, 60-61, 117

Small-for-gestational Age, 1, 73

Super-obesity, 172-173, 179-180

T
Theoretical Domains Framework, 94, 96, 104, 106, 162

Twin Gestations, 60-61, 68, 70

Twin Pregnancies, 60-62, 65, 67-68, 70-71, 135

U
Umbilical Artery, 24, 118

V
Vaginal Delivery, 38-39, 42, 44, 51, 57, 116-117, 121-122

W
Weight Gain, 1-3, 5, 7-12, 19-22, 24, 27-36, 45, 47-49, 53-63, 65-71, 75-77, 84-86, 91-93, 95, 97, 103, 105-115, 124-125, 130-132, 134-157, 160, 162-171, 178-179, 187-188, 196-197

Women's Perceptions, 28, 31, 34, 98